# INSTRUMENTED FUSION
# OF THE DEGENERATIVE LUMBAR SPINE

## STATE OF THE ART, QUESTIONS, AND CONTROVERSIES

# Instrumented Fusion of the Degenerative Lumbar Spine

## State of the Art, Questions, and Controversies

Editors

**Marek Szpalski, M.D.**
Orthopaedic Surgeon
Senior Consultant
Centre Hospitalier
Molière Longchamp
Brussels, Belgium

**Robert Gunzburg, M.D., Ph.D.**
Orthopaedic Surgeon
Senior Consultant
Brugmann University Hospital
Brussels, Belgium

**Dan M. Spengler, M.D.**
Orthopaedic Surgeon
Professor and Chairman
Vanderbilt University
Nashville, Tennessee

**Alf Nachemson, M.D., Ph.D.**
Orthopaedic Surgeon
Professor and Chairman
Göteburg University
Göteburg, Sweden

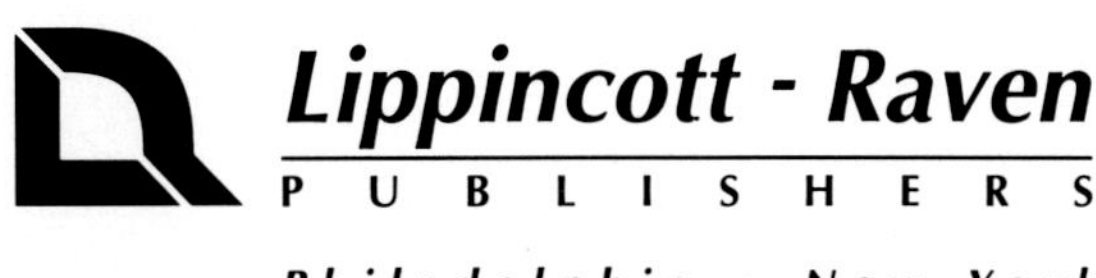

**Lippincott-Raven Publishers, 227 East Washington Square, Philadelphia, Pennsylvania 19106**



Made in the United States of America.

Instrumented fusion of the degenerative lumbar spine: state of the art, questions, and controversies/editors, Marek Szpalski . . . [et al.].
    p.    cm.
  ISBN 0-397-51801-3
  1. Lumbar vertebrae—Surgery. 2. Spinal fusion. 3. Spinal implants. 4. Backache—Surgery. I. Szpalski, Marek.
  [DNLM: 1. Lumbar Vertebrae—surgery. 2. Spinal Fusion—instrumentation. 3. Internal Fixators. 4. Low Back Pain—therapy.
WE 750 I59 1996]
RD768.I54 1996
617.3′75059—dc20
DNLM/DLC
for Library of Congress          96-16765
                                     CIP



9  8  7  6  5  4  3  2

# Introduction

Instrumented fusion in degenerative disorders of the lumbar spine is a fascinating topic. The subtitle of this book, State of the Art, Questions, and Controversies, enables us to highlight a number of the interesting aspects of this subject.

*State of the Art:* Many technically elegant instrumentation devices have been developed to enhance fusion in the lumbar spine. The diversity of techniques and principles, however, shows the lack of an ideal solution. This leads to questions.

*Questions:* Questions are numerous, the foremost being whether there is a place for fusion in the treatment of common degenerative lumbar disorders, considering the high incidence of this (radiologic) condition in totally symptom-free individuals. This, in turn, leads to controversies.

*Controversies:* Recently, controversies have arisen, especially in the United States, concerning the use of some fusion devices. This controversy has spread from the medical community to the general public and the media. The high cost of instrumented procedures leads to further controversies because no undisputed proof of efficacy in degenerative disorders has been given.

There is only one correct way to clarify these points, and that is by prospective randomized studies. For this to be realized, we must all agree to speak the same language and use the same measurement instruments. To achieve this, outcome variables and statistical methods must be agreed on. Only at this cost will we be able to shed light on instrumented fusion of the lumbar spine and avoid criticism, not only from within the medical community but, perhaps more important, from government and health-financing institutions.

*Marek Szpalski, M.D.*
*Robert Gunzburg, M.D., Ph.D.*

# Foreword

M. Szpalski and R. Gunzburg have taken the initiative to bring together an outstanding faculty, not only to describe many techniques of surgical management of degenerative low back pain but also to discuss the validity of this approach. Many authors in this book propose their own approaches with different types of instrumentation. Other disciplines involved in lumbar spine problems discuss the biomechanical aspects and the imaging techniques used to evaluate fusion with spinal implants. New knowledge of physiopathology of pain and of the methodologic and statistical criteria of validity of surgical treatment has provided a basis for the scientific arguments needed to specify more accurately the indications for surgical management, which remain the focal point for discussion.

It is generally accepted that intervention is required for stabilization of major spinal deformities, tumors, unstable fractures, painful spondylolisthesis, and postsurgical instability. For back pain, some evidence (5,7,13) suggests that a number of conditions can be successfully treated with fusion. For example, in spondylolisthesis in young patients, spinal decompression with simultaneous spinal fusion yields better results than laminectomy alone. The role of fusion is debatable when degenerative changes such as osteoarthrosis cause low back pain, and no one can predict the results of surgery and its influence on neighboring spinal segments (6).

Modern developments in immunochemistry and molecular biology have allowed the formulation of new theories about the aging disc, but unfortunately they cannot explain why one degenerative lumbar disc induces pain whereas another does not. We know that in asymptomatic subjects, MRI will demonstrate a 30–40% incidence of pathologic findings (4). The principle of fusion is based on the principle of the painful motion segment (3,8). Therefore, suppression of intervertebral motion should eliminate pain. It must be remembered, however, that in most chronic conditions pain is not always caused by mechanical constraints only. Chemical and inflammatory factors at the nociceptor level also play a role, and the results of fusion are not always those that had been anticipated (12).

One cause of pain may be a torn annulus (7,9) (so-called discogenic pain), and removal of the annulus seems logical. It is now clear that repeated minor injuries in a motion segment produce tears in the annulus (9). The outer layer of the annulus has a rich sensory innervation and the disc has a poor healing potential.

Wiltse (12) reported that many patients whose posterolateral fusion was unquestionably solid still experienced severe pain. This might result from persistent disabling discogenic pain provoked by neovascularization and by inflammatory cell infiltration of the anterior annulus, or it might be caused by a residual relative mobility of the anterior part of the vertebrae.

The true origin of back pain remains an enigma to the surgeon, and the decision to fuse is always difficult to make in cases of degenerative lumbar disc, knowing that there is a risk for failure or even for worsening of the previous condition.

Approximately 80% of the population will suffer low back pain in their lifetimes, and it is generally agreed that most patients are best treated conservatively. Unfortunately, there seems to be a direct relation between the amount of spinal surgery performed in a given geographic region and the number of orthopaedic and neurosurgeons practicing in that area (2). About eight times as many spinal surgical procedures are carried out in the United States per capita as in the United Kingdom. That means that the final results depend on many factors that we do not control well enough. The clinical outcomes of most "surgical inventors" appear good enough to convince them to continue application of their own ideas and techniques.

Turner et al. (10) report that of all papers they reviewed on the subject of spinal fusion for back pain, only 47 described adequate follow-up, although 68% of patients reported in these papers had a satisfactory outcome from fusion. The success rates ranged from 16 to 95%. There are so many different approaches to treatment, selection, assessment of patients, and objective criteria that it is impossible to compare results and to draw conclusions about fusion for back pain.

A multicenter, randomized, prospective clinical trial is difficult and cumbersome to perform. However, only such a study will answer definitive questions about the efficacy of spinal fusion. With the help of statisticians, we should validate our criteria. There is an urgent need for an internationally accepted consensus of standardized patient evaluation, taking in account such factors as psychological disturbances, workplace problems, and litigation issues, which are common causes of failure.

Most implants and instrumentations have been designed for spinal deformities, trauma, and spinal tumors. They provide powerful tools for stabilization and manipulation of the spine, and they probably increase fusion rates. However, these implants are now used for treatment of the degenerative lumbar spine, even without evidence of instability.

Spinal implants should be assessed by cyclic loading tests to establish their mechanical capacities and should respond most accurately to realistic forces and bending moments. Fortunately, in the United States and the European Union, all devices must be certified by an administrative office after verification of the essential requirements: safety of the device and its performance according to the manufacturer's claims (5). All of the systems presented in this book appear to fulfill those criteria.

Although pedicle screws with plates or rods are used in many devices, the use of instrumentation to achieve fusion remains a matter of controversy. In an independently reviewed comparative study of uninstrumented and instrumented lumbar fusion, Bernhardt et al. (1) showed no benefit from instrumentation. This was confirmed by our clinical outcome in 1991 (11). Zdeblick (14), however, reported in 1993 a 65% fusion rate in the uninstrumented group as opposed to 95% in the instrumented group. Nevertheless, stress concentration on the disc above and below the stabilized segments and stress protection in the fused area, with secondary osteoporosis, may become an even greater problem than when spine fusion was achieved only by the use of bone grafts.

The various modalities of fusion in themselves represent a controversial issue. Some authors claim that, to achieve fusion, relative elasticity of the instrumentation yields better results than rigid instrumentation. Others are convinced that bone graft to replace the disc, with or without cages, offers a greater guarantee of stability and a painless segment. Still others claim that the highest rate of fusion is obtained with a circle arthrodesis of the anterior and posterior columns of the motion segments. Because we know there is a relationship between the final clinical outcome and the quality of fusion, these questions are important.

Only when conservative measures have failed should surgery be considered. Inadequate surgical training, poor surgical technique, and incorrect diagnosis will lead to failure and are no longer acceptable. With the right selection, right diagnosis, and right technique, fusion can be indicated in the treatment of painful chronic lesions even if, over the long term, the results are the same as those of conservative approaches and natural history, because we can often influence and reduce the period of evolution of back pain.

The aim of this book is to provide a better understanding of the problem of low back pain and the potential for treating it successfully with surgery. There is an urgent need for an internationally accepted consensus to develop a method for standardized patient evaluation, and we hope that, just as total hip replacement has replaced hip fusion, we will find new procedures for treatment of patients with back pain.

*André Vincent, M.D.*
*Professor and Chairman*
*Department of Orthopaedics*
*and Traumatology*
*Cliniques Universitaires St. Luc*
*Brussels, Belgium*

## References

1. Bernhardt M, Swartz DE, Clothiaux PL, Crowell RR, White AA III. Posterolateral lumbar and lumbarsacral fusion with and without pedicle screw internal fixation. *Clin Orthop* 1992;284:109–15.
2. Cherkin D, Deyo R, Loeser J, Bush T. *An international comparison of back surgery rates*. Marseilles: International Society for the Study of the Lumbar Spine, 1993.
3. Farfan HF, Kirkaldy-Willis WH. The treatment of lumbar intervertebral joint disorders. *Clin Orthop* 1981;158:198–214.
4. Jensen MC, Brant-Zawadski MN, Obuchowski N, Modic MT, Malkasian D, Roos JS. Magnetic resonance imaging of lumbar spine in people without back pain. *N Engl J Med* 1994;331:69–73.
5. Mulholland RC. Pedicle screw fixation in the spine. *J Bone Joint Surg* 1994;76B:517–9.
6. Nachmenson AL. Evaluation of results in lumbar spine surgery. *Acta Orthop Scand* 1993(suppl 251):130–3.
7. O'Brien JP. Anterior spinal tenderness in low-back pain syndromes. *Spine* 1979;4:85–8.
8. O'Brien JP, Mc Donald JW. Controversy in management of spinal fusion. *BMJ* 1996;312:38–40.
9. Park WM, McCall I, O'Brien JP, Webb JK. Fissuring of the posterior annulus fibrosus in the lumbar spine. *Br J Radiol* 1979;52:382–7.
10. Turner TA, Ersek M, Herron L, Hasselkorn J, Kent D. Patient outcome after lumbar spinal fusion. *JAMA* 1992;19:907–12.
11. Vincent A, Dubuc JE, De Nayer P, Delloye Ch. Étude comparative d'arthrodèse lombo-sacrée postéro-latérale et postérieure avec et sans ostéosynthèse. *Acta Orthop Belg* 1991;5(suppl I):228–41.
12. Wiltse LL. Surgery for intervertebral disc disease of lumbar spine. *Clin Orthop* 1977;129:22–45.
13. Wolf MW, Palafox AI, Levet BM. Instrumented lumbar fusion of 103 consecutive patients [Abstract]. In: Whitecloud TS III, ed. *Proc Scoliosis Res Soc* 1993;146.
14. Zdeblick TA. A prospective, randomized study of lumbar fusion: preliminary results. *Spine* 1993;18:983–91.

# Contents

# Contributors

**Michael A. Adams, Ph.D.**   *Senior Research Fellow, Department of Anatomy, University of Bristol, Bristol, England*

**Selcuk Babacan, M.D.**   *Neurosurgeon, Dr. Horst Schmidt Clinic, Wiesbaden, Germany*

**Pietro Bartolozzi, M.D.**   *Professor and Head, Department of Orthopaedic Surgery, Policlinico di Borgo-Roma, Verona, Italy*

**Michel Benoist, M.D.**   *Consultant Rheumatologist of Paris Hospitals, University of Paris VII, Paris, France*

**Emanuele Boero, M.D.**   *Orthopedic Surgeon, Policlinico di Borgo-Roma, Verona, Italy*

**Rémy Cavagna, M.D.**   *Orthopaedic Surgeon, Clinique du Ter, Lorient, France*

**Marco Cassini, M.D.**   *Orthopaedic Surgeon, Policlinico di Borgo-Roma, Verona, Italy*

**Filip Deckers, M.D.**   *Registrar, Department of Radiology, Antwerp University Hospital, University of Antwerp, Antwerp, Belgium*

**Joël Delécrin, M.D.**   *Orthopaedic Surgeon, Hotel Dieu, Nantes, France*

**Arthur M. De Schepper, M.D., Ph.D.**   *Professor and Head, Department of Radiology, Antwerp University Hospital, University of Antwerp, Antwerp, Belgium*

**Vijay K. Goel, Ph.D.**   *Professor, Department of Biomedical Engineering, The University of Iowa, Iowa City, Iowa*

**Charles C. Greenough, M.D., M.Chir., F.R.C.S.**   *Consultant Orthopaedic Surgeon, Middlesbrough General Hospital, Middlesbrough, England*

**Michael Grevitt, F.R.C.S.**   *Spine Fellow, Centre for Spinal Studies and Surgery, Queens Medical Centre, Nottingham, England*

**Peter Griss, M.D.**   *Professor and Head, Department of Orthopaedic Surgery, Philipps University, Marburg, Germany*

**Robert Gunzburg, M.D., Ph.D.**   *Senior Consultant, Department of Orthopaedic Surgery, Brugman University Hospital, Brussels, Belgium*

**Monica Harris, R.N.**   *Research Sister, Centre for Spinal Studies and Surgery, Queens Medical Centre, Nottingham, England*

**Jean-Pierre Hayez, M.D.**   *Head, Department of Orthopaedics Surgery, Centre Hospitalier Moliére Longchamps, Brussels, Belgium*

**Jean Huppert, M.D.**   *Orthopaedic Surgeon, Clinique du Parc, Castelnau le Lez, France*

**Rabbi Khazim, F.R.C.S.**   *Spine Fellow, Centre for Spinal Studies and Surgery, Queens Medical Centre, Nottingham, England*

**Patrick Kluger, M.D.**   *Orthopaedic Surgeon, Ulm University, Ulm, Germany*

**Andreas Korge, M.D.**   *Orthopaedic Surgeon, Ulm University, Ulm, Germany*

**Hein J. A. Kruls, M.D.**   *Orthopaedic Surgeon, Ignatius Ziekenhuis, Breda, The Netherlands*

**Stephen D. Kuslich, M.D.**   *Assistant Clinical Professor, Department of Orthopaedic Surgery, University of Minnesota; and Spinal Surgeon, St. Croix Orthopaedics, Stillwater, Minnesota*

**Philippe Lapresle, M.D.**   *Orthopaedic Surgeon, Clinique Arago, Paris, France*

**Christian Louis, M.D.**   *Orthopaedic Surgeon, Hôpital de la Conception, Marseille, France*

**René Louis, M.D.**   *Professor and Head, Department of Orthopaedics, Hôpital de la Conception, Marseille, France*

**Eduardo R. Luque, M.D.**   *Chief and Director, Department of Orthopaedic Surgery, Germán Díaz Lombardo Hospital, Mexico City, Mexico*

**Thierry Marnay, M.D.**   *Orthopedic Surgeon, Clinique du Parc, Castelnau le Lez, France*

**Christian Mélot, M.D., Ph.D.**   *Associate Professor of Medicine, Department of Intensive Care, Erasmus University Hospital; and Professor of Biostatistics, Free University of Brussels, Brussels, Belgium*

**Christiane Melzer**   *Dr. Horst Schmidt Clinic, Wiesbaden, Germany*

**Michael Melzer**   *Dr. Horst Schmidt Clinic, Wiesbaden, Germany*

**Gilles Missenard, M.D.**   *Orthopaedic Surgeon, Clinique Arago, Paris, France*

**Alf Nachemson, M.D., Ph.D.**   *Professor and Chairman, Department of Orthopaedic Surgery, Göteborg University, Göteborg, Sweden; and Research Professor, Georgetown University, Washington, D.C.*

**Lutz P. Nolte, Ph.D.**   *Head, Biomechanics, Maurice Mueller Institute of Biomechanics, Bern, Switzerland*

**Margareta Nordin, R.P.T., Dr. Sci.**   *Research Associate Professor, School of Medicine, New York University; and Director, Occupational and Industrial Orthopaedic Center, Hospital for Joint Diseases, New York University Medical Center, New York, New York*

**Nicolas R. Panaro, M.D.**   *Department of Rehabilitation Medicine, Rusk Institute, New York, New York*

**Paul M. Parizel, M.D., Ph.D.**   *Adjunct Head, Department of Radiology, Antwerp University Hospital, University of Antwerp, Antwerp, Belgium*

**Dario Pasquetto, M.D.**   *Orthopaedic Surgeon, Policlinico di Borgo-Roma, Verona, Italy*

**Norbert Passuti, M.D.**   *Professor, Department of Orthopaedic Surgery, Hotel Dieu, Nantes, France*

**Gilles Perrin, M.D.**   *Professor of Neurosurgery, Hôpital Neurologique, Lyon, France*

**Michael Pfeiffer, M.D.**   *Orthopaedic Surgeon, Department of Orthopaedic Surgery, Philipps University, Marburg, Germany*

**Charles D. Ray, M.D.**   *Neurosurgeon; Emeritus Director, Institute for Low Back and Neck Care, Minneapolis, Minnesota; and Director of Research and Development, Spinal Research and Education Foundation, Norfolk, Virginia*

**Carlton Reckling, M.D.**   *Spine Fellow, Centre for Spinal Studies and Surgery, Queens Medical Centre, Nottingham, England*

**Abraham Rogozinski, M.D.**   *Orthopaedic Surgeon, Rogozinski Orthopedic Clinic, Jacksonville, Florida*

**Chaïm Rogozikski, M.D.**   *Orthopaedic Surgeon, Rogozinski Orthopedic Clinic, Jacksonville, Florida*

**Robert Schönmayr, M.D.**   *Professor and Chief, Department of Neurosurgery, Dr. Horst Schmidt Clinic, Wiesbaden, Germany*

**Dan M. Spengler, M.D.**   *Professor and Chairman, Department of Orthopaedics, Vanderbilt University, Nashville, Tennessee*

**Reinhard Steffen, M.D.**   *Associate Professor, Department of Orthopaedics, St. Josef Hospital, Ruhr University, Bochum, Germany*

**Marek Szpalski, M.D.** *Senior Consultant, Department of Orthopaedic Surgery, Centre Hospitalier, Molière Longchamp; Stagemmeester in Manual Therapy, Vrij Universiteit Brussel, Brussels, Belgium; Adjunct Assistant Professor of Orthopaedics and Rehabilitation, Vanderbilt University, Nashville, Tennessee; and Senior Scientist, Hospital for Joint Diseases, New York University Medical Center, New York, New York*

**Shinobu Takahashi, M.D.** *Associate Professor, Department of Orthopaedic Surgery, Hotel Dieu, Nantes, France*

**Pieter F. van Akkerveeken, M.D., Ph.D.** *Orthopaedic Surgeon, RugAdviesCentra Nederland, Zeist, The Netherlands*

**Ad F. A. van Beurden, M.D.** *Orthopaedic Surgeon, Ignatius Ziekenhuis, Breda, The Netherlands*

**Luc van der Hauwe, M.D.** *Resident, Department of Radiology, Antwerp University Hospital, University of Antwerp, Antwerp, Belgium*

**Johan W. van Goethem, M.D.** *Resident, Department of Radiology, Antwerp University Hospital, University of Antwerp, Antwerp, Belgium*

**André Vincent, M.D.** *Professor and Chairman, Department of Orthopaedic Surgery, Cliniques Universitaires St. Luc, Brussels, Belgium*

**John Webb, F.R.C.S.** *Consultant Spine Surgeon, Centre for Spinal Studies and Surgery, Queens Medical Centre, Nottingham, England*

**Friedrich Weidt, M.D.** *Department of Orthopaedics, Ulm University, Ulm, Germany*

**Roland E. Willburger, M.D.** *Orthopaedic Surgeon, St. Josef Hospital, Ruhr University, Bochum, Germany*

**Ralf H. Wittenberg, M.D.** *Associate Professor, Department of Orthopedic Surgery, St. Josef Hospital, Ruhr University, Bochum, Germany*

*Instrumented Fusion of the Degenerative Lumbar Spine: State of the Art, Questions, and Controversies,* edited by M. Šzpalski, R. Gunzburg, D. M. Spengler, and A. Nachemson. Lippincott–Raven Publishers, Philadelphia © 1996.

# 1

# Biomechanics of Spinal Implants

## M. A. Adams

*Comparative Orthopaedic Research Unit, Department of Anatomy, University of Bristol, Bristol BS2 8EJ, England*

Spinal implants are used to treat a wide variety of painful and disabling spinal disorders. Although a "successful" implant is one that relieves pain and disability, regardless of its mechanical characteristics, it is widely believed that a successful surgical outcome should be associated with reduced mechanical stress or strain (deformation) in certain pain-sensitive structures. The surgeon must therefore anticipate how a given implant will affect mechanical loading of the structure presumed to be responsible for the patient's pain.

Recent anatomic and clinical studies suggest that severe and chronic low back pain most often originates from the annulus fibrosus and, to a lesser extent, the apophyseal joints (24,25,43,47,59–61). This chapter therefore concentrates on stress distributions within these structures and how they might be affected by spinal implants. The emphasis is on spinal mechanics rather than specific implant designs.

As a secondary purpose, this chapter offers some general guidelines for the design and testing of new implants. None of the devices currently in use is effective for all patients, so it is inevitable that new devices will be introduced as our understanding of spinal pain and spinal mechanics improves.

## BIOMECHANICS OF THE LUMBAR SPINE

### Distribution of Compressive Load Among Intervertebral Discs, Ligaments, and Apophyseal Joints

Most of the compressive forces on the lumbar spine is resisted by the intervertebral discs, the exact proportion being reflected by the hydrostatic pressure (intradiscal pressure) within the nucleus pulposus (16). For the same applied compressive force, intradiscal pressure increases by up to 100% in flexed postures (16) as a result of tension generated in stretched intervertebral ligaments (Fig. 1A). Conversely, postures that preserve or increase the lordosis of the osteoligamentous lumbar spine increase loading of the apophyseal joints and decrease intradiscal pressure by up to 40% (16) (Fig. 1B).

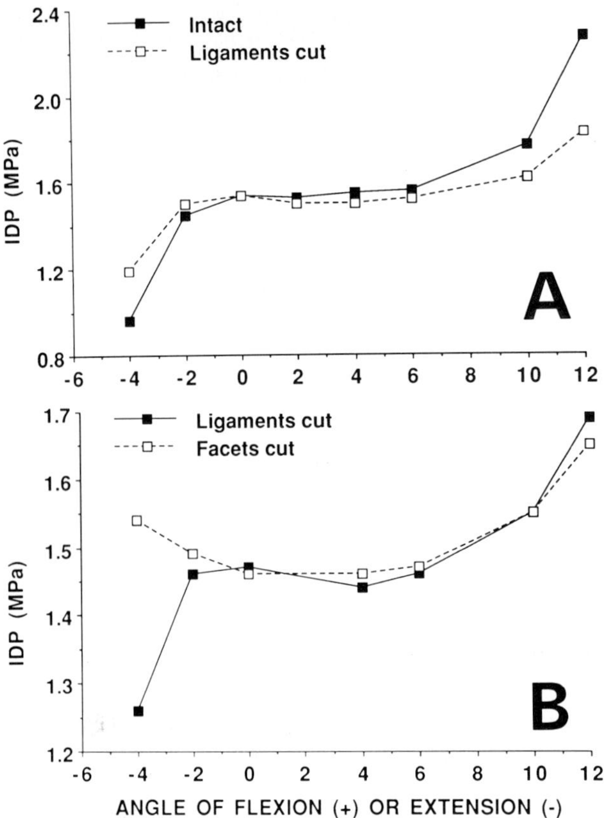



**FIG. 1.** Intradiscal pressure (IDP) varies with the angle of flexion and extension, even when the applied compressive force is constant (2 kN). **A:** Cutting all of the ligaments of the neural arch reduces IDP in flexion, indicating that ligament tension increases the compressive force on the disc in flexed postures. **B:** Removing the bony surfaces (facets) of the apophyseal joints increases IDP in extension, indicating that these surfaces relieve the disc of compressive load in extended postures. Male, 49 years old, L4–5. Adapted from Adams et al. (16).

Sustained ("creep") loading also affects the distribution of compressive load in the lumbar spine. Creep expels water from intervertebral discs (11) and reduces the vertical separation of adjacent vertebrae. As a result, ligament tension in flexed postures is reduced (5) and apophyseal joint loading in lordotic postures is increased (8,35).

### Distribution of Compressive Stress Within Intervertebral Discs

It is possible to measure stress distributions throughout the disc using a miniature pressure transducer, side-mounted in a 1.3–mm-diameter needle (44,45). In regions of the disc that do not exhibit a hydrostatic pressure, the transducer measures the average compressive stress acting perpendicular to its surface. Typical stress profiles for a mature disc (grade 2 on degeneration scale of 1–4) are shown in Fig. 2. In younger discs, the hydrostatic region extends throughout the inner and middle annulus. In the outermost 3–5 mm of annulus there is insufficient proteoglycan gel to exhibit much compressive stress, and it may be no coincidence that this is the only region of the disc in which nerve endings are found (20,25,69). According to a mathematical model (41) and some cadaver experiments (7,27), the outer annulus acts as a tensile "skin" that contains the hydrostatic region and that resists bending and twisting of the disc.

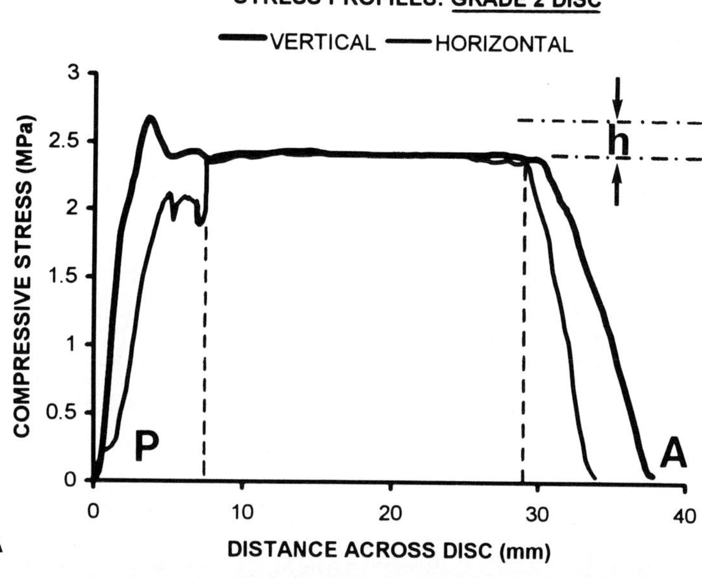


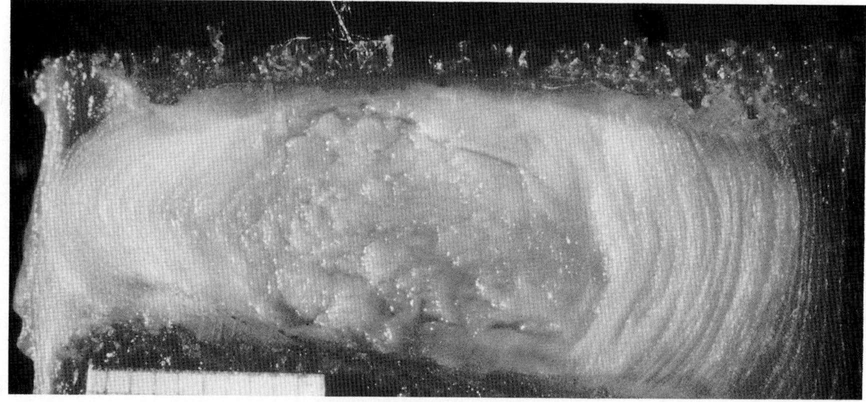


**FIG. 2. A:** Distribution of horizontal and vertical compressive stress along the sagittal midline of a nondegenerated intervertebral disc loaded to 2 kN in the neutral posture. Male, 40 years old, L2–3. The central region between the dotted lines exhibits a hydrostatic pressure in which stress does not vary with direction or location. The height of stress "peaks" (h) referred to in the text is measured relative to nuclear pressure. P, posterior; A, anterior. **B:** A midsagittal section through a similar disc.

## Effect of Age and Degeneration on Intradiscal Compressive Stress

With increasing age and degeneration, the central hydrostatic region shrinks and peaks of compressive stress appear in the middle of the annulus, especially posterior to the nucleus (16–18,44). Stress peaks can become particularly large after creep loading (15,44) and in lordotic postures (16). Damage to a vertebral body endplate allows more space for the nucleus. This causes an immediate drop in intradiscal pressure of up to 50% (18) and a transfer of stress from nucleus to annulus (Fig. 3A). The resulting stress peaks in the annulus therefore become so large that they can cause the annulus to collapse in toward the depressurized nuclear cavity (19), as

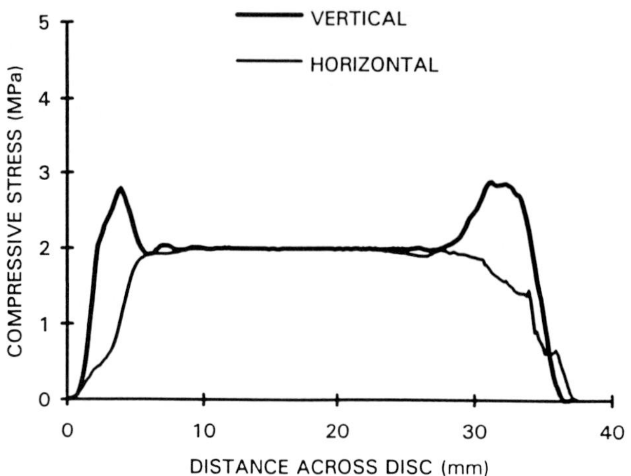

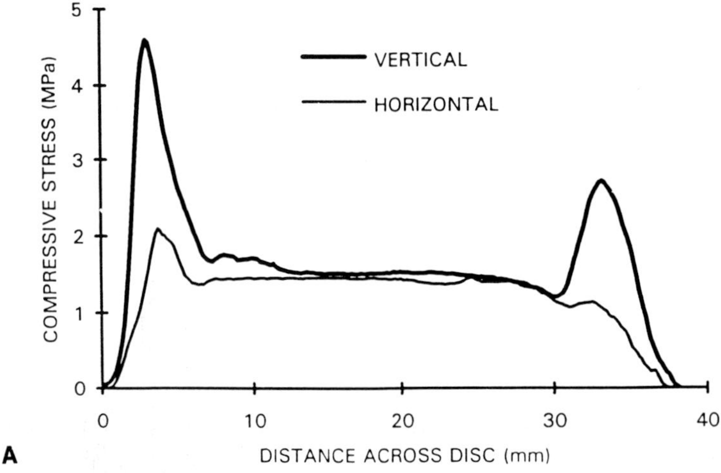

5
4
3
2
1
0
COMPRESSIVE STRESS (MPa)
VERTICAL
HORIZONTAL
0    10    20    30    40
DISTANCE ACROSS DISC (mm)
A

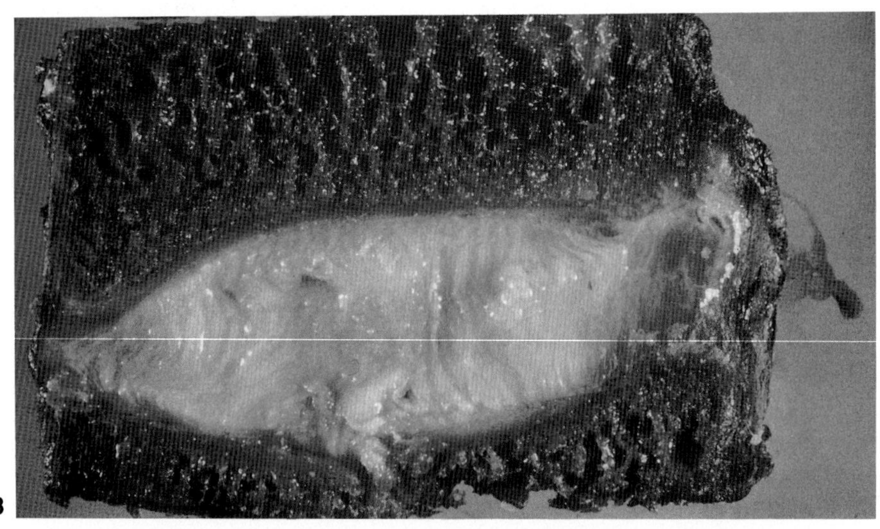

B

shown in Fig. 3B. Disc prolapse also depressurizes the nucleus and transfers compressive stress onto the annulus. Structural damage to the annulus and vertebral endplates probably explains the irregular stress distributions commonly found in degenerated discs (Fig. 4). It may be of particular relevance to spinal fixation that moderately degenerated discs from middle-aged cadavers sometimes show evidence of incomplete failure of the posterior annulus (17), as shown in Fig. 4. Multiple stress peaks suggest some structural disruption in an annulus that has not collapsed entirely but is continuing to resist as several separate units. Stress distributions such as this have been recorded in vivo from patients undergoing spinal fusion operations (62), and they are painful. An association between incomplete failure of the posterior annulus and pain is consistent with the findings of provocation discography (47). One might speculate that complete failure of the posterior annulus causes a marked reduction in disc height and increased loading of the apophyseal joints, which then "stress-shield" the painful posterior annulus. This may explain why there is such poor correspondence between back pain and the degree of disc degeneration.

### Bending Stresses Acting on the Spine

The above discussion has considered compressive (axial) loading of the spine, but it is becoming apparent that bending and torsional stresses are of equal or greater importance in the etiology of spinal disorders. Forward bending movements are resisted primarily by the back muscles, so that in the fully flexed toe-touching position, the bending stress (bending "moment") acting on the osteoligamentous spine is approximately 20 Nm (3), which is only 33% of that required to damage it (3,13,14). The protective action of the back muscles may be reduced, however, during dynamic movements and after muscle fatigue. At the spine's elastic limit, the interspinous ligament is the first structure to be damaged (14). The bending moment acting on the disc is then only 14 Nm on average, which is less than half of that required to damage it (7), so the disc is protected by the ligaments just as the ligaments are protected by muscles (Fig. 5). The maximal tensile force that can act in each ligament is reflected by its tensile strength, for which typical values are shown in Fig. 6. Note that the anterior longitudinal ligament and capsular ligaments are particularly strong and that the posterior longitudinal ligament is particularly weak. Hyperflexion beyond the range permitted by the ligaments eventually tears the peripheral posterior annulus fibrosus, usually at mid-height (7). When high compressive forces are combined with high bending moments, disc prolapse can occur, either in a sudden injury (10) or as a result of fatigue failure of the annulus (12,38).

Backwards bending of the lumbar spine is resisted primarily by the neural arch (6,39). A combination of severe backwards bending and compression, applied repetitively, can cause posterior "hairpin" bulging of the posterior annulus or anterior disc prolapse (6). In some cadaveric specimens, a combination of low compressive

---

**FIG. 3. A:** Distribution of compressive stress along the sagittal midline of a lumbar intervertebral disc, before (top) and after (bottom) one of the vertebral endplates was damaged by compressive overload. Endplate damage decompresses the nucleus and generates high stress peaks in the annulus. Male, 30 years old, L4–5, posterior on left, loaded at 2 kN in 2° of extension. Adapted from Adams (2). **B:** Stress peaks in the annulus as shown in *A* can cause the annulus to collapse into the nucleus during subsequent cyclic loading.

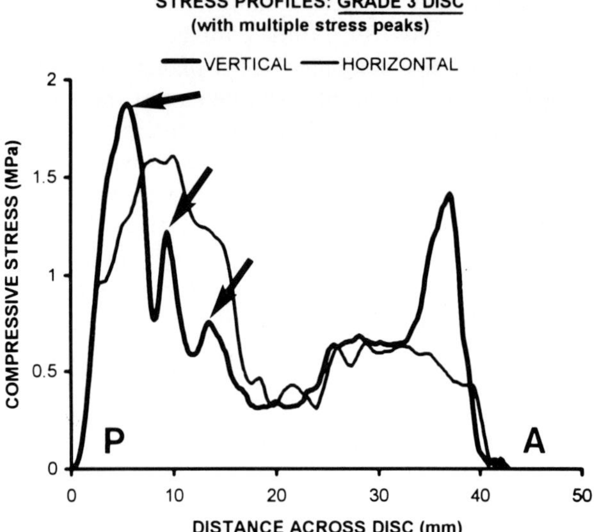


**FIG. 4.** Distribution of compressive stress along the sagittal midline of a moderately degenerated lumbar disc (grade 3 on a scale of 1–4). Multiple stress peaks within the posterior annulus suggest that its structure is disrupted but not destroyed. Discs such as this may be painful. Male, 47 years old, L3–4, posterior on left, loaded at 2 kN in 4° of extension.

loading and high backwards bending can lead to the posterior annulus being stress-shielded by the apophyseal joints (Adams 1995, unpublished results). Hyperextension causes the descending inferior articular processes to be deflected rearwards by the lamina below. This may be a cause of spondylolysis (39), and the facet tip may damage the inferior margins of the joint capsule (68).

Lateral bending of the lumbar spine is strongly resisted by the disc (58) because its lateral diameter is 50% greater than its sagittal diameter. A combination of lateral and forward bending is particularly harmful to the annulus because it concentrates tensile stress in one of the posterolateral corners (10,12). However, the lateral bending component is often confused with torsion.

### Torsion

Torsion or twisting of the lumbar spine occurs about a center of rotation in the posterior annulus (9,28) so that the peripheral anterior annulus is most affected. This may explain how "peripheral rim tears" (52) are formed. The posterior annulus is well protected by the apophyseal joint surfaces, and torsion does not cause posterior disc prolapse (9,36) unless it is accompanied by substantial bending and compression (38).

### Shear

In standing postures, the lower lumbar discs are inclined at a considerable angle to the horizontal, so a substantial forward "shear" force is acting in the plane of the disc. The shear force can reach 760 N during activities such as marching with a heavy

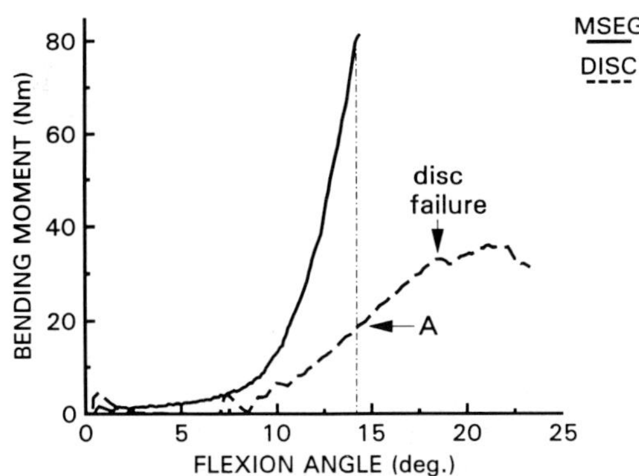


**FIG. 5.** When a cadaveric motion segment is flexed under the combined influence of compression and bending, the applied bending moment rises rapidly near the elastic limit of flexion (*vertical dashed line*). If the ligaments of the neural arch are cut through, then the intervertebral disc can be flexed several degrees more before failing. This illustrates the protective role of the ligaments. Male, 28 years old, L4–5. Adapted from Adams et al. (7).

backpack (29), but much of it may be resisted by the back muscles (57). Shear forces cause each lower lumbar vertebra to move forward over the one below, until the apophyseal joint surfaces prevent further movement. The inferior articular processes can be bent backwards about the pars interarticularis, and fractures resembling spondylolysis can occur if the shear force rises to approximately 2 kN in a single loading cycle (32) or to 760 N during cyclic "fatigue" loading (29). Intervertebral discs merely "creep away" from sustained or repetitive shear forces (31), so removal of one or both facet joints can lead to axial rotation or forward translation of the upper vertebra relative to the one below.

## PREVENTING INTERVERTEBRAL MOVEMENT

Many spinal implants attempt to prevent intervertebral movement so as to promote bony union between adjacent vertebral bodies. It is assumed that this will reduce pain from intervertebral discs, ligaments, nerve roots, and joint capsules that are deformed by spinal movements. Physiologic spinal movements involve combinations of translations and rotations, so that there are no fixed centers of rotation, but the instantaneous center of rotation during flexion and extension (see Fig. 6) stays close to the nucleus pulposus (55), and in axial rotation it lies in the posterior annulus fibrosus (9,28). Therefore, it might be expected that spinal movements would be limited most severely by implants, such as pedicle screw fixators and anterior plating systems, that lie at some distance from these regions of the disc. Interbody fusion devices appear to be less suitable for this particular purpose because they lie at the "fulcrum" or pivot point and are therefore likely to be disrupted by high forces arising from muscles pulling on the neural arch, which acts as a long lever.

However, this analysis is probably too simplistic because interbody fusion devices may be able to obtain additional stability from the strong intervertebral ligaments that lie farther from the center of rotation. Normally, intervertebral ligaments do little to restrict small spinal movements because most of them are slack for a considerable range of flexion (14) and extension (6), especially in degenerated "unstable" spines (46). During a fusion operation, this slack can be taken up, and stability increased, simply by distracting the vertebral bodies as the implant is inserted between them. Distraction of between 2 mm and 5 mm would be sufficient to remove the slack in the capsular ligaments and generate a tensile force of 300–1,000 N in them (30). If the apophyseal joints were osteoarthritic, then only 2 mm of distraction would have a similar effect (30). A high ligament force would help to stabilize the adjacent disc because it would act to oppose any flexion movements of the spine. It may be matched by a similar force in the anterior longitudinal ligament (Fig. 6). It should be possible to take practical advantage of this mechanism by increasing the amount of distraction when interbody devices are inserted until the desired degree of ligament tension is achieved. Changes in ligament tension probably explain why motion segments become more resistant to bending after a saline injection into the disc (22) and why bending stiffness falls markedly after disc creep (5).

## UNLOADING THE INTERVERTEBRAL DISC?

A secondary and quite distinct purpose of some spinal implants appears to be to protect the intervertebral discs from high compressive force. However, it is not enough simply to provide an alternative pathway through the neural arches by means of some rigid fixator (Fig. 7), because the disc has such a high compressive stiffness

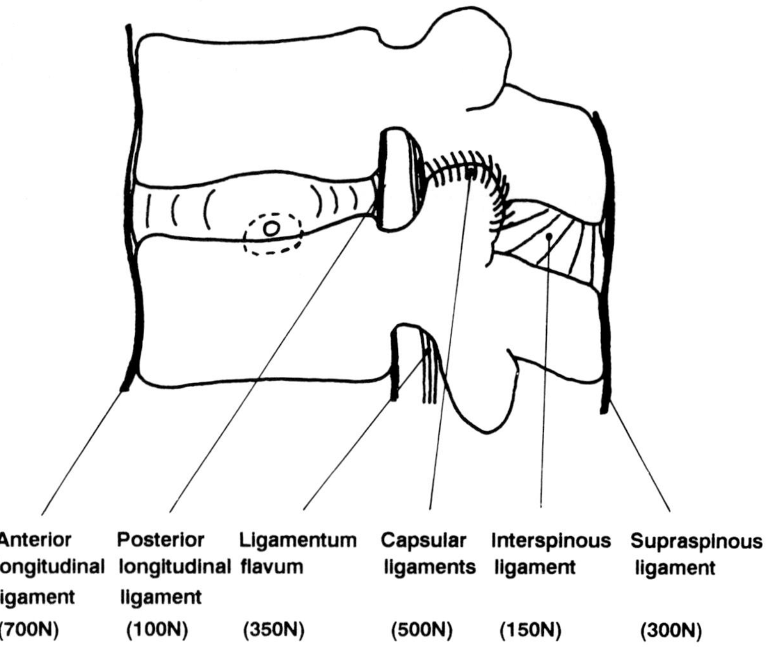



**FIG. 6.** Flexion and extension of a lumbar motion segment take place about a moving center of rotation (O) which lies near the center of the intervertebral disc (55). The restraint to movement that each ligament can provide is proportional to the ligament strength (shown in Newtons) and the distance of the ligament from O. Data from refs. 14, 30, and 49. From Adams (1).

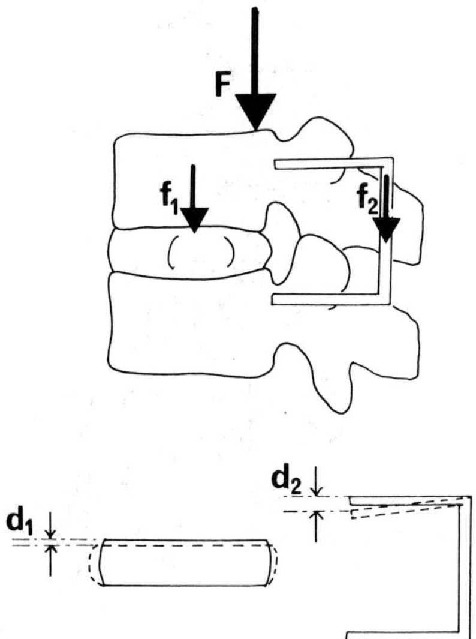



**If d₁ < d₂ then f₁ > f₂**

**FIG. 7.** When a compressive force F acts on an instrumented motion segment, part of the force is resisted by the disc (f₁) and part by the fixator (f₂). The relative sizes of f₁ and f₂ depend on the relative deformability of the disc (d₁), and the fixator–neural arch construct (d₂). Any loosening of the fixator screws will make d₂ large and f₂ small.

that only a small compressive deformation is required to generate high compressive stresses within it. Typically, a compressive deformation of only 1 mm generates a compressive force of 1 kN on the disc (8). In principle, rigid spinal instrumentation systems could re-route compressive force around a painful disc. In practice, however, they are unlikely to prevent small vertical deformations of 1 mm or less, which are all that is required to load the disc. Fixators can bend, and movements can occur at the fixator–screw or screw–bone interfaces, especially after cyclic loading. This may explain why anterior plates failed to prevent deterioration of surgically disrupted discs in an animal model of disc degeneration (48). It should not be claimed that a spinal fixation system unloads the disc unless this can be demonstrated by measurements of intradiscal pressure.

## FUSION IN FLEXION OR EXTENSION?

Although it would be difficult to remove much compressive loading from the entire disc, it is a simple matter to alter the internal distribution of stress within the disc so that load is shifted away from a particular pain-sensitive region. Approximately 4° of flexion is sufficient to remove peaks of compressive stress from the posterior annulus and generate an even distribution of compressive stress across the entire disc (16). Flexion also removes vertical loading of the apophyseal joint surfaces (8,16,35). Conversely, 4° of extension reduces intradiscal pressure and transfers load from the central region of the vertebral endplate to the apophyseal joints (8,16,39).

Obviously, the angle of flexion or extension must be chosen with care because it has a major effect on the distribution of forces in the fused spine. The choice should not be influenced by vague notions of what is "natural" or normal, because there is no such thing as a "normal" lumbar curvature. Standing erect involves approximately 12–15° of lumbar extension (from L1 to S1) relative to the curvature of an excised cadaver spine (6), whereas unsupported sitting involves approximately 30° of flexion (21,33). Because both postures are equally "normal," other criteria should be used to justify this important detail of surgical procedure.

## EVALUATION OF SPINAL IMPLANTS

This section comprises a short summary of a more comprehensive review of methodology in mechanical testing of the spine (2).

### Animal Model, Mathematical Model, or In Vitro Experiment?

Animal models can be used to demonstrate biologic (cell-mediated) principles, such as a tissue's response to altered mechanical loading or to foreign materials or wear debris. Structural failure cannot be reliably predicted on the basis of experiments on small animals because of the "cube square law" that states, in effect, that structures become weaker as they are "scaled up" in size unless stronger materials are employed to construct them.

Analytic mathematical models can be used to assess the feasibility of a design implant, but little more. Although finite element models have greater potential and are increasing in importance (37), at present they suffer from several limitations. The first is the variability and poor quality of experimental data concerning the mechanical properties of complex spinal tissues such as the annulus fibrosus. This obliges the modeler to make simplifying assumptions and arbitrary choices regarding the behavior of the materials. Other problems confronting the modeler are the difficulty in simulating loosening at the bone–screw and screw–fixator interfaces and the fact that contact forces across adjacent neural arches depend greatly on the shape of the individual vertebrae on which the model is based. These difficulties reduce the predictive power of finite element models and prevent them from being an adequate substitute for experimental testing of spinal implants. However, models are suitable for optimizing existing implant designs.

For the immediate future, it will be necessary to evaluate spinal implants by performing mechanical experiments on human and animal tissues. If the implant design relies on the precise anatomy of the neural arch, then human cadaveric spines should be used. Implants that fix adjacent vertebral bodies or depend on pedicle screws are less sensitive to interspecies differences in anatomy, so it may be more appropriate to evaluate them on animal spines of similar size. Animal spines may even be preferable when the only human material available is old and osteoporotic (66), or when comparisons between several different fixators demand large numbers of similar specimens (70).

### What Forces and Moments Should Be Applied?

When a spinal implant is evaluated in the laboratory, the spine–implant construct must be subjected to realistic forces and bending moments. Spinal tissues are "nonlinear," which means that they are stiffer at high loads (see Fig. 5). They are also "viscoelastic," which means that they are stiffer if loaded rapidly (4,51,67). The nonlinear viscoelastic properties of spinal tissues ensure that the distribution of loading among different structures depends on the magnitude of load applied and on the rate at which it is applied. Therefore, mechanical loading regimens applied to instrumented spines in vitro must resemble those encountered in vivo, and this means high and rapid loading. If specimens are loaded rapidly, they also recover rapidly, and reliable comparisons can therefore be made among repeated tests on the same specimen.

Everyday movements, such as bending forward, standing up, or sitting down, take approximately 0.5–5 s to complete, and loading cycles applied in vitro should therefore be of similar duration. The compressive force acting on the spine in life varies from 500 N when standing, to 700 N when sitting, and to 2 kN during light manual work in an erect or slightly stooped posture (50). Lifting weights of 10–30 kg from the ground generates peak compressive forces of 3–6 kN in healthy young men (34,56). The sagittal plane bending moment acting on the lumbar spine usually lies in the range of 10–20 Nm during similar lifting activities (3,34). Torques acting on the lumbar spine in life have never been quantified, but a torque of 20 Nm will damage some lumbar motion segments (9), therefore, 10–15 Nm may represent the normal physiologic range.

### Motion Segments or Whole Lumbar Spines (L1–S1)?

The size of some implants requires them to be tested in large multisegment specimens. Large specimens have the additional advantage of preserving those ligaments that span more than one vertebra, and they ensure that the intermediate vertebrae are loaded by means of the disc on both their superior and inferior surfaces (54). However, large specimens have a considerable disadvantage also. In the absence of muscle support, they buckle in response to high compressive loading, as shown in Fig. 8. The problem is that movements of the intermediate "floating" vertebrae are restrained neither by muscles, as they would be in life, nor by the apparatus, as they would be in a motion segment experiment.

### Should Separate "Muscle Forces" Be Applied?

It is not always necessary to simulate the action of individual muscles in the laboratory, because any number of forces acting on a rigid body in a given plane can be summed and represented by a single force (2). The major back muscles act at small angles to the sagittal plane (26) and are symmetrical about that plane, so their out-of-plane components can be ignored for most purposes. Likewise, the vertebrae are stiffer than the intervertebral soft tissues, especially at low to moderate load levels, so the rigid body approximation is often acceptable. Separate "muscle forces" would be valuable, however, in any cadaver experiment that seeks to examine deformations of the vertebrae themselves, and apparatus capable of simulating these forces has recently been described and evaluated (64). The major effect of muscle forces thus far reported (65) is to apply a compressive preload to the specimen at the same time as bending, but this can be done with much simpler apparatus (2,14).

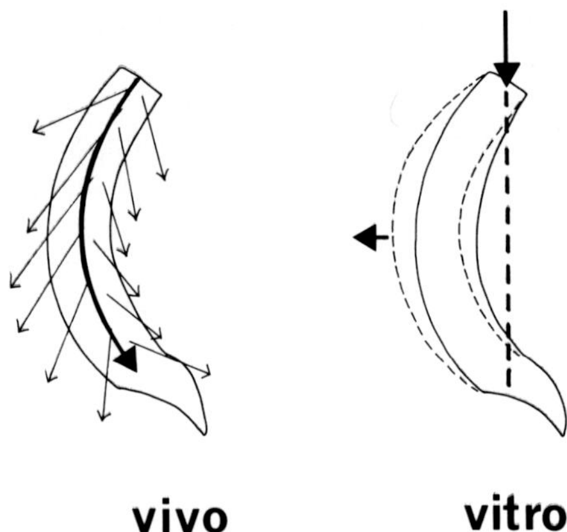


**FIG. 8.** In vivo, the lumbar spine is loaded by many muscle attachments such that the resultant spinal compressive force passes through each intervertebral disc. If a whole lumbar spine is loaded in vitro by means of a single applied force, then this force will not pass through all of the discs and the spine will tend to buckle. Buckling can be minimized by testing short sections of spine.

### Complex Loading or "Pure" Compression and Bending?

In life, the spine is rarely subjected to simple loading in compression, bending, or torsion. Instead, it is subjected to several components at the same time, and the spine's response to one component depends on the presence of the others. For example, the spine's bending stiffness increases with increasing compressive preload (3,42), and torsional stiffness increases in the presence of bending (40). In addition, intervertebral discs can be made to prolapse in response to high bending and compressive loads, but only if these loads are applied at the same time (10,12,38). Laboratory experiments should therefore endeavor to reproduce the complex spinal loading typically seen in life.

### Suggested Experimental Protocol for Evaluating Spinal Implants

1. Measure the load deformation characteristics of the (noninstrumented) spine specimen in compression, axial rotation, flexion, lateral bending, and hyperextension, using loads and loading rates discussed above.
2. Apply the spinal implant and repeat test 1.
3. Apply 10,000 cycles of loading in compression and bending, and then repeat test 1 again
4. Compress the instrumented specimen to failure to determine the strength of the spine–implant construct.

A comparison of results from tests 1 and 2 will indicate the stabilizing effect of the implant. Test 3 will reveal any marked tendency to loosen, migrate, or fail in "fatigue" *in the short term*. (Long-term failure mechanisms are clearly outside the scope of cadaver experiments.) The strength determined in test 4 could be compared to the strength of noninstrumented spines to gauge the weakening effect of the implant.

When the implant's ability to unload the disc is of primary concern, this should be checked during the tests by measuring intradiscal pressure. Suitable transducers can now be bought for only a few hundred pounds (44,45). Several recent publications contain additional advice concerning spinal implant testing (23,53,63,64,66,70).

## DISCUSSION

The past few years have seen rapid progress in our understanding of the tissue origins of back pain (25,43) and in the investigative procedures required for accurate diagnosis (47,59–62). This progress has been matched by detailed information concerning the distribution of mechanical stress within the intervertebral discs, ligaments, and apophyseal joints of (noninstrumented) lumbar spines (15–18,35). If the effects of spinal implants on these stress distributions can be characterized, then it should be possible to devise a logical rationale for the design and use of spinal implants. The surgeon would be able to identify, with a reasonable degree of certainty, just what structure is painful, what loads are provoking it, and what implant is most likely to protect it. Of course, the success or otherwise of any treatment depends more on psychosocial factors than on mechanical factors, but it is nevertheless important to try to get the mechanics right and to base all surgical interventions on sound scientific principles.

## ACKNOWLEDGMENT

The work of the author is supported by the Arthritis and Rheumatism Council of Great Britain.

## REFERENCES

1. Adams MA. Biomechanics of the lumbar motion segment. In: Boyling JD, Palastanga N, eds. *Grieve's modern manual therapy—the vertebral column.* Edinburgh: Churchill Livingstone, 1994: 109–30.
2. Adams MA. Mechanical testing of the spine: an appraisal of methodology, results and conclusions. *Spine* 1995;20:2151–6.
3. Adams MA, Dolan P. A technique for quantifying bending moment acting on the lumbar spine in-vivo. *J Biomech* 1991;24:117–26.
4. Adams MA, Dolan P. Time dependent changes in the lumbar spine's resistance to bending. *Clin Biomech* [*in press*].
5. Adams MA, Dolan P, Hutton WC. Diurnal variations in the stresses on the lumbar spine. *Spine* 1987;12:130–7.
6. Adams MA, Dolan P, Hutton WC. The lumbar spine in backward bending. *Spine* 1988;13:1019–26.
7. Adams MA, Green TP, Dolan P. The strength in anterior bending of lumbar intervertebral discs. *Spine* 1994;19:2197–203.
8. Adams MA, Hutton WC. The effect of posture on the role of the apophyseal joints in resisting intervertebral compressive force. *J Bone Joint Surg* 1980;62-B:358–62.
9. Adams MA, Hutton WC. The relevance of torsion to the mechanical derangement of the lumbar spine. *Spine* 1981;6:241–8.
10. Adams MA, Hutton WC. Prolapsed intervertebral disc. A hyperflexion injury. *Spine* 1982;7:184–91.
11. Adams MA, Hutton WC. The effect of posture on the fluid content of lumbar intervertebral discs. *Spine* 1983;8:665–71.
12. Adams MA, Hutton WC. Gradual disc prolapse. *Spine* 1985;10:524–31.
13. Adams MA, Hutton WC. Has the lumbar spine a margin of safety in forward bending? *Clin Biomech* 1986;1:3–6.
14. Adams MA, Hutton WC, Stott JRR. The resistance to flexion of the lumbar intervertebral joint. *Spine* 1980;5:245–53.

15. Adams MA, McMillan DW, Green TP, Dolan P. Sustained loading generates stress concentrations in lumbar intervertebral discs. *Spine* 1996;21:434–8.
16. Adams MA, McNally DM, Chinn H, Dolan P. Posture and the compressive strength of the lumbar spine. International Society of Biomechanics Award Paper. *Clin Biomech* 1994;9:5–14.
17. Adams MA, McNally DS, Dolan P. Stress distributions inside intervertebral discs: the effects of age and degeneration. *J Bone Joint Surg Br* [*in press*].
18. Adams MA, McNally DS, Wagstaff J, Goodship AE. Abnormal stress concentrations in lumbar intervertebral discs following damage to the vertebral body: a cause of disc failure. European Spine Society (Acromed) Award Paper. *Eur Spine J* 1993;1:214–21.
19. Adams MA, Morrison HP, Dolan P. Internal disruption of an intervertebral disc can be caused by previous minor damage to an adjacent vertebral body. Presented to the International Society for the Study of the Lumbar Spine, Helsinki, Finland, June, 1995.
20. Ahmed M, Bjurholm A, Kreicbergs A, Schultzberg M. Neuropeptide Y, tyrosine hydroxylase and vasoactive intestinal polypeptide-immunoreactive nerve fibers in the vertebral bodies, discs, dura mater, and spinal ligaments of the rat lumbar spine. *Spine* 1993;18:268–73.
21. Andersson GBJ, Murphy RW, Ortengren R, Nachemson AL. The influence of backrest inclination and lumbar support on lumbar lordosis. *Spine* 1979;4:52–8.
22. Andersson GBJ, Schultz AB. Effects of fluid injection on mechanical properties of intervertebral discs. *J Biomech* 1979;12:453–8.
23. Ashman RB, Bechtold JE, Edwards WT, et al. In-vitro spinal arthrodesis implant mechanical testing protocols. *J Spinal Dis* 1989;2:274–81.
24. Beaman ND, Graziano GP, Glover RA, Wojtys EM, Chang V. Substance P innervation of lumbar spine facet joints. *Spine* 1995;18:1044–9.
25. Bogduk N. The innervation of the intervertebral discs. In: Boyling JD, Palastanga N, eds. *Grieve's modern manual therapy—the vertebral column.* Edinburgh: Churchill Livingstone, 1994:149–62.
26. Bogduk N, Macintosh JE, Pearcy MJ. A universal model of the lumbar back muscles in the upright position. *Spine* 1992;17:897–913.
27. Brinckmann P, Grootenboer H. Change of disc height, radial disc bulge and intradiscal pressure from discectomy: an in-vitro investigation on human lumbar discs. *Spine* 1991;16:641–6.
28. Cossette JW, Farfan HF, Robertson GH, Wells RV. The instantaneous centre of rotation of the third lumbar intervertebral joint. *J Biomech* 1971;4:149–53.
29. Cyron BM, Hutton WC. The fatigue strength of the lumbar neural arch in spondylolysis. *J Bone Joint Surg* 1978;60-B:234–8.
30. Cyron BM, Hutton WC. The tensile strength of the capsular ligaments of the apophyseal joints. *J Anat* 1981;132:145–50.
31. Cyron BM, Hutton WC, Stott JRR. Spondylolysis—the shearing stiffness of the lumbar intervertebral joint. *Acta Orthop Belg* 1979;45:459–69.
32. Cyron BM, Hutton WC, Troup JDG. Spondylolytic fractures. *J Bone Joint Surg* 1976;58-B:462–6.
33. Dolan P, Adams MA, Hutton WC. Commonly adopted postures and their effect on the lumbar spine. *Spine* 1988;13:197–201.
34. Dolan P, Earley M, Adams MA. Bending and compressive stresses acting on the lumbar spine during lifting activities. *J Biomech* 1994;27:1237–48.
35. Dunlop RB, Adams MA, Hutton WC. Disc space narrowing and the lumbar facet joints. *J Bone Joint Surg* 1984;66-B:706–10.
36. Farfan HF, Cossette JW, Robertson GH, Wells RV, Kraus H. The effects of torsion on the lumbar intervertebral joints: the role of torsion in the production of disc degeneration. *J Bone Joint Surg* 1970;52-A:468–97.
37. Goel VK, Gilbertson LG. Applications of the finite element method to thoracolumbar spinal research—past, present, and future. *Spine* 1995;20:1719–27.
38. Gordon SJ, Yang KH, Mayer PJ, Mace AH, Kish VL, Radin EL. Mechanism of disc rupture—a preliminary report. *Spine* 1991;16:450–6.
39. Green TP, Allvey JC, Adams MA. Spondylolysis: bending of the inferior articular processes of lumbar vertebrae during simulated spinal movements. *Spine* 1994;19:2683–91.
40. Gunzburg R, Hutton W, Fraser R. Axial rotation of the lumbar spine and the effect of flexion. *Spine* 1991;16:22–9.
41. Hukins DWL. Disc structure and function. In: Ghosh P, ed. *The biology of the intervertebral disc,* Vol. I. Boca Raton, FL: CRC Press, 1988:24–7.
42. Janevic J, Ashton-Miller JA, Schultz AB. Large compressive preloads decrease lumbar motion segment flexibility. *J Orthop Res* 1991;9:228–36.
43. Kuslich SD, Ulstrom CL, Michael CJ. The tissue origin of low back pain and sciatica. *Orthop Clin North Am* 1991;22:181–7.
44. McNally DS, Adams MA. Internal intervertebral disc mechanics as revealed by stress profilometry. *Spine* 1992;17:66–73.
45. McNally DS, Adams MA, Goodship AE. Development and validation of a new transducer for intradiscal pressure measurement. *J Biomed Eng* 1992;14:495–8.

46. Mimura M, Panjabi MM, Oxland TR, et al. Disc degeneration affects the multidirectional flexibility of the lumbar spine. *Spine* 1994;19:1371–80.
47. Moneta GB, Videman T, Kaivanto K, et al. Reported pain during lumbar discography as a function of annular ruptures and disc degeneration. *Spine* 1994;19:1968–74.
48. Moore RJ, Latham JM, Vernon-Roberts B, Fraser RD. Does plate fixation prevent disc degeneration after a lateral annulus tear? *Spine* 1994;19:2787–90.
49. Myklebust JB, Pintar F, Yoganandan N, et al. Tensile strength of spinal ligaments. *Spine* 1998;13:526–31.
50. Nachemson A. Disc pressure measurements. *Spine* 1981;6:93–7.
51. Neumann P, Keller TS, Ekstrom L, Hansson T. Effect of strain rate and bone mineral on the structural properties of the human lumbar anterior longitudinal ligament. *Spine* 1994;19:205–11.
52. Osti OL, Vernon-Roberts B, Fraser RD. Annulus tears and intervertebral disc degeneration: an experimental study using an animal model. *Spine* 1990;15:762–7.
53. Panjabi MM. Biomechanical evaluation of spinal fixation devices: I. A conceptual framework. *Spine* 1988;13:1129–34.
54. Panjabi MM, Oxland TR, Yamamoto I, Crisco JJ. Mechanical behavior of the human lumbar and lumbosacral spine as shown by three-dimensional load-displacement curves. *J Bone Joint Surg* 1994;76-A:413–24.
55. Pearcy MJ, Bogduk N. Instantaneous axes of rotation of the lumbar intervertebral joints. *Spine* 1988;13:1033–41.
56. Potvin JR, McGill SM, Norman RW. Trunk muscle and lumbar ligament contributions to dynamic lifts with varying degrees of trunk flexion. *Spine* 1991;16:1099–108.
57. Potvin JR, Norman RW, McGill SM. Reduction in anterior shear forces on the L4/L5 disc by the lumbar musculature. *Clin Biomech* 1991;6:88–96.
58. Schultz AB, Warwick DN, Berkson MH, Nachemson AL. Mechanical properties of human lumbar spine segments. Part 1. Response in flexion, extension, lateral bending and torsion. *J Biomech Eng* 1979;101:46–52.
59. Schwarzer AC, Aprill CN, Bogduk N. The sacroiliac joints in chronic low back pain. *Spine* 1995;20:31–7.
60. Schwarzer AC, Aprill CN, Derby R, et al. Clinical features of patients with pain stemming from the lumbar zygapophyseal joints. *Spine* 1994;19:1132–7.
61. Schwarzer AC, Aprill CN, Derby R, Fortin J, Kine G, Bogduk N. The prevalence and clinical features of internal disc disruption in patients with chronic low back pain. *Spine* 1995;20:1878–83.
62. Shackleford IM, McNally DS, Mulholland RC, Goodship AE. The relationship between lumbar disc internal biomechanics and pain as provoked by discography. Presented to the International Society for the Study of the Lumbar Spine, Helsinki, Finland, June, 1995.
63. Strauss PJ, Novotny JE, Wilder DG, Grobler LJ, Pope MH. Multidirectional stability of the Graf system. *Spine* 1994;19:965–72.
64. Wilke H-J, Claes L, Schmitt H, Wolf S. A universal spine tester for in vitro experiments with muscle force simulation. *Eur Spine J* 1994;3:91–7.
65. Wilke H-J, Wolf S, Claes L, Arand M, Wiesend A. Stability increase of the lumbar spine with different muscle groups. A biomechanical *in vitro* study. *Spine* 1995;20:192–8.
66. Wittenberg RH, Shea M, Swartz DE, Lee KS, White AA III, Hayes WC. Importance of bone mineral density in instrumented spine fusions. *Spine* 1991;16:647–52.
67. Yahia LH, Audet J, Drouin G. Rheological properties of the human lumbar spine ligaments. *J Biomed Eng* 1991;13:399–406.
68. Yang KH, King AI. Mechanism of facet load transmission as a hypothesis for low back pain. *Spine* 1984;9:557–65.
69. Yoshizawa H, O'Brien JP, Smith WT, Trumper M. The neuropathology of intervertebral discs removed for low-back pain. *J Pathol* 1980;132:95–104.
70. Zdeblick TA, Warden KE, Zou D, McAfee PC, Abitbol JJ. Anterior spinal fixators. A biomechanical *in vitro* study. *Spine* 1993;18:513–7.

*Instrumented Fusion of the Degenerative
Lumbar Spine: State of the Art, Questions,
and Controversies,* edited by M. Szpalski,
R. Gunzburg, D. M. Spengler, and
A. Nachemson. Lippincott–Raven
Publishers, Philadelphia © 1996.

# 2

# The Surgical Approach to the Lumbar Spine

## Robert Gunzburg, *Marak Szpalski, and *Jean-Pierre Hayez

*Brugmann University Hospital, 1020 Brussels, Belgium; and *Centre
Hospitalier, Molière Longchamp, 1180 Brussels, Belgium*

It is essential for spine surgeons to be able to approach the lumbar spine through either an anterior or a posterior approach so that pathology to all its structures can be dealt with. Surgery of the degenerative lumbar spine often requires bone grafting. Most approaches can avoid the need for a separate incision over the ilium.

### POSTERIOR APPROACH

The posterior approach is the most widely used and allows procedures involving the posterior elements of the spine (spinous processes, laminae, facet joints, and pedicles) as well as the cauda and the intervertebral discs.

Positioning of the patient is very important. In the prone position, supports are required under the anterior iliac crests and at the chest level. Care must be taken to avoid pressure on the lateral femoral cutaneous nerve, breasts, and nipples, It is essential that the abdomen lies free so as to reduce pressure on the inferior vena cava (Fig. 1), thus keeping venous plexus filling around the dura to a minimum. Incorrect positioning may result in excessive bleeding, difficult surgery, and unsatisfactory results. Although the patient may also be positioned on the side, this is rarely required in surgery for degenerative conditions.

The landmarks that guide the incision are easily palpable. Even in obese patients the spinous processes can easily be felt. The L4–L5 interspace is usually level with the posterosuperior iliac crest. The incision is carried until the spinous processes are reached. At this point, two options are possible.

### Midline Approach

On either side of the spinous processes, the paraspinal muscles can be detached subperiostally using a Cobb elevator. The midline structures comprising the spinous processes, as well as their ligamentous attachments (inter- and supraspinous liga-

*17*

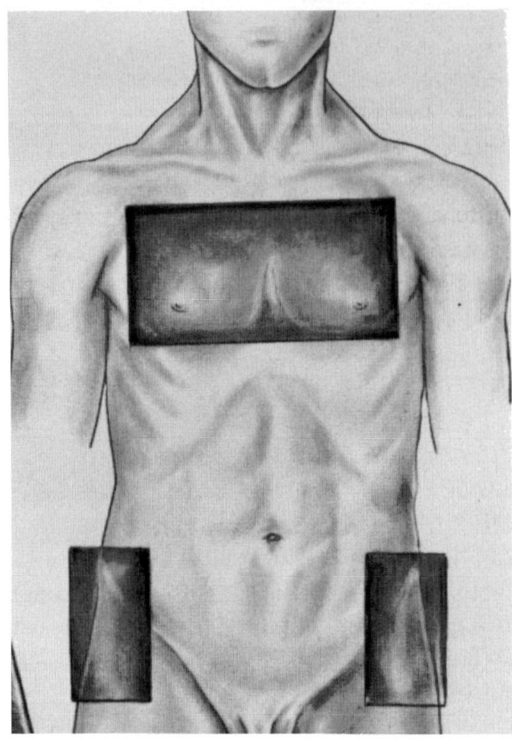

**FIG. 1.** Positioning for the posterior approach. Support and padding is necessary over the anterior superior iliac crests and thorax. (From ref. 2 with permission.)

ments) remain unaltered. The dissection is carried down along the laminae and yellow ligaments towards the facet joints. If necessary, the facet joint capsule can be stripped of its muscle attachments (Fig. 2). Medially, the dissection involves the descending facet and more laterally the ascending facet. If necessary, the dissection can be continued laterally over the ascending facet up to the transverse process. Care must be taken not to damage the intratransverse ligament. Just cranial to the facet joints, at the level of the transverse processes, the segmental vessels supplying the paraspinal muscles often bleed profusely, and careful cauterization must therefore be performed. Pedicular screws can be inserted at this point.

Further dissection toward the canal is possible by removing the ligamentum flavum from its attachments to the laminae. If necessary, partial resection of the superior or inferior lamina (or both) can be performed (partial laminectomy). Blunt dissection lateral to the dura will allow exploration of the anterior aspect of the spinal canal. This approach can be extended by simply lengthening the skin incision cranially or caudally as required.

### Paraspinal Approach

An alternative route has been described by Wiltse et al. (3). After skin and subcutaneous fat incision, the dissection is carried out bilaterally and superficial to the lumbar fascia. At the level of the spinous process of L4, approximately 3 cm from the midline, a vertical incision is made through both the lumbar and the muscle fascia. An intermuscular fascia can easily be recognized, allowing dissection toward the lateral aspect of the facet joints and the medial aspect of the transverse processes. In

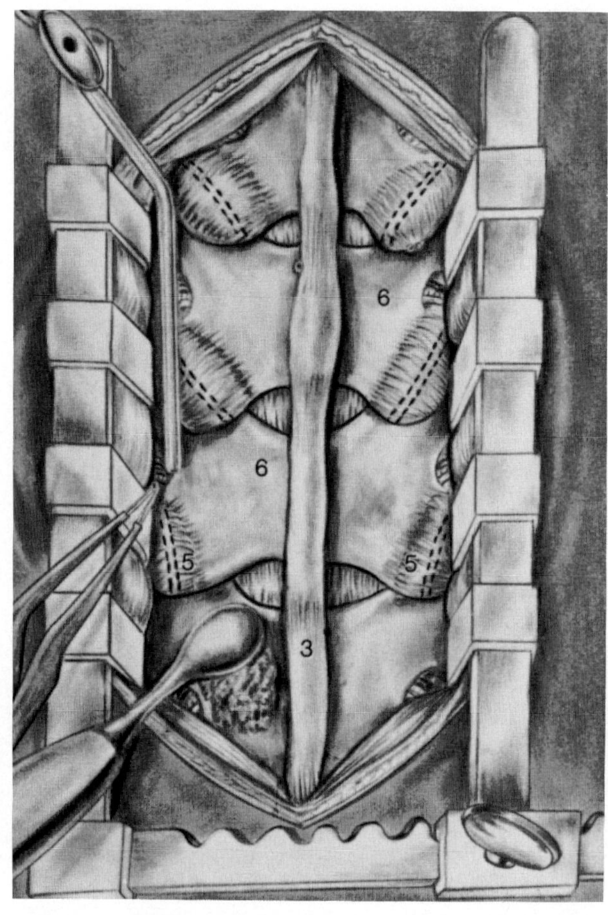

**FIG. 2.** Bilateral exposure up to the facet joints. Spinous process (3), facet joints (5), lamina (6). (From ref. 2 with permission.)

this way, surgery can be performed at the level of the facet joints and transverse processes without detaching the muscles from the midline. Pedicular screwing and posterolateral bone grafting can be carried out. Both sides are closed over a suction drain, and the muscle fascia and lumbar fascia are sutured with a resorbable thread. Between the lumbar fascia and the subcutaneous fat layer, the virtual space should also be drained and can be reduced by attaching the subcutaneous tissues to the midline.

If additional canal decompression is required, a third incision can be carried out. After careful subperiosteal dissection along one side of the spinous processes, an osteotomy of these structures is performed with a sharp osteotome. The spinous process, with its contralateral muscle attachments, is retracted and a flavectomy with partial laminectomy can be performed. It is essential to leave a laminar bridge so that after completion of the canal surgery the spinous processes can be replaced in their original position. This approach respects the mechanical midline structures while keeping muscle stripping to a minimum.

Both techniques allow harvesting of bone grafts from the iliac crest. The skin incision is extended to the sacrum and, at the level of L5–S1, careful dissection is realized towards one side. With the midline approach, the dissection is carried out superficial to the dorsal lumbar fascia. With the paraspinal approach, the iliac crest can be reached either superficial to the dorsal lumbar fascia or between the muscle fascia.

The posterior aspect of the iliac crest overlies the sacrum, from which generous quantities of cancellous bone can be harvested. Care must be taken not to damage the insertion of the iliolumbar ligaments.

## ANTERIOR AND ANTEROLATERAL APPROACHES

The anterior aspect of the lumbar spine can be reached retroperiotoneally, transperitoneally, or, with newer techniques, laparoscopically. The patient is placed in a supine position, making sure that the necessary area(s) remains free for the incision(s). The most obvious landmarks are the umbilicus, the symphysis pubis, the anterior superior iliac crest, and the inferior border of the rib cage.

### Anterolateral (Retroperitoneal) Approach

For this approach, the patient can be positioned in a semilateral position or in the supine position. When an instrumented fusion must be carried out, the latter position is preferred. In the supine position, a pad must be placed under the left buttock to facilitate harvesting of iliac crest bone grafts. After this procedure the pad must be removed to avoid lumbar tilting during the instrumentation surgery.

An oblique incision is carried out, starting at the posterior half of the twelfth rib on the left side and extending down towards the lateral edge of the rectus abdominis muscle, about halfway between the umbilicus and the symphysis pubis. Here, two options are available.

### *Transmuscular Approach*

The external oblique, internal oblique, and transversus abdominis muscle are divided in line with the skin incision. After the initial incision has been deepened through the subcutaneous fat, the aponeurosis of the external oblique appears. Its muscle fibers are in line with the incision. Now the internal oblique appears, with its fibers perpendicular to the skin incision. After their division, the transversus abdominis appears. Its muscle fibers are also divided in line with the skin incision. Sectioning of these two deep muscle layers causes some denervation, but if the muscle is closed carefully postoperative hernias can be reduced to a minimum. With gentle blunt finger dissection, the peritoneum is detached from the abdominal wall and retracted medially. The ureter is not disturbed and is carried forward with the peritoneum. Progressively, the psoas muscle appears. At the level of the vertebral bodies, just medial to the psoas muscle, the aorta and vena cava appear. After division of the segmental lumbar arteries and veins, the aorta and vena cava can be mobilized to the right (Fig. 3). At this point, Steinman pins can be inserted into the vertebral bodies to facilitate retraction by providing good exposure. If necessary, the segmental level can be verified with fluoroscopy.

During the dissection it is important to avoid damage to the sympathetic chain that is located over the medial aspect of the psoas muscle and the lateral aspect of the vertebral body. The genitofemoral nerve overlies the anterior surface of the psoas

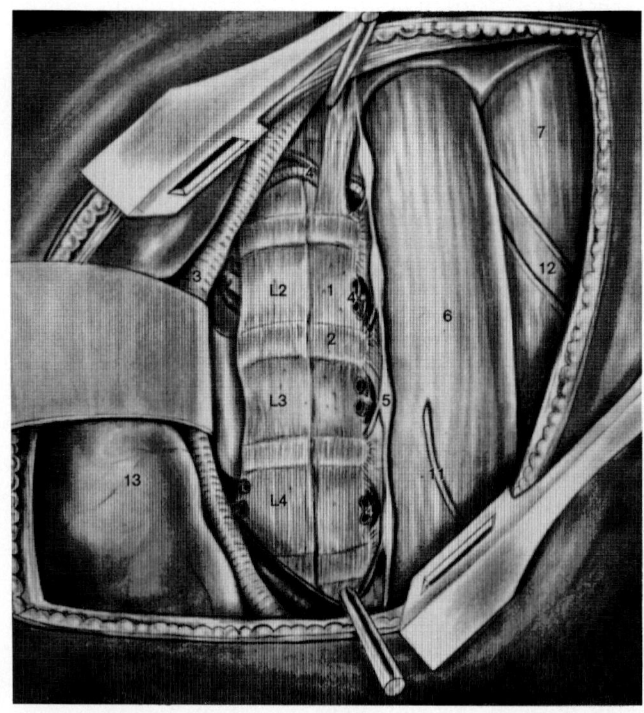

**FIG. 3.** Wide exposure of the lumbar spine. Vertebral body (1), intervertebral disc (2), aorta (3), segmental arteries and veins (4), sympathetic chain (5), psoas muscle (6), quadratus lumborum muscle (7), genitofemoral nerve (11), iliohypogastric nerve (12), peritoneum (13). (From ref. 2 with permission.)

and should also be left unaltered. At the end of the operation the different layers are closed with a resorbable suture. It is seldom necessary to drain the site.

### Anterolateral Muscle-Splitting (Retroperitoneal) Approach

This approach was described by Fraser (1). The positioning and skin incision are the same. However, after division of the external oblique muscle an alternative route is taken to avoid dividing the deep muscle layers perpendicular to the direction of their fibers. The medial part of the external oblique is retracted medially to expose the rectus muscle over most of its length. The rectus sheath is divided at about 2 cm from its lateral edge, and the incision is extended both upwards and downwards. The lateral border of the rectus muscle is gently retracted medially and, with careful blunt finger dissection at the level of the semilunar line, the peritoneum is detached from the posterior aspect of the posterior rectus sheath. Progressively, it is in turn divided at 1–2 cm from its lateral edge. Slowly the peritoneum comes free, and further dissection and surgery can proceed as described above. In closing the surgical wound, first the posterior rectus sheath is sutured, then the anterior rectus sheath, followed by the external oblique. With this approach, no muscle fiber has to be divided, and the different deep layers present incisions perpendicular to one another, thus reducing the risk for abdominal wall herniation. Here also, it is seldom necessary to place a suction drain.

With both approaches it is possible to harvest iliac crest bone grafts through the same skin incision. After division of the external oblique muscle, the iliac crest is approached between the external and internal oblique muscles. Care must be taken to remain at about four fingers' width from the anterior superior iliac crest to avoid damage to the lateral femoral cutaneous nerve.

## Anterior Approach

The pure anterior approach is usually reserved for surgery at the L5–S1 disc. For some cases in which the retroperitoneal approach cannot be used, this approach can also be considered for higher levels. However, it involves mobilization of the major vessels. The approach is transperitoneal and can be performed open or laparoscopically. When surgery is performed carefully, there is usually no need to drain the site.

The patient is placed in the supine position with a varying degree of Trendelenburg. If bone grafts are required, a separate incision must be carried out over one of the iliac crests.

### *Open Transperitoneal Approach*

The landmarks for the incision are easily recognized. The umbilicus normally projects at the level of the L3–L4 disc space. In obese patients, however, this may vary. The pubis or symphysis can usually be recognized. The incision is midline and longitudinal, and extends from just below the umbilicus to just above the symphysis. If necessary, the incision can be extended cranially.

The skin incision is deepened through the subcutaneous fat up to the fibrous separation between the left and the right rectus sheaths, and the two rectus muscles are gently separated with the fingers in the lower half. Cranially, the incision extends in line with the skin incision through the linea alba. The peritoneum is now exposed. It is in turn incised, taking care not to interfere with the underlying viscera. The peritoneal incision is extended both cranially and caudally, taking care not to damage the dome of the bladder, which is emptied by an in situ catheter. The peritoneum is again incised at the level of the promontorium and further dissection is performed towards the L5–S1 disc. The sacral artery and vein run over the disc and down the anterior surface of the sacrum, and must be ligated. The presacral sympathetic nerves must be avoided as much as possible, as damage to these structures in men may result in retrograde ejaculation and/or impotence. Injecting saline into the area of the presacral plexus may help to identify and thus preserve this neural structure. The bifurcation of the aorta and vena cava inferior lies at the level of L5, and normally the full L5–S1 disc can be exposed without interfering with the vessels (Fig. 4).

L4–L5 can also be exposed, but this requires a larger dissection and mobilization of the large vessels. The sigmoid colon is retracted toward the right and the vessels are mobilized towards the left. To do this, the fifth and sometimes the fourth lumbar arteries and veins must be ligated. This must not be done flush with the major vessel, because it may effectively create a hole that is difficult to close. Care must be taken not to damage the left ureter, which runs over the left common iliac vessels. Touching it gently will cause peristaltism, a helpful characteristic during the dissection. In cases that present with a high bifurcation, it is sometimes possible to dissect upwards, retracting the common iliac vessels cranially and laterally. Unlike the configuration on the right side, the left common iliac vein lies more caudal than the left common iliac artery, making dissection of the left side potentially more dangerous because the vein is more fragile than the artery.

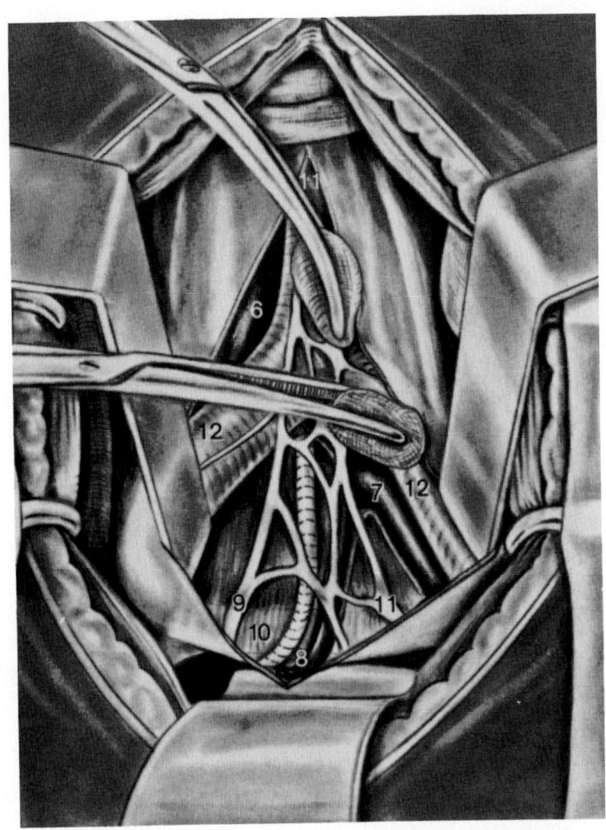

**FIG. 4.** Retroperitoneal presacral structures. Vena cava inferior (6), common iliac vein (7), medial sacral vein (8), superior hypogastric nerves (9 and 11), medial sacral artery (10), common iliac arteries (12). (From ref. 2 with permission.)

## *Laparascopic Transperitoneal Approach*

This approach is reserved for the L5–S1 disc, although experienced surgeons may wish to use it at the L4–L5 level. To perform laparascopic surgery of the lumbar spine, six portals must be placed. A portal for the scope is created through the umbilicus. A straight or preferably a 30° camera should be used. Abdominal gas filling is gradually obtained with $CO_2$ up to a pressure of 15 mm Hg. On either side of this portal, even slightly more cranially, additional portals of 15 mm are inserted for the dissection instruments. Just medially from but at the level of the anterior superior iliac crest, two more portals are inserted for the retracting instruments. The sigmoid colon and sometimes the uterus must be retracted during the operation at the L5–S1 level. Further laparoscopic surgery through the posterior peritoneum is identical to the surgery described in the open procedure. In line with the L5–S1 disc, a sixth large (18-mm) portal is created, through which the specific spinal instruments can be inserted.

## REFERENCES


1. Fraser R. A wide muscle splitting approach to the lumbosacral spine. *J Bone Joint Surg* 1982;64-B:44–6.
2. Louis R. *Chirurgie du rachis. Anatomie chirurgicale et voies d'abord.* Springer-Verlag: Berlin, 1982.
3. Wiltse LL, Bateman JG, Hutchinson RH, Nelson WE. The paraspinal sacrospinalis-splitting approach to the lumbar spine. *J Bone Joint Surg* 1968;50A:919.

*Instrumented Fusion of the Degenerative Lumbar Spine: State of the Art, Questions, and Controversies*, edited by M. Szpalski, R. Gunzburg, D. M. Spengler, and A. Nachemson. Lippincott–Raven Publishers, Philadelphia © 1996.

# 3

# Imaging of Spinal Implants and Radiologic Assessment of Fusion

Paul M. Parizel, Johan W. Van Goethem, Luc van den Hauwe, Filip Deckers, *Robert Gunzburg, and Arthur M. De Schepper

*Department of Radiology, Universitair Ziekenhuis Antwerpen, University of Antwerp, B-2650 Edegem, Belgium; and *Department of Orthopedic Surgery, Eeuwfeestkliniek, B-2018 Antwerpen, Belgium*

Spinal fixation devices are used to stabilize the spine, reduce deformities and fractures and replace abnormal vertebrae (8,18–20). Bone fusion is usually attempted, along with placement of surgical instrumentation materials (18,20). The spine is inherently unstable, and early operative intervention improves mobilization and rehabilitation. A variety of fusion methods are now in use. Surgical procedures usually consist of posterior (posterior elements) and/or anterior (vertebral body) fixation. Persistent lumbar instability is a clinical problem. It is often the cause of recurrent low back pain in patients who have undergone lumbar fusion (12).

Determining the solidity of the fusion is a difficult problem. It was widely accepted at one time that the only way to determine the solidity of lumbar fusion was to explore it surgically (4). This principle is known as Bosworth's dictum (1,2,4,5), and was undoubtedly inspired by the limited possibilities of imaging techniques half a century ago and by the inconsistent and often unreliable results provided by plain x-rays. Routine reexploration of the surgical fusion is impractical, however, because of the expense and morbidity involved (4). Therefore, it is important to find a radiologic imaging technique that will reliably assess the status of the lumbar fusion.

A variety of radiologic methods have been used to image the postoperative spine. Imaging modalities include x-rays (plain x-rays, polytomograms, biplane bending films, stereophotogrammetry, myelography, and CT myelography), computed tomography (CT), radionuclide bone scans, and magnetic resonance imaging (MRI). Medical imaging studies can be divided into two categories, depending on whether they assess the functional or structural integrity of fusions. Most modalities assess structural integrity (x-rays, tomograms, CT scan, MRI). The purpose of these techniques is essentially to identify the bony continuity of the fusion mass. Conversely, imaging studies that assess functional integrity include any type of bending films. The purpose here is to demonstrate motion between vertebral segments. These studies depend heavily on patient cooperation and may fail to show abnormal motion because of muscle guarding, spasm, or internal fixation (4).

This chapter focuses on imaging strategies and imaging findings, and underscores the need for radiologists to familiarize themselves with the surgical procedures performed at their institution.

## CONVENTIONAL X-RAYS

Any discussion regarding imaging strategies in the lumbar spine after fusion should start with conventional x-rays. Plain x-rays obtained in two projections (anteroposterior and lateral) remain the mainstay of implant evaluation; oblique projections are sometimes needed (8,19,20). Plain radiographs demonstrate the position of the spinal elements, hardware, graft material, and evidence of complications. Plain radiographs judge the structural integrity and do not assess the functional integrity as do flexion–extension radiographs. Recent literature data suggest that, with static two-dimensional radiographs, the presence or absence of arthrodesis can be predicted in approximately 69% of cases (1). These are based on the overall agreement between radiographic assessment of fusion and actual surgical results in reintervention. However, in one of five cases, plain radiographs underestimate the degree of fusion (1,22). The reason for this is believed to be that premineralized osteoid may be functionally fused but may appear radiolucent on radiographic film (1). The calcification of osteoid takes many months. It is generally accepted that 6 to 9 months after surgery are necessary for development of solid fusion to be seen radiographically (8,18–20). In the first months after surgery, it can therefore be hazardous to diagnose a nonunion unless there is evidence of failure of hardware (e.g., broken screws) or loss of correction.

An important feature in conventional x-ray examination of the postoperative lumbar spine is the possibility of obtaining bending films. Motion between bone elements should be demonstrated to confirm nonunion or pseudarthrosis. It has been reported that bending films have low specificity but high sensitivity. Their percentage of false-negatives is low and they are least likely to miss a solid fusion (4).

Conventional polytomography, a technique that has largely been replaced by CT, retains some usefulness in imaging of the postoperative spine. However, in routine clinical practice the technique is used less frequently, largely because most major radiology departments have replaced complex motion tomographic units with CT scanners. Some authors have emphasized that, together with CT scans, polytomography was the most specific examination in the postfusion lumbar spine (specificity values of 86 and 84, respectively). This implies that CT and polytomography had the lowest level of false-positive results and are least likely to show solid fusion if pseudarthrosis has developed (4). Sensitivity values are highest for plain radiographs (sensitivity 89) and bending films (sensitivity 96) (4).

Some authors have advocated the use of roentgen stereophotogrammetric analysis to determine the presence or absence of mobility between vertebral segments (11). This technique implies making simultaneous exposures by using two roentgen tubes, with an angle of 40° between the central rays (11). The patient is examined in supine and erect positions. The films are then analyzed by a photogrammetric instrument and intervertebral translations between supine and erect positions are determined.

## COMPUTED TOMOGRAPHY

Computed tomography studies play a limited role in patients in whom metallic instrumentation devices have been used, because of the streak artifacts (beam hardening) associated with these devices. Streak artifacts due to metallic spinal fusion devices grossly degrade axial CT images and obscure anatomic details of soft tissues, thereby rendering image interpretation virtually impossible. The effects of streak artifacts can be limited by the use of a high-quality CT scanner, thin slices, wide window settings, and artifact reduction reconstruction algorithms.

Bony structures suffer less from such image degradation, especially when thin slices are used in combination with wide window bone settings and artifact-reduction reconstruction algorithms. When thin sections are used, multiplanar re-formations in the sagittal and coronal planes can be of use to complete the examination (14).

Three-dimensional CT with multiplanar re-formations can provide greater information than the direct axial images. Multiplanar reconstructions are of particular interest in evaluating vertical alignment, lateral neural foramen compromise, and articular facet and pars interarticularis integrity (23). Literature data indicate that reformatted CT images demonstrated fusion pseudarthrosis more frequently than axial CT images or conventional radiographs (14). This is because three-dimensional reconstructions are helpful in demonstrating the complex anatomy of the fusion and in visualizing sites of vertebral integrity, consequences of previous surgery, solidity and anatomy of fusion, and points of instability (23). Therefore, they can be helpful in preoperative planning as well as intraoperative localization (14).

A useful application of axial CT images is the visualization of the path of the pedicle screws as they pass through the pedicle and into the vertebral body (e.g., Steffee plates and pedicle screws in the lumbosacral region) (19,20). The use of pedicle screws enables surgeons to reduce degenerative deformities of the lumbar spine and to maintain accurate positional control of the motion segment in anatomic alignment and in normal sagittal and coronal plane balance (3). However, correct placement of pedicle screws is difficult, even with fluoroscopic guidance (7,22). The assessment of pedicle screw placement is becoming an increasingly important indication for CT scanning. In 1987, the Scoliosis Research Society morbidity committee found that there was a 3.2% incidence of neurologic injury from pedicle screw instrumentation (7). Plain radiographs alone do not accurately reveal pedicle screw placement (7). Thin-section CT scans should be used to evaluate postoperative neurologic deficits in patients with pedicle screws (Fig. 1). Compared with plain x-rays, CT detects a much larger number of screws medial to the pedicles (lateral recess) (7).

If compression of the dural sac or nerve root sleeves is suspected, myelography can be of help. Multiple views are needed to project the suspected level of abnormality away from the metallic surgical implants. CT myelography may be of use unless large metallic implants are present, in which case the CT images will be degraded by streak artifacts.

## MAGNETIC RESONANCE IMAGING

Magnetic resonance imaging has become the modality of choice for imaging the spine. In the preoperative assessment of the patient undergoing fusion, MRI is useful

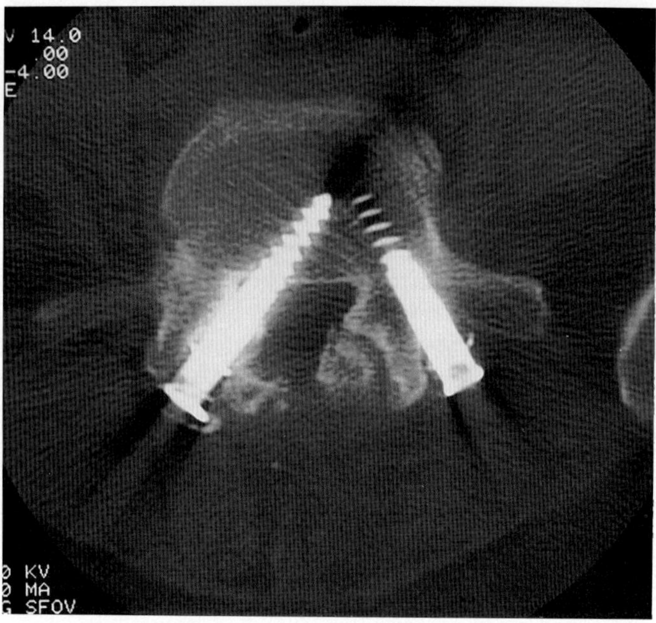

**FIG. 1.** Assessment of pedicle screws with CT. Axial CT image through the L5 vertebral body in 51-year-old woman with bilateral pedicle screws. The left pedicle screw is correctly positioned. Conversely, the right pedicle screw is in part medial to the pedicle and traverses the right lateral recess of the spinal canal.

for detection of disc degeneration in the levels above or below the intended fusion (13). In MRI, the presence of foreign metal objects such as spinal fixation devices gives rise to local magnetic field distortion (16). If the material is ferromagnetic (e.g., stainless steel), a large distortion of the magnetic field deforms the image appearance and may render interpretation of anatomic structures completely impossible (Fig. 2). This artifact is more pronounced with ferromagnetic materials than with nonferromagnetic materials (e.g., titanium), when MRI is performed at higher field strengths, and when gradient echo sequences (e.g., FLASH) are used. On a physical level, the metal artifact in MRI is explained by the occurrence of a non-negligible local gradient compared with the frequency-encoding gradient. When the implants are made of nonferromagnetic materials (e.g., titanium or tantalum), distortion of the magnetic field is less severe but still obscures normal anatomy (16). In clinical practice, the presence of large metallic spinal fixation devices renders MRI of the involved region of the spine virtually impossible. Even in the absence of metallic fusion devices, small fragments of metal sheared from instruments during surgery can give rise to ovoid areas of decreased signal intensity overlying the operated region (17). This is occasionally encountered in patients with metal artifacts at the site of discectomy or corporectomy (17). These artifacts vary in size from small, which mimics a small anterior extradural defect, to large, which obscures the fusion mass and contents of the spinal canal. Often these metal artifacts are seen with MRI, even when x-ray or CT do not reveal metallic density in this region. Posterior fixation procedures in the spine [e.g. cervical wiring, Steffee plates (21), Harrington rods (10)] are defined by the metal artifacts they produce. Gradient-echo images are more susceptible to metal artifacts than spin-echo or turbo–spin-echo images (16). Metal artifacts are more pronounced when MRI is performed at higher field strengths (16).

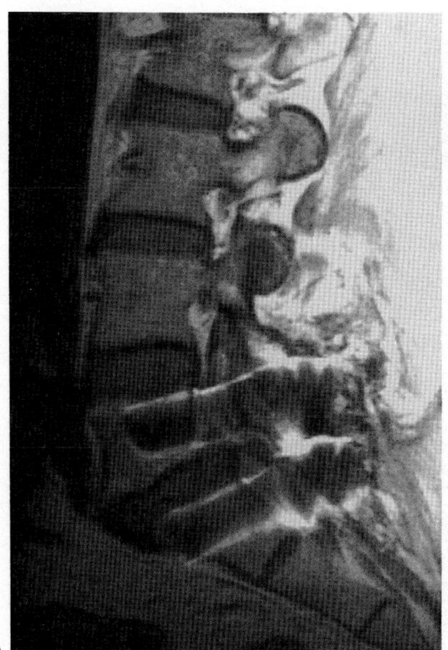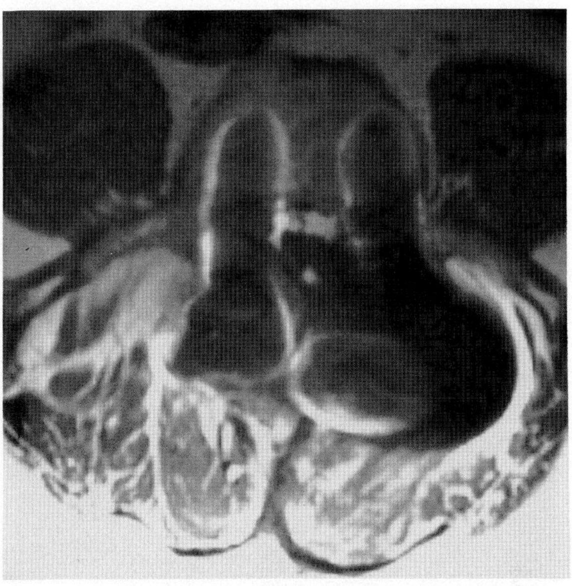

A B

**FIG. 2. A,B:** MR image distortion by pedicle screws. Sagittal and axial $T_1$-weighted MR images in 38-year-old man with L5 and S1 pedicle screws. Metal artifacts, due to local magnetic field distortion, obscure and deform anatomic structures, thereby rendering image interpretation virtually impossible.

A promising application of MRI is in the postoperative evaluation of patients treated with interbody fusion bone grafts to document posterior or posterolateral graft extrusion into the neural canal or failure of interbody fusion (6). In large series, the approximate incidence of graft extrusion is estimated at 2% of cases (6). Posterolateral extrusion of a graft can cause direct nerve root compression, usually characterized by immediate and severe radicular pain. Axial CT slices may yield confusing and even contradictory results, depending on the exact level and orientation of the axial slice relative to the implants (bone graft, plug, cage). Thanks to its multiplanar imaging capability, MRI provides direct sagittal and coronal images that define the exact position of the bone graft (cage) (Fig. 3). Moreover, MRI is useful in revealing associated pathology in the spinal canal. Accurate assessment of the degree and direction of plug dislocation is important because it is directly related to the clinical symptomatology and can therefore determine the need for reintervention.

## RADIOGRAPHIC SIGNS OF FUSION

The value of plain radiographs of the spine in the patient after fusion is unclear. It has been suggested that plain radiography underestimates the rate of pseudarthrosis compared with surgical exploration, particularly when a hairline pseudarthrosis is present (9,15).

Conversely, other authors have indicated that plain radiographs may underestimate the degree of fusion. The referring clinician is sometimes faced with the puzzling contradiction that the radiology examination does not show evidence of fusion in a patient who is doing well clinically. The reason for this apparent contradiction

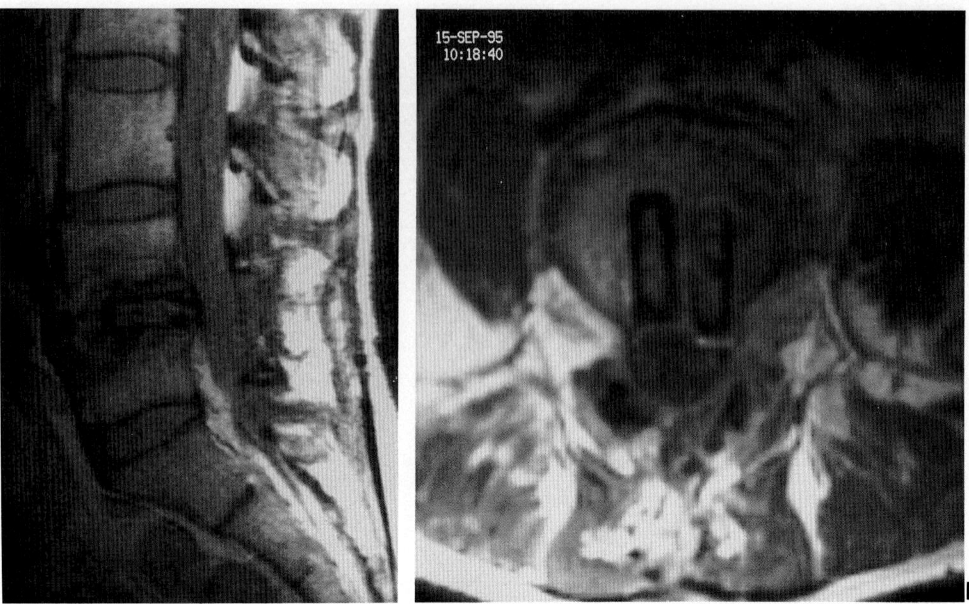

**FIG. 3. A,B:** Postoperative MR imaging of interbody fusion with cages. Sagittal and axial $T_1$-weighted MR images in a 47-year-old man treated with interbody fusion grafts (cages) at L4-L5. The axial MR image through the L4-L5 disc level shows correct positioning of the right cage, and slight posterior extrusion of left cage into the spinal canal. Because of its multiplanar imaging capability, MRI can accurately define the exact position of the bone graft or cage.

is believed to be that premineralized osteoid may be functionally fused but may appear radiolucent on radiographic film (1). The calcification of osteoid takes many months. As a rule of thumb, it is accepted that 6 to 9 months are necessary for development of solid fusion to be seen radiographically after the time of surgery (8,19,20).

After mineralization of the osteoid, the bone in the fusion area may appear radiographically denser than the adjacent vertebral bone. As mature bone trabeculae develop, they bridge the fusion area. This leads to obliteration of the cortical vertebral endplates and thus to a loss of the so-called "graft–host" interface between the implant bone and the normal vertebral bone. In some instances, a dense line of sclerotic bone may be an indicator of fusion. The ossification of the graft sometimes progresses in an anterior direction within the intervertebral disc space. A well-known sign that indicates solid bony fusion is resorption of spondylotic spurs (although this may take several months). Likewise, fusion of the facet joints is a reassuring sign of functional fusion of two segments. The radiographic signs of fusion are summarized in Table 1 (3).

## PSEUDARTHROSIS AND OTHER COMPLICATIONS

There are several causes of possible complications that may be observed by imaging procedures in patients treated with fixation devices or with interbody bone grafts. An unfortunate cause of unsatisfactory outcome after surgery is erroneous

**TABLE 1.** *Radiographic signs of fusion*

| |
|---|
| Bone in the fusion area is radiographically more dense and more mature than was originally achieved in surgery |
| Loss of "graft–host interface" between donor bone and vertebral bone (sclerotic line also indicates fusion) |
| Mature bony trabeculae bridging the fusion area with obliteration of the cortical endplates |
| Resorption of anterior vertebral traction spurs |
| Anterior progression of the graft within the disc space |
| Fusion of the facet joints |
| "Ring" phenomenon on CT |

preoperative diagnosis or inaccurate level identification. This can occur in patients with lumbosacral transitional vertebrae, in whom mislabeling of vertebral segments may result in surgery at a wrong level. Intraoperative complications include:

Injury of the nerve roots of the cauda equina (or the spinal cord at higher levels)

Laceration or tearing of the dural sac. This can lead to the formation of a postoperative (pseudo)meningocele, presumably caused by laceration of the dura and leakage of cerebrospinal fluid through the defect

Injury to blood vessels (leading to hemorrhage). The presence of intradural blood may cause arachnoiditis, which is characterized on imaging studies (myelography, CT myelography, or MRI) by thickening, clumping, and matting of nerve roots in the dural sac

Intraoperative surgical damage to the soft tissues can lead to the development of epidural fibrosis, a well known cause of "failed back surgery syndrome"

Incorrect choice or malpositioning of hardware may occur (see above).

Complications during the immediate postoperative period include hematoma and infection (19). Infection in the operated disc space leads to spondylodiscitis, with symmetric involvement of two adjacent vertebral bodies from one infected disc space. These infections are difficult to treat by conventional antibiotic treatment and may become chronic. Late postoperative complications include migration, dislodgement, or fracture of implant material. This may contribute to complications such as instability (caused by failure to fuse, pseudarthrosis), failure of fusion, and pain, with possible neurologic damage (19). On MRI, the presence of an intermediate signal intensity gap on $T_1$-weighted images is an indicator of pseudarthrosis (9). An overview of the radiographic signs of pseudarthrosis is given in Table 2 (3,6,9,19). Bone graft material can migrate or hypertrophy, resulting in impingement on the spinal canal or neural foramen. Rarely, the bone adjacent to the operated level may fracture, especially in osteoporotic patients.

**TABLE 2.** *Radiographic signs of pseudarthrosis*

| |
|---|
| Collapse of the construction with loss of disc space height despite apparent rigid posterior fixation with pedicle screws |
| Vertebral slippage |
| Posterior or posterolateral bone graft extrusion into the spinal canal |
| Broken screws (due to pseudarthrosis with continued stress on implant) |
| Resorption of the bone graft; decrease of bone density |
| Major lucency or gap visible in the fusion area (2 mm or more around the entire periphery of the graft or cage) |
| Presence of an intermediate signal intensity gap on $T_1$-weighted images |

## CONCLUSIONS

In postoperative assessment of a patient after lumbar fusion, comparison with previous radiographic documents is required to detect subtle changes that may indicate fusion or may herald an impending complication. Subtle changes on plain x-rays may become more evident with flexion–extension views or with thin-section CT images (including three-dimensional reformatted images). It is important to inform the radiologist performing the examination about any previous surgical procedure(s). This may affect the imaging strategy to be followed, and it is important when radiographs are evaluated and imaging studies are considered. For the postoperative patient with a normal clinical course, routine re-exploration of the spine is probably not recommended (1,4). In problem patients (e.g., persistent inexplicable pain, symptoms suggesting pseudarthrosis) surgical re-exploration can be justified (4).

Radiologists should be familiar with the procedures and equipment used by the surgeons at their institution. Obviously, a meaningful postoperative radiologic evaluation can be accomplished only when indications for surgical techniques, their radiologic appearance, and possible complications are known (8). Radiologists face continual changes in both surgical technique and instrumentation and should be knowledgeable about the devices available and the biomechanical principles that direct their use. Knowledge of spinal fixation devices and surgical techniques is required for identification of evolving complications. Radiologic findings should be discussed in close collaboration with the surgical colleagues.

## REFERENCES


1. Blumenthal SL, Gill K. Can lumbar spine radiographs accurately determine fusion in postoperative patients? Correlation of routine radiographs with a second surgical look at lumbar fusions. *Spine* 1993;18:1186–9.
2. Bosworth DM. Techniques of spinal fusion: pseudarthrosis and method of repair. *AAOS Instructional Course Lecture V* 1948:295–313.
3. Brantigan JW. Pseudarthrosis rate after allograft posterior lumbar interbody fusion with pedicle screw and plate fixation. *Spine* 1994;19:1271–80.
4. Brodsky AE, Kovalsky ES, Khalil MA. Correlation of radiologic assessment of lumbar spine fusions with surgical exploration. *Spine* 1991;16:S261–5.
5. Cleveland M, Bosworth DM, Thompson FR. Pseudarthrosis in the lumbosacral spine. *J Bone Joint Surg* 1948;30A:302–12.
6. Coughlan JD. Extrusion of bone graft after lumbar fusion: CT appearance. *J Comput Assist Tomogr* 1986;10:399–400.
7. Farber GL, Place HM, Mazur RA, Jones DEC, Damiano TR. Accuracy of pedicle screw placement in lumbar fusions by plain radiographs and computed tomography. *Spine* 1995;20:1494–9.
8. Foley MJ, Calenoff L, Hendrix RW, Schafer MF. Thoracic and lumbar spine fusion: post-operative radiologic evaluation. *Am J Roentgenol* 1983;141:373–80.
9. Ghazi J, Golimbu CN, Engler GL. MRI of spinal fusion pseudarthrosis. *J Comput Assist Tomogr* 1992;16:324–6.
10. Harrington PR. The history and development of Harrington instrumentation. *Clin Orthop* 1973;93:110–2.
11. Johnson R, Selvik G, Strömqvist B, Sundén G. Mobility of the lower lumbar spine after posterolateral fusion determined by roentgen stereophotogrammetric analysis. *Spine* 1990;15:347–50.
12. Lang Ph, Chafetz N, Genant HK, Morris JM. Lumbar spinal fusion. Assessment of functional stability with magnetic resonance imaging. *Spine* 1990;15:581–8.
13. Lang Ph, Genant HK, Chafetz NI, Hedtmann A, Norman D, Krämer J. Magnetresonanztomographie bie Spondylolyse und Spondylolisthese. *Z Orthoped* 1988;126:651–7.
14. Lang Ph, Genant HK, Steiger P, Chafetz NI, Morris JM. Dreidimensionale Computertomographie und multiplanare CT-Reformationen bei lumbalen Spondylodesen. *Fortschr Röntgenstr* 1988;148:524–9.

15. McMaster MJ, James JIP. Pseudarthrosis after spinal fusion for scoliosis. *J Bone Joint Surg* 1976; 58B:305–12.
16. Parizel PM. The influence of field strength on magnetic resonance imaging (a comparative study in physicochemical phantoms, isolated brain specimens and clinical applications). PhD Thesis, University of Antwerp, Wilrijk, 1994.
17. Ross JS, Hueftle MG. Postoperative spine. In: Modic MT, Masaryk TJ, Ross JS, eds. *Magnetic resonance imaging of the spine*. Chicago: Year Book Medical Publishers, 1989.
18. Slone RM, MacMillan M, Montgomery WJ. Spinal fixation. Part 1. Principles, basic hardware, and fixation techniques for the cervical spine. *Radiographics* 1993;13:341–56.
19. Slone RM, MacMillan M, Montgomery WJ, Spinal fixation. Part 3. Complications of spinal instrumentation. *Radiographics* 1993;13:797–816.
20. Slone RM, MacMillan M, Montgomery WJ, Heare M. Spinal fixation. Part 2. Fixation techniques and hardware for the thoracic and lumbosacral spine. *Radiographics* 1993;13:521–43.
21. Steffee AD, Biscup RS, Sitkowski DJ. Segmental spine plates with pedicle screw fixation: a new internal fixation device for disorders of lumbar and thoracolumbar spine. *Clin Orthop* 1986;203:45–53.
22. Weinstein JN, Spratt KN, Spengler D, Brick C, Reid S. Spinal pedicle fixation: reliability and validity of roentgenogram-based assessment and surgical factors on successful screw placement. *Spine* 1988; 13:1012–8.
23. Zinreich SJ, Long DM, Davis R, Quinn CB, McAfee PC, Wang H. Three dimensional CT imaging in postsurgical "failed back" syndrome. *J Comput Assist Tomogr* 1990;14:574–80.

*Instrumented Fusion of the Degenerative Lumbar Spine: State of the Art, Questions, and Controversies,* edited by M. Šzpalski, R. Gunzburg, D. M. Spengler, and A. Nachemson. Lippincott–Raven Publishers, Philadelphia © 1996.

# 4

# Spinal Fusion: A Rheumatologist's Point of View

Michel Benoist

*University of Paris VII, 75116 Paris, France*

This discussion of spine fusion is limited to the lumbosacral arthrodesis. Indications of fusion where loss of substance is involved, such as tumors or traumas, are beyond the scope of this presentation. Surgical treatment in these patients aims at obtaining alignment and stabilization of the lumbar spine, at improving the neurologic status, and at allowing early mobilization. The indications and technique of fusion depend on the fracture patterns and on the anatomic extent and type of spinal tumor. Healing of vertebral and paravertebral septic lesions, as well as control of spinal instability and deformity in lumbar spine sepsis, may require open surgical procedures and fusion, although many cases develop spontaneous interbody arthrodesis. Indications of surgery for idiopathic scoliotic deformities in adolescence or adult life is a special topic and is presented in another chapter. This chapter is devoted to fusion for low back pain of degenerative and mechanical origin.

In France, most chronic low back patients are first seen by rheumatologists, who are usually rather conservative, and very few patients undergo spinal fusion for degenerative disc disease. However, there is a subgroup of chronic sufferers who experience persistent pain despite aggressive and appropriate nonsurgical treatment. This subset of patients is growing in industrialized countries and is responsible for most of the costs of the health services (20). When confronted with this type of patient, and after having tried the useful therapies, the rheumatologist is tempted to refer the patient to the spinal surgeon but hesitates because of the relative uncertainty of the results. The experience of the rheumatologist has sometimes been disappointing, and there may be doubt about the results of the published studies, especially the variations in the different series, despite the use of the same techniques. The rheumatologist may question the validity of the outcome assessments. As stated in 1973 by de Sèze and Kahn (54), ''a good proportion of fused low back patients are better after surgery despite the progress in imaging and in surgical technique.'' The same authors acknowledge that the rheumatologist is in a better position to see the bad results that need further medical treatment, because the satisfied patients will be lost to follow-up or will be followed by the surgical team.

More than 20 years have passed, imaging of the lumbar spine has tremendously improved, and techniques of fusion have multiplied with all sorts of new methods for internal fixation. Can this pessimistic opinion of arthrodesis for low back pain of degenerative and mechanical origin be radically changed?

The concept of fusion of an abnormal functional spinal unit is based on the idea that suppression of movement of a pathologically unstable segment will eliminate the nociceptive input. Mechanical stimulation of the nociceptive system is the most frequent generating mechanism for low back and radicular pain. In the case of low back pain, the local receptors are located in the annulus, ligaments, and facets. In sciatica, the nociceptive message starts from the inflamed nerve root and ganglion. The inciting mechanical and physical stimulus, e.g., compression or instability, is associated with inflammatory, chemical, and neurogenic factors, which in turn sensitize the local receptors that perpetuate the nociceptive message at a low level of stimulation. It is believed that elimination of motion will relieve the mechanical constraints, suppress the other activating factors of this complex network, and bring relief of pain. However, it must be remembered that the nociceptive message is transmitted through the dorsal horn of the spinal cord to the ascending pathways and high centers, with ultimate cortical processing. Therefore, in discussing fusion for chronic low back pain, it is important to consider not only the peripheral nociception but also the role of the central nervous system which, in chronic conditions, is sensitized by a complex cascade of chemical, cellular, and molecular events (7).

Recent technical progress in lumbar fusion, including various devices for internal fixation, has increased the possibility of correcting and stabilizing the mechanical deformities and of obtaining a solid fusion. It is hoped that in the near future the use of osteoinductive growth factors will considerably enhance the process of posterolateral intertransverse fusion, as already demonstrated in experimental animals (2). Unfortunately, the technical success of fusion is not always parallel with the clinical improvement, and appropriate patient selection remains the most important factor of success (56).

## SELECTION OF PATIENTS

In clinical rheumatology, low back pain, with or without sciatica, is one of the most common causes of consultations. Most attacks of acute or subacute back pain resolve rapidly with or without health care services. However, chronic or recurring back pain develops in a small group of patients who do not respond to a wide variety of conservative treatments including orthodox or heterodox techniques. Which patients of this chronic group are appropriate candidates for arthrodesis? Fundamental to answering this question is a knowledge of the cause of the pain. In other words, an anatomic lesion must be identified and localized as the source of pain. This lesion is presumed to produce a continuous hyperstimulation of the nociceptors. Stabilization by complete elimination of movement is therefore advisable. Obviously, this may be the case when a lumbar segmental instability is clearly demonstrated.

### Spondylolisthesis

Isthmic spondylolisthesis is a good example of segmental instability. Persistence of mechanical low back and/or leg pain in a child or an adult with a progressive slip despite appropriate conservative treatment is generally accepted as an indication for lumbar fusion. This is especially true in an adult with pain and progressive olisthesis at the L4–L5 level. The clinical results of surgical intervention in the spondylolisthesis group are usually good, approaching 80% if a solid fusion is obtained (59). However, as emphasized by Thomasen (59), if concomitant problems of the lumbar spine, such as disc degeneration at other levels, are associated, the clinical improvement is significantly decreased. Consequently, a careful imaging study of the lumbar spine should be performed before surgery. Even in a young adult, the level above the slip may be degenerated. On the other hand, associated psychosocial factors and compensation problems may also be associated and should be considered as significant prognostic factors. The influence of these factors in the clinical outcome of lumbar fusion is discussed later in this chapter.

### Degenerative Instabilities

There are a few other conditions in which instability can be identified as a source of repetitive nociceptive stimulation. These conditions are included in the group of so-called degenerative instabilities (21) secondary to degenerative changes of the discs and of the facets. The ill-defined notion of instability or lack of stability implies an abnormal motion of a spinal unit under load, capable of stimulating the nociceptive system and of threatening the neural elements (21). Degenerative spondylolisthesis or acquired degenerative scoliosis is a good example of degenerative instability. The former condition is a frequent cause of stenosis. If surgery is required, fusion after decompression is advisable if the lesion is focal and if extensive sacrifice of one or both facets has been necessary to adequately decompress the neural structures (5,16,37,51). Degenerative scoliosis is another example of spinal malalignment. Progressive rotational deformities with lateral deviation may also require spinal fusion if back pain and symptoms of spinal stenosis are not relieved by nonoperative treatment (26,34,40).

In clinical practice, most chronic low back pain patients have no obvious radiologic signs of spinal malalignment and instability. Clinical symptoms and physical signs often proposed as suggestive of instability have been proved to be nonspecific (21,49). Similarly, the radiographic confirmation is very often doubtful. Degenerative changes, even traction spurs, are not reliable indicators (38). Flexion and extension radiographs, as proposed by Dupuis et al. (11), sometimes demonstrate an obvious translational or retrolisthetic instability. However, the many studies conducted on this subject have shown the variation in the measurements because of intra- and interobserver errors (27,36). The normal physiologic displacement is not precisely known and varies according to age (12,62). Motion of the degenerated disc is often decreased and the functional flexion–extension radiographs are rarely useful and demonstrative (13). Preoperative radiographs have also disclosed a complete inhibition of translational movements, whereas at surgery an abnormal intervertebral mobility was found (39). Rotational instability, as often observed in degenerative spondylolithesis, can be suspected on AP radiographs that demonstrate a misalignment of the spinous process. Many years ago, Kirkaldy-Willis and Farfan (32) proposed dynamic computed tomography (CT) scans with rotational stresses. Increased movement and gaping of the facet joints could be considered a sign of rotational instability. However, the validity of this technique, recently revived by Graf (24), has not yet been confirmed by a study on normal subjects. An alternative method of identifying segmental instability has been to limit the mechanical constraints by bracing and then to study the response of pain to immobilization. However, it is now well known that no type of brace can achieve a complete elimination of motion in a particular motion segment, with the exception of one and one-half hip spica (15). A few authors have studied the pain response to immobilization by the use of external fixators, as originally proposed by Olerud et al. (14,45,47). This dramatic method is extremely aggressive, uncomfortable for the patient, and has a potential risk for complications. Moreover, fusions performed according to the data obtained by this method have not been followed by more successful clinical results (9).

The search for some kind of instability remains negative in many cases of degenerative disc disease (33,42). Therefore, in the majority of these chronic back pain patients, the exact cause of nociception remains unknown. It is possible that, as stated by Kirkaldy-Willis and Farfan (32), very subtle displacements and minor mechanical perturbations can cause pain. On the other hand, it has been shown that the degenerated nucleus pulposus has inflammatogenic properties capable of inducing lesions of the nerve roots (48). Similarly, the chemical irritating effect might stimulate the nociceptors located in the annulus and ligaments. Minor displacements of the facets associated with chemical and inflammatory factors are another possible source of nociception originating from the facets. In this context, arthrodesis of a degenerated lumbar segment could be compared to arthrodesis of the hip for osteoarthritis, before the era of prosthesis, in which bony fusion of the joint was able to suppress the source of the mechanical and chemical factors responsible for the peripheral nociception.

### Degenerative Disc Disease

Degeneration of a spinal unit is defined by changes on plain radiographs including disc narrowing and osteophyte formation on the margins of the vertebral bodies. Narrowing of the facets joints and osteophytosis are, in the early phase of degeneration, better viewed on CT. Clear radiologic evidence of disc degeneration on plain radiographs is not always obtained (19). Until recently, discography was used as a diagnostic criterion (44). The discogram, which can be assisted by CT, provides reliable imaging of degeneration as opposed to the classical image of normal discs. The volume of the dye accepted by the disc, which normally does not exceed 1 ml, is another source of information. Degenerated discs usually become painful when injected with the dye, and in some cases the injection can accurately reproduce the patient's symptoms. However, reproducibility of the pain often remains doubtful. Therefore, utilization of discography as an imaging tool and to pinpoint the exact source of the pain is still controversial (43). For that reason and because of the painful character of the procedure, MRI is now largely replacing discography to assess disc degeneration as a determinant of the fusion levels. Changes in the signals on $T_2$-weighted images mirror the degree of hydration of the disc and consequently of its degeneration. However, it has been shown that the data obtained by MRI do not always correlate with those of discography. An abnormal discogram may contrast with a normal MRI, and vice versa (8,23,29,53).

Which individuals of this degenerative disease group, without apparent instability, should be referred to the surgeon? The answer to this question is not easy and must be modulated. First, a long period of properly performed medical management must be achieved. Chronic low back pain is classically but artificially defined as back pain lasting for more than 3 months. Obviously, persistence of pain over 3 months does not automatically call for surgical intervention. Before surgery is considered, reassurance, explanation of symptoms, and functional restoration programs are mandatory. Second, surgery should not be considered if more than two levels are degenerated (10). Risk of failed fusion in multiple-level arthrodesis has been demonstrated by many studies (6,9,27). Third, age, obesity, concomitant organic diseases, and severe osteoporosis are risk factors that contraindicate surgery in some instances. It has also been shown that cigarette smoking significantly decreases the rate of successful fusion (3).

One group of patients remains, with a long history of pain nonresponsive to nonoperative treatment, with no major general contraindication, and with imaging studies exhibiting one or two degenerated low lumbar levels. In theory, the patients in this group are appropriate candidates for fusion. At this point, the clinician must clearly explain the results to be expected, the risks, and the possibility of complications. The decision will ultimately be made by the patient after weighing the benefit–risk factors. However, before advising fusion the clinician must evaluate additional variables that may determine successful results, i.e., the psychosocial factors.

## RESULTS OF FUSION

The expected results of arthrodesis must be divided into technical results, i.e., the rate of fusion, and clinical results i.e., the outcome of pain and the functional capacity. The technical results depend on the type of operation and on the quality of the operative technique. In this regard, the role of the rheumatologist, who often chooses the surgeon and takes part in discussion of possible techniques, is not negligible. Pseudoarthrosis depends largely on the minutiae of the technique and of the technique itself. The various operative approaches and techniques, their expected rate of fusion, and their complications and results are discussed in other chapters. However, in my opinion the anterior approach has a higher risk for morbidity, including vascular and neurologic complications and sexual dysfunction. The posterolateral approach has a lower risk for complications. In addition, when it is necessary to decompress the nerve roots during surgery, the posterior approach is obviously indicated. Internal fixation appears to be justified if there is an associated, radiologically demonstrated instability.

The clinical results are dependent in part on the technical results. However it has been shown in a number of studies that pseudarthrosis can be painless and that all solid bony fusions are not synonymous with successful clinical results (27). It should also be pointed out that assessment of fusion is sometimes difficult, especially when a rigid instrumentation device has been used (27). In fact, when the usual high rate of sound fusion in properly performed surgery is considered, the expected clinical results depend mostly on patient selection. As stated earlier, chronic pain is characterized by hyperexcitability of the nociceptors and by sensitization of the central nervous system. In addition, chronic pain can induce neurotic symptoms such as depression. This is especially true in patients who have been treated by several physicians and are not better, sometimes worse, and often in distress. It is now relatively easy to assess the degeneration of the spinal unit presumably responsible for the nociception, but there is no way to assess the participation of the central nervous system and to appreciate their respective roles in pain. However, it is easier to evaluate the role of the third component, i.e., the psychological status. This aspect is particularly important. A large consensus emerges from published studies that psychological disturbances, problems in the workplace, litigation, and compensation are the most frequent causes of failure (61). It is therefore of paramount importance to include a careful assessment of the psychosocial factors in the preoperative work-up of a candidate for fusion. The case history includes interrogation of the patient and evaluation of the history and of other adverse parameters such as duration of work loss, problems in the workplace, or litigation or compensation. It also includes a search for other accompanying symptoms, such as sleep difficulties, extreme fatigue, and sexual dysfunction. Interrogation of family and friends is sometimes very useful. This evaluation is often sufficient to determine the severity of the disability and the influence of psychosocial factors. In many instances, referral for psychological or psychiatric evaluation status is justified. At this point, as emphasized by Frymoyer and Nachemson (22), it is important to differentiate two patient groups: those with symptoms of chronic back pain without a noticeable psychosocial overlay and those with severe disability, a long period of work loss, problems in the workplace, and compensation. Patients in the former group are the best candidates for fusion. However, some of these apparently normal individuals may have nonobvious psychosomatic problems. Therefore, caution remains necessary. It is often useful to include, before the surgical decision, a trial of tricyclic agents. These drugs have analgesic properties and improve sleep. Their antidepressant effect may also improve the subclinical depression that is often secondary to chronic pain. Some studies have shown the efficacy of tricyclic agents in chronic low back pain (1,50).

The second subset includes patients with a long period of work loss and disability, the presence of compensation, and sometimes abuse of drugs and alcohol. Many studies have shown that the clinical success of fusion is strikingly decreased in this group with severe psychosocial problems and that surgery is usually not the solution. Fusion may be decided on only after failure of intensive rehabilitation multidisciplinary programs if a certain and severe peripheral cause of pain is present. Some of these patients will return to function, but a low rate of return to work can be expected, especially in workers who perform heavy manual labor (9,58,60).

As mentioned above, in this group of "degenerated discs," the overall clinical results reported in the literature are extremely variable, according to the series more than according to the techniques used. For example, the positive results of anterior fusion range from more than 80% in some studies (18,52) to 50% or less in others (17,57). The causes of this discrepancy may be related to technical failure of union. However, the incidence of pseudarthrosis does not appear to be a major determinant in the clinical end results. Pseudarthrosis is not always painful, especially in patients with degenerative disc disease. Other technical causes of persistent pain in spite of solid fusion, such as graft source and structure, number of levels fused, painful soft tissues, and persistence of degenerated disc tissue must also be considered. However, it appears that the discrepancy of results among the various series, which makes overall appreciation of the efficacy of fusion difficult, is essentially determined by the selection of patients and by methodologic criteria and outcome assessment (27,41). In many series, patients are not homogeneous and include conditions other than low back pain for lumbar spine degenerative disc disease without making the differentiation. Moreover, the psychosocial parameters that are such significant prognostic factors are not always carefully identified preoperatively, and patient groups are not presented separately. Furthermore, it has been clearly demonstrated that the percentage of good results depends on whether or not the assessment has been performed by an independent observer, and by the questionnaire design and the rating criteria of results (30).

These problems of methodology are crucial. For example, in a recent study of anterior fusion, striking differences were observed between the objective and the subjective results. Only 40% of the patients fell into the good or excellent category using a low back outcome score, whereas when using a subjective assessment, 68% rated themselves as having complete relief or a good deal of relief (25). In addition to relief of pain, which should be expected in correctly selected patients, the ability to return to work is a most important criterion for judging the efficacy of treatment. The rate of return to work depends not only on pain relief but also on the patient's motivation, on conditions in the workplace, and on the duration of work loss (58,60). The type of social security system is also involved. For example, in a series from Hong Kong (35), 113 of 126 patients with anterior fusion for idiopathic low back pain returned to work and only 10 patients changed their jobs. Seven of 50 workers changed from heavy manual work to lighter jobs because of their back problems. In contrast, in a French series of 155 anterior fusions for the same indication, only 30 of 76 who performed heavy manual labor returned to their original work after surgery; 79 of 97 moderate or light workers did not change their jobs, and 28 did not return to work (58). In a Scandinavian study, the working capacity remained unchanged in only 53% of the cases, and the pension rate because of low back pain was one-third higher than before the operation (59).

These examples clearly indicate the importance of occupational and social factors in the clinical results and the rate of return to work. Therefore, I agree with Deburge's opinion (9) that return to work is a very debatable outcome criterion for assessing improvement achieved by treatment aimed principally at suppressing pain. In patients engaged in heavy manual work, return to the original work cannot be warranted. For this category of patients, it is advised to include in the preoperative program changing to a lighter job when possible. In some instances a change of workplace is sufficient to alleviate the pain and eliminate the need for surgery.

## FUSION AFTER DISCECTOMY FOR DISC HERNIATION AND IN MANAGEMENT OF FAILED BACK SYNDROME

Neural decompression for disc herniation is usually achieved by the posterior approach and usually does not create instability. Fusion as an adjunct procedure was performed routinely in the early years to avoid recurrent disc herniation and persistent low back pain. However, many studies have shown that the majority of disc excisions are not complicated by chronic low back pain and that accompanying fusion is not necessary. In a few instances, persistence of symptoms may require later stabilization. In these cases, the indications are similar to those described for the degenerative disc disease group. Less invasive procedures, such as chemonucleolysis or percutaneous discectomy, may also be followed by postoperative low back pain. In my experience of over 1,500 cases of chemonucleolysis, cases with symptoms requiring later arthrodesis have been exceptional. Moreover it has been shown by experimental and clinical studies that instability is not a complication of chemonucleolysis (10,31,55).

The majority of the studies devoted to management of the failed back syndrome

(FBS) emphasize the efficiency of posterolateral fusion associated with canal reexploration in the symptomatic, multiply-operated back patient (4). A different approach to the FBS problem has also been advocated. This method entails distraction and fusion without opening the spinal canal. It aims at restoring the normal lumbar spine height, thus reopening the foramina and alleviating nerve root compression. Different procedures have been described: the posterior approach by Zielke and Strempel (63), using a special device to provide distraction of the low back area, combined with a transverso-alar fusion; the anterior interbody fusion, which reopens the collapsed disc space, as proposed by Hirabayashi et al. (28); and, finally, a combined operation proposed by O'Brien and Holte (46), using both anterior and posterior instrumentation. The operative results were considered satisfactory by O'Brien and Holte in 60% of 150 patients and by Zielke and Strempel in 49%. Unfortunately, patients are not homogeneous, and the exact number of FBS patients treated in these two studies is not mentioned.

## CONCLUSIONS

At the beginning of this chapter I questioned whether the rather pessimistic view of fusion in degenerative lumbar disc disease that prevailed among rheumatologists 20 years ago could be changed. The answer must be modulated, and the following conclusions can be drawn.

First, the results of fusion for low back pain and sciatica depend primarily on correct selection of patients. When an unstable lesion, e.g., spondylolisthesis, is identified in a patient with a normal psychological status, suppression of the abnormal motion is logical and gives acceptable outcome.

Second, in older patients with degenerative malalignments, such as degenerative spondylolisthesis or scoliosis, instability is usually associated with stenosis. Progressing deformities and threats to neural structures may require decompression with fusion.

Finally, fusion is more often considered in chronic patients with "degenerative discs" or "failed backs" without apparent instability. The clinical success depends primarily on good selection of patients. This requires careful evaluation of the severity of the pain and disability and of the quality and duration of nonoperative treatment. Psychosocial factors, including compensation status, workplace conditions, workers' perceptions of the job, and time of sick-listing must be accurately assessed. If these causes of poor results are avoided and if good technique can achieve a solid fusion, satisfactory pain relief can be expected in patients with one or two degenerated discs. However even in this ideal group, the success range remains uncertain, and further controlled studies with rigorous objective and subjective rating criteria are still needed to appreciate more accurately the clinical results with regard to presently used multiple techniques.

## REFERENCES


1. Alcoff J, Jones E, Rust P, et al. Controlled trial of Imipramine for chronic low-back pain. *J Fam Pract* 1982;14:841–6.
2. Boden SD, Shimandle JH, Damien JJ, et al. In vivo evaluation of a resorbable osteoconductive composite as a graft substitute for lumbar spinal fusion. Presented at the 22nd Annual Meeting of I.S.S.L.S., Helsinki, Finland, June, 1995.
3. Brown CW, Orme TY, Richardon JD. The rate of pseudarthrosis in patients who are smokers and patients who are nonsmokers. A comparison study. *Spine* 1986;11:942–3.

4. Cauchoix J, Benoist M. Management of the failed back syndrome. In: Floman Y, ed. *Disorders of the lumbar spine*. Rockville, MD: Aspen Publishers, 1990:421–45.
5. Cauchoix J, Benoist M, Chassaing V. Degenerative spondylolisthesis. *Clin Orthop* 1976;115:122–9.
6. Cleveland M, Bosworth DM, Thompson F. Pseudarthrosis in the lumbar spine. *J Bone Joint Surg* [*Am*] 1948;30:302–11.
7. Codere TJ, Katz J, Vacarrino AL, et al. Contribution of central neuroplasticity to pathological pain. *Pain* 1993;52:259–85.
8. Colhoun E, McCall IW, Williams L, et al. Provocation discography as a guide to planning operations on the spine. *J Bone Joint Surg* [*Br*] 1988;70B:267–71.
9. Deburge A. La chirurgie des lombalgies. *Gazette Med* 1994;101:20–4.
10. Delecourt C, Zakine S, Lassale B. Devenir dynamique du disque lombaire chemonucléolysé [Personal communication].
11. Dupuis PR, Young-Hing K, Cassidy JD, Kirkaldy-Willis WH. Radiologic diagnosis of degenerative spinal instability. *Spine* 1985;10:262–76.
12. Dvorak J. Normal motion of the lumbar spine as related to age and gender. *Eur Spine J* 1995;4:18–25.
13. Dvorak J, Panjabi MM, Novotny JE, et al. Clinical validation of functional flexion–extension roentgenograms of the lumbar spine. *Spine* 1991;16:943–50.
14. Esses SI, Bradford DJ, Kostuik JP. The role of external skeletal fixation in the assessment of low-back disorders. *Spine* 1989;14:594–601.
15. Fidler MW, Plasmans CM. The effect of four types of support on the segmental mobility of the lumbo-sacral spine. *J Bone Joint Surg* [*Am*] 1983;65:943–7.
16. Fitzgeral JA, Newman PH. Degenerative spondylolisthesis. *J Bone Joint Surg* [*Br*] 1976;58:184–92.
17. Flynn JC, Hoque MA. Anterior fusion of the lumbar spine. End result study with long term follow up. *J Bone Joint Surg* [*Am*] 1979;61A:1143–50.
18. Freebody D, Bendall R, Taylor RD. Anterior transperitoneal lumbar fusion. *J Bone Joint Surg* [*Br*] 1971;53:617–27.
19. Frymoyer JW, Newberg A, Pope MH, et al. Spine radiographs in patients with low-back pain. *J Bone Joint Surg* [*Am*] 1984;66:1048–55.
20. Frymoyer JW. Back pain and sciatica. *N Engl J Med* 1988;318:291–300.
21. Frymoyer JW. Segmental instability. Overview and classification. In: Frymoyer JW, ed. *The adult spine. Principles and practice*. New York: Raven Press, 1991:1873–90.
22. Frymoyer JW, Nachemson A. Natural history of low-back disorders. In: Frymoyer JW, ed. *The adult spine. Principles and practice*. New York: Raven Press, 1991:1537–48.
23. Gibson MJ, Buckley JJ, Mawhinney R, et al. MRI and discography in the diagnosis of disc degeneration. *J Bone Joint Surg* 1986;68B:369–73.
24. Graf H. Instabilité vertébrale. Traitement à l'aide d'un systèm souple. *Rachis* 1992;4:12–128.
25. Greenough C, Taylor L, Fraser RD. Anterior lumbar fusion: results, assessment techniques and prognostic factors. *Eur Spine J* 1994;3:225–30.
26. Grubb SA, Lipscomb HJ, Coonrad RW. Degenerative adult onset scoliosis. *Spine* 1988;13:241–5.
27. Hanley EN, Phillips ED, Kostuik JP. Who should be fused? In: Frymoyer JW, ed. *The adult spine. Principles and practice*. New York: Raven Press, 1991:1893–915.
28. Hirabayashi K, Ukai S, Toyama Y, et al. Anterior spinal body fusion as the salvage operation for failed back. *J West Pacif Orthop Assoc* 1985;22:17–24.
29. Horton WC, Daftari TK. Which disc is actually a source of pain? A correlation between magnetic resonance imaging and discography. *Spine* 1992;17:164–71.
30. Howe J, Frymoyer JW. The effects of questionnaire design on the determination of end results in lumbar spinal surgery. *Spine* 1985;10:804–5.
31. Kahanovitz N, Arnoczky S, Kummer F. The comparative biochemical histologic and radiographic analysis of canine lumbar discs treated by surgical excision or chemonucleolysis. *Spine* 1985;10:178–83.
32. Kirkaldy-Willis WH, Farfan HF. Instability of the lumbar spine. *Clin Orthop* 1982;165:110–23.
33. Knutson F. The instability associated with disc degeneration. *Acta Radiol* 1944;25:593–609.
34. Kostuik JP. Recent advances in the treatment of painful adult scoliosis. *Clin Orthop* 1980;147:238–52.
35. Leong CY. Anterior spinal fusion for low-back syndrome. In: Floman Y, ed. *Disorders of the lumbar spine*. Rockville, MD: Aspen Publishers, 1990:463–502.
36. Lindahl O. Determination of the sagittal mobility of the lumbar spine. *Acta Orthop Scand* 1966;37:241–54.
37. Lombardi JS, Wiltse LL, Reynolds J, et al. Treatment of degenerative spondylolisthesis. *Spine* 1985;10:821–7.
38. MacNab I. The traction spur: an indicator of segmental instability. *J Bone Joint Surg* 1971;53:663–70.
39. Morscher EW. Lumbar spine instability. In: Floman Y, ed. *Disorders of the lumbar spine*. Rockville, MD: Aspen Publishers, 1990:447–62.
40. Nachemson A. Adult scoliosis and back pain. *Spine* 1979;4:513–7.
41. Nachemson A. Fusion for low-back pain and sciatica. *Acta Orthop Scand* 1985;56:285–6.

42. Nachemson A. Lumbar spine instability. A critical update and symposium summary. *Spine* 1985;10: 290–1.
43. Nachemson A. Editorial comment: lumbar discography. Where are we today? *Spine* 1989;14:555–7.
44. North American Spine Society. Position statement on discography. *Spine* 1988;13:1343.
45. North A, Wilde P, Mulholland A, et al. External fixation of the lumbar spine as a predictor of the outcome of spinal fusion. Presented at the annual meeting of the International Society for the Study of the Lumbar Spine, Kyoto, Japan, 1989.
46. O'Brien JP, Holte DC. Simultaneous combined anterior and posterior fusion. *Eur Spine J* 1992;1:2–6.
47. Olerud S, Sjostrom L, Karlstrom G, et al. Spontaneous effect of increased stability of the lower spine in cases of severe chronic back pain. The answer of an external transpeduncular fixation test. *Clin Orthop* 1986;203:67–74.
48. Olmarker K, Blomquist MS, Stromberg MS, et al. Inflammatogenic properties of nucleus pulposus. *Spine* 1995;20:665–9.
49. Paris SV. Physical signs of instability. *Spine* 1985;10:277–9.
50. Pheasant H, Bursk A, Goldfarb J, et al. Amitriptyline and chronic low-back pain: a randomized double blind cross-over study. *Spine* 1983;8:552–7.
51. Reynolds JB, Wiltse LL. Surgical treatment of degenerative spondylolisthesis. *Spine* 1977;4:148–9.
52. Sacks S. Anterior interbody fusion of the lumbar spine. *Clin Orthop* 1966;44:163–70.
53. Schneiderman G, Flannigan B, Kingston S, et al. MRI in the diagnosis of disc degeneration. Correlation with discography. *Spine* 1987;12:276–81.
54. Seze S de, Kahn MF. Symposium sur le traitement chirurgical des lombalgies. *Rev Rhum Mal Osteoartic* 1973;40:721–5.
55. Spencer DL, Miller JA, Schultz AB. The effects of chemonucleolysis on the mechanical properties of the canine lumbar disc. *Spine* 1985;10:555–61.
56. Spengler DM, Freeman C, Westbrook R, et al. Low-back pain following multiple spine procedures: failures of initial selection. *Spine* 1980;5:356–60.
57. Stauffer RN, Coventry MB. Anterior interbody lumbar spinal fusion. *J Bone Joint Surg [Am]* 1972; 54:756–68.
58. Symposium sur le Traitement Chirurgical des Lombalgies. *Rev Rhum Mal Osteoartic* 1973;40:745–67.
59. Thomasen E. Intercorporeal lumbar spondylodesis, 312 patients followed for 2–20 years. *Acta Orthop Scand* 1985;56:287–93.
60. Waddell G, Kummel EG, Lotto WN, et al. Failed lumbar disc surgery and repeat surgery following industrial injuries. *J Bone Joint Surg [Am]* 1979;61:201–7.
61. Wing PC, Wilfling FJ, Kokan PJ. Psychological demographic and orthopaedic factors associated with prediction of outcome of spinal fusion. *Clin Orthop* 1973;90:153–60.
62. Woody J, Lehmann T, Weinstein J, et al. Excessive translation on flexion–extension radiographs in asymptomatic population. Presented at the meeting of I.S.S.L.S., Miami, Florida, 1988.
63. Zielke K, Strempel J. Posterior lateral distraction spondylodesis using the two-fold sacral bar. *Clin Orthop* 1986;203:151–8.

*Instrumented Fusion of the Degenerative
Lumbar Spine: State of the Art, Questions,
and Controversies,* edited by M. Szpalski,
R. Gunzburg, D. M. Spengler, and
A. Nachemson. Lippincott–Raven
Publishers, Philadelphia © 1996.

# 5

# Outcome Assessment of Lumbar Spinal Fusion

Charles G. Greenough

*Middlesbrough General Hospital, Middlesbrough,
Cleveland, TS5 5AZ, England*

The published results of fusion operations for low back pain have shown a wide variation of "good" results, ranging from 16 to 95% (17). The cause of this variation remains incompletely explained, but for spinal surgeons it is of vital importance. Throughout the world, increasing pressure on budgets is causing the purchasers of health care to examine more closely the effectiveness of treatments offered. Surgeons must provide sound evidence of the value of fusion if funding for this treatment is to continue. This chapter examines possible causes for the observed variations in results and outlines some principles for the measurement of outcome after spinal fusion.

When outcome assessment is considered, it is important to distinguish between two quite different results. The *technical outcome* is the answer to the question, "Has the surgeon achieved what he or she set out to achieve?" In this context, a successful technical result is a solid bony fusion. The *clinical outcome* is the answer to the question, "Has the patient benefited from the procedure?"

A successful technical result does not necessarily mean a successful clinical result, and vice versa. It is wrong, therefore, to include measurements of technical success in composite outcome scores.

## TECHNICAL OUTCOME

The measurement of bony fusion is in itself not easy. The introduction of increasingly sophisticated assessment tools has, in turn, cast doubt on the accuracy of previous techniques. Thus, Stauffer and Coventry (16) relied on the demonstration of trabeculae crossing the fusion site. Later, Pearcy and Borough (12), using an accurate biplanar radiologic technique in flexion and extension, demonstrated significant motion between the vertebrae in six of 10 patients who had the appearance of trabeculae crossing the fusion site. Moreover, Laasonen and Soini (10) found in a group of 25 patients with nonunion demonstrated on computed tomography (CT) scanning that assessment with plain films and flexion–extension views falsely indicated union in 16 cases.

The introduction of internal fixation has rendered the assessment of fusion by plain films more difficult and by CT scanning almost impossible. Recent evidence suggests that radiologic assessment of fusion in instrumented cases is only 68% accurate overall and is worst at the L4–L5 level, at which the false-positive rate was 28% (9). Therefore, the use of instrumentation, which renders more accurate assessment methods difficult, may result in significant overestimation of the technical results.

### Back Pain Clinic

Please mark on the line below how much pain you have had from your back on average over the past week:

0  1  2  3  4  5  6  7  8  9  10

No pain                     Maximal pain
at all                        possible

Please check the answer that most closely describes you on each of the following six sections:

| | | |
|---|---|---|
| At present, are you working? | Full time at your usual job | (9) |
| | Full time at a lighter job | (6) |
| | Part time | (3) |
| | Not working | (0) |
| At present, can you undertake household chores or odd jobs? | Normally | (9) |
| | As much as usual but slowly | (6) |
| | A few, not as many as usual | (3) |
| | Not at all | (0) |
| At present, can you undertake sports or active pursuits (e.g., dancing)? | As much as usual | (9) |
| | Almost as much as usual | (6) |
| | Some, much less than usual | (3) |
| | Not at all | (0) |
| Do you have to rest during the day because of pain? | Not at all | (6) |
| | A little | (4) |
| | Half the day | (2) |
| | Over half the day | (0) |
| How often do you have a consultation with a doctor or have any treatment (e.g., physiotherapy) for your pain? | Never | (6) |
| | Rarely | (4) |
| | About once a month | (2) |
| | More that once a month | (0) |
| How often do you have to take painkillers for your pain? | Never | (6) |
| | Occasionally | (4) |
| | Almost every day | (2) |
| | Several times each day | (0) |

Please check the box that best describes how much your back pain affects each of the following six activities:

| | No effect | Mildly/ not much | Moderately/ difficult | Severely/ impossible |
|---|---|---|---|---|
| Sex life | (6) | (4) | (2) | (0) |
| Sleeping | (3) | (2) | (1) | (0) |
| Walking | (3) | (2) | (1) | (0) |
| Sitting | (3) | (2) | (1) | (0) |
| Traveling | (3) | (2) | (1) | (0) |
| Dressing | (3) | (2) | (1) | (0) |

**FIG. 1.** The Low-Back Outcome Score as given to the patient. Scoring for the pain scale: 7–10 = 0; 5–6 = 3; 3–4 = 6; 0–2 = 9.

**TABLE 1.** *Diagnosis by compensation group*

| Diagnosis | Compensation | Noncompensation | All patients |
|---|---|---|---|
| Discogenic pain | 71 | 58 | 129 (45%) |
| Disc prolapse | 17 | 25 | 42 (15%) |
| Facet arthropathy | 17 | 26 | 43 (15%) |
| Soft tissue strain | 21 | 11 | 32 (10%) |
| Spondylolisthesis | 9 | 10 | 19 (7%) |
| Other | 10 | 12 | 22 (8%) |

Finally, the assessment of fusion should be performed on a patient basis, i.e., a pseudarthrosis at only a single level in a multiple-level operation still represents a technical failure for that patient.

## CLINICAL OUTCOME

Assessment of the clinical results of spinal surgery has been complicated by the large number of assessment techniques used in the literature. Howe and Frymoyer (8) used 14 different published outcome assessments in a group of over 200 patients who had undergone lumbar intervertebral disc excision more than 10 years previously. These authors found that the proportion of "successes" was significantly influenced by the outcome measure used, ranging from 97 to 60%. Subjective measures, e.g., the patients' opinions of the operation, gave a higher proportion of "successful" results compared to objective measures, such as return to original employment. Therefore, the choice of assessment technique alone can determine whether an operative procedure is described as a success or a failure. The most important methods of clinical outcome assessment are clinical examination (or degree of physical impairment), the patient's subjective opinion of the operation, and the use of a disability score.

Physical examination suffers from a number of significant difficulties. Some attributes are affected by psychological disturbance (14). Some physical measurements display a considerable diurnal variation (13). Interobserver error is a problem (11). Intraobserver error is also possible over the long period of follow-up required. Observer bias exists. Furthermore, even using "hard" signs, such as the loss of a reflex or weakness of a single motor group, the presence of nerve root dysfunction at presentation has not been shown to correlate with disability at review (1,3).

The patient's subjective opinion varies according to the questioner. There is no agreed format for a questionnaire of patient opinion. What questions should be asked? An agreed format would at least allow comparison of the results of one study

**TABLE 2.** *Factors with a significant influence on outcome*

| | |
|---|---|
| Compensation claim | $p < 0.0001$ |
| Psychological disturbance at presentation | $p < 0.002$ |
| Time off work | $p < 0.02$ |
| Age at injury | $p < 0.005$ |
| Sex | $p < 0.02$ |
| Socioeconomic status | $p < 0.01$ |
| Twisting or jerking injury | $p < 0.05$ |

**TABLE 3.** *Factors with no significant influence on outcome*

Diagnosis
Severity of injury
Length of follow-up
Neurologic deficit
Migrant status
Smoking
Interval between injury and initial consultation
Timing of first therapy
Marital status

with those of another. The following format has been used in two published series (6,7) but requires further validation in other studies:

Excellent: Very satisfied, complete or almost complete relief
Good: Fairly satisfied, a good deal of relief
Fair: Not very satisfied, only a little relief
Poor: Failure, no relief or worse than before

Most disability measures are in the form of patient self-report questionnaires and few studies have directly compared one scale with another. One such study compared the Oswestry Disability Index, the Disability score of Waddell, and the Low-Back Outcome Score (4). The Low-Back Outcome Score uses 13 different items, totaling 75 points, and the items are weighted for pain and the energy involved (Fig. 1). The three scores were assessed in a group of patients who underwent follow-up after conservative therapy for low back pain. The Low-Back Outcome Score proved to be more discriminating, particularly in the patients with better results, and was also the most comprehensive in explaining the variance of the outcome of the patients.

## CONFOUNDING FACTORS

In addition to the treatment, many patient-related factors contribute significantly to the observed results and must be analyzed in detail. The importance of these factors has been demonstrated in a number of studies of conservative, surgical, and rehabilitation treatment.

### Conservative Treatment

Greenough (3), in a carefully controlled retrospective study, defined a group of 300 patients complaining of low back pain after injury. Of this group, 150 patients were

**TABLE 4.** *Patients undergoing spinal fusion*

| Patient population | Anterior | Posterolateral |
| --- | --- | --- |
| Men | 67 | 65 |
| Women | 69 | 78 |
| Compensation | 93 | 67 |
| Noncompensation | 43 | 76 |
| Age at surgery | 41 (17–62) | 43 (22–79) |
| Follow-up (months) | 40 (22–82) | 35 (27–52) |

**TABLE 5.** *Indications for surgery*

| Indication | Anterior | Posterolateral |
| --- | --- | --- |
| Discogenic pain | 87 | 84 |
| Failed surgery | 34 | 15 |
| Spondylolysis/listhesis | 11 | 23 |
| Instability | 3 | 19 |

claiming compensation for their injury and 150 were not. All patients related the onset of their back pain to an identifiable incident, but fractures and dislocations were excluded. All patients were of working age at the time of the injury. These patients were all treated conservatively and at follow-up, 274 (91%) patients were reviewed at a median follow-up of 50 months (range 13–300 months) for the compensation patients and 52 months (range 9–332 months) for the noncompensation patients. The diagnosis (Table 1) was made by a single orthopedic specialist who treated only spinal conditions, and was confirmed by radiologic investigations where appropriate.

An injury severity score was allocated to each patient. At presentation, two psychometric instruments were administered to each patient: the Pain Drawing (15) and the inappropriate signs of Waddell (18). These were scored according to published criteria, and when either of the scores was positive the patient was defined as disturbed. Social group was allocated from the Ann Daniel Scale (2).

At review, each patient completed the Low-Back Outcome Score. Multiple regression analysis was performed using the Outcome Score as the dependent variable with sixteen independent variables. The total variance explained ($r_2$) was 48.3%. The variables examined and their significance appear in Tables 2 and 3.

The two variables of compensation and psychological disturbance at presentation accounted for 35% of the variance, or more than half of the explained variance.

Despite the fact that the diagnosis was made by a single experienced practitioner using consistent criteria, the diagnostic classification employed could not be shown to have any prognostic significance. Because specific diagnoses were not prognostic, specific treatments based on this classification may also not be as effective as had been hoped. The results of therapy in this study group have been investigated (5). A number of therapies, including educational classes, exercises, facet injections, and epidural nerve blockade, were used. Only educational classes were shown to have a significant effect, and then only in a small subset of patients. Interestingly, whereas noncompensation patients improved after facet injection, compensation patients became worse! Thus, in this carefully constructed population, patient-related factors outside the control of the treating practitioner had far more influence on the outcome than diagnosis or treatment.

**TABLE 6.** *Number of levels fused*

| Fusion | Anterior | Posterolateral |
| --- | --- | --- |
| Four-level fusion | 0 | 2 |
| Three-level fusion | 1 | 16 |
| Two-level fusion | 56 | 69 |
| One-level fusion | 79 | 68 |

**TABLE 7.** *Technical results: radiologic fusion*

| Findings | Anterior | Posterolateral |
|---|---|---|
| Fusion | 100 (74%) | 108 (78%) |
| Pseudarthrosis | 35 (26%) | 14 (10%) |
| Indeterminate | | 16 (12%) |

## Surgical Treatment

The results of two consecutive series of spinal fusions performed by the same surgeon have been reported (5,6). In the first series, 151 anterior lumbar fusions were performed by the senior author (RDF) and in the second 152 posterolateral fusions stabilized with Steffee plates were undertaken. Independent review of 136 (90.1%) of the first series and 137 (90.1%) of the second series was completed (Tables 4–6).

Fusion was assessed by an independent observer using plain films, and in the anterior series CT scanning was also used in cases of uncertainty (Table 7).

Interestingly, in the anterior series the technical results were influenced by compensation status; 60 of 93 compensation patients fused compared with 39 of 43 noncompensation patients ($p < 0.01$).

There was no significant difference in the subjective assessments of the two series (Table 8), but there was a marked difference in the results as assessed by the Low-back Outcome Score (Table 9).

Therefore, when assessed using a subjective method, the results of the two techniques appear similar and satisfactory, with 67% and 63% of patients achieving a good or excellent result. When measured objectively, there is a twofold difference in good or excellent results between the two techniques (40 and 18%, respectively), and the overall results are less satisfactory. The results of the instrumented posterolateral fusion were very disappointing, with almost 50% falling into the "poor" category.

No influence of radiologic fusion could be demonstrated on the clinical results (Table 10), demonstrating that the technical results do not necessarily influence the clinical results.

In both series, compensation status significantly affected the results at review (Table 11).

Psychological disturbance at presentation did not significantly influence the outcome in the patients studied. However, psychological disturbance at review was very strongly associated with poor results (Table 12).

## Rehabilitation

Multiple regression analyses on a group of 96 patients followed up at a minimum of 12 months from completion of an educational rehabilitation program confirmed the

**TABLE 8.** *Subjective assessment of the two series at follow-up[a]*

| Assessment | Anterior | Posterolateral |
|---|---|---|
| Very satisfied, almost complete relief | 30 (24%) | 36 (27%) |
| Fairly satisfied, good deal or relief | 54 (43%) | 48 (36%) |
| Not very satisfied, a little relief | 27 (22%) | 32 (24%) |
| Failure, no relief or worse than before | 13 (11%) | 16 (12%) |

[a] Nonsignificant.

**TABLE 9.** *Objective assessment of the two series at follow-up[a]*

| Assessment | Anterior | Posterolateral |
| --- | --- | --- |
| Excellent >65 | 21 (17%) | 7 (5%) |
| Good 50–64 | 29 (23%) | 18 (13%) |
| Fair 30–49 | 44 (35%) | 45 (33%) |
| Poor <30 | 31 (25%) | 67 (49%) |

[a] $p = 0.001$.

**TABLE 10.** *Influence of radiologic fusion on results at follow-up (compensation cases only)[a]*

| Location | Fusion | No fusion | |
| --- | --- | --- | --- |
| Anterior | | | |
| Outcome score | 43 (3–75),45 | 34 (14–75),25 | n.s. |
| Satisfaction | 6 (1–10),41 | 5 (0–10),24 | n.s. |
| Pain | 5 (0–8),46 | 5 (1–10),26 | n.s. |
| Posterolateral | | | |
| Outcome score | 25 (7–67),47 | 25 (10–72),12 | n.s. |
| Satisfaction | 2 (0–3),46 | 2 (0–3),12 | n.s. |
| Pain | 6 (0–10),47 | 6 (2–10),12 | n.s. |

[a] n.s., nonsignificant.

**TABLE 11.** *Influence of compensation on results at follow-up[a]*

| Location | Compensation | Noncompensation | |
| --- | --- | --- | --- |
| Anterior | | | |
| Outcome score | 42 (1–75),85 | 55 (14–75),40 | $p < 0.01$ |
| Satisfaction | 6 (0–10),81 | 8 (1–10),41 | n.s. |
| Pain | 5 (0–10),89 | 3 (0–8),42 | $p < 0.05$ |
| Posterolateral | | | |
| Outcome score | 25 (7–72),61 | 35 (7–75),76 | $p < 0.001$ |
| Satisfaction | 2 (0–3),60 | 2 (0–3),72 | $p < 0.02$ |
| Pain | 6 (1–10),61 | 5 (0–10),75 | $p < 0.05$ |

[a] n.s., nonsignificant.

**TABLE 12.** *Influence of psychological disturbance at review[a]*

| Location | Disturbed | Not disturbed | |
| --- | --- | --- | --- |
| Anterior | | | |
| Compensation | | | |
| Outcome score | 28 (3–55),36 | 50 (1–75),48 | $p < 0.0001$ |
| Satisfaction | 5 (0–8),35 | 7 (2–10),46 | $p < 0.0001$ |
| Pain | 6 (2–10),36 | 4 (0–10),51 | $p < 0.0001$ |
| Noncompensation, n.s. | | | |
| Posterolateral | | | |
| Compensation | | | |
| Outcome score | 22 (5–47),40 | 33 (14–65),23 | $p < 0.0001$ |
| Satisfaction | 2 (0–3),38 | 2 (0–3),23 | n.s. |
| Pain | 6 (2–9),37 | 5 (1–9),23 | $p < 0.02$ |
| Noncompensation | | | |
| Outcome score | 22 (4–63),22 | 44 (17–75),47 | $p < 0.0001$ |
| Satisfaction | 1 (0–3),21 | 3 (0–3),47 | $p < 0.0001$ |
| Pain | 7 (2–10),22 | 3 (0–8),47 | $p < 0.0001$ |

[a] n.s., nonsignificant.

importance of compensation status and psychological disturbance to the results of treatment. In addition, this group of patients was studied prospectively and it was found that the most important prognostic factor was the disability score at presentation ($p < 0.0001$) (Greenough, unpublished data).

## CONCLUSIONS

In summary, the patient population and initial disability, the assessment technique, and confounding factors all have a major role in determining the "results" of a treatment such as spinal fusion. Indeed, these factors may explain more of the variance of the outcome than the condition or treatment itself. In future studies a number of points must be considered:

1. The population must be adequately described before the intervention. This should include data on socioeconomic status as well as compensation status, initial psychological distress, duration of symptoms, age, and sex.
2. The intervention itself must be described clearly enough to be reproduced by another surgeon.
3. Outcome must be measured using a recognized instrument that is discriminating and comprehensive. This instrument must be used before surgery to provide a measure of initial severity.
4. Technical results should be described separately. The limitations of the accuracy of current techniques of assessment, particularly in instrumented fusions, must be acknowledged.
5. Subjective results should be reported using a standard format. This type of assessment should not be used alone, because the method discriminates poorly.
6. Confounding factors must be explicitly included in the analysis.

## REFERENCES


1. Currey HLF, Greenwood RM, Lloyd GG, Murray RS. A prospective study of low back pain. *Rheumatol Rehab* 1979;18:94–104.
2. Daniel A. *Power, privilege and prestige*. Longman Cheshire Publishers: Melbourne, 1983:197–206.
3. Greenough CG. Recovery from low back pain. 1–5 year follow-up of 287 injury-related cases. *Acta Orthop Scand* 1993;64(suppl)254:1–34.
4. Greenough CG, Fraser RD. Assessment of outcome in patients with low-back pain. *Spine* 1992;17:36–41.
5. Greenough CG, Fraser RD. Aetiology, diagnosis and treatment of low back pain. *Eur Spine J* 1994;3:22–7.
6. Greenough CG, Peterson MD, Hadlow S, Fraser RD. Instrumented posterolateral lumbar fusion. Society for Back Pain Research, Aberdeen, April, 1995.
7. Greenough CG, Taylor LJ, Fraser RD. Anterior lumbar fusion: results, assessment techniques and prognostic factors. *Eur Spine J* 1994;3:225–30.
8. Howe J, Frymoyer JW. The effects of questionnaire design on the determination of end results in lumbar spine surgery. *Spine* 1985;10:804–5.
9. Kant AP, Daum WJ, Dean SM, Uchida T. Evaluation of lumbar spine fusion: plain radiographs versus direct surgical exploration and observation. *Spine* 1995;20:2313–7.
10. Laasonen EM, Soini J. Low back pain after lumbar fusion. Surgical and computed tomographic analysis. *Spine* 1989;14:210–3.
11. McCombe PF, Fairbank JCT, Cockersole BC, Pynsent PB. Reproducibility of physical signs in low-back pain. *Spine* 1989;14:908–18.
12. Pearcy M, Burrough S. Assessment of bony union after interbody fusion of the lumbar spine using a biplanar radiographic technique. *J Bone Joint Surg [Am]* 1982;64B:228–32.
13. Porter RW, Trailescu IF. Diurnal changes in straight leg raising. *Spine* 1990;15:103–6.

14. Rae PS, Waddell G, Venner RM. A simple technique for measuring lumbar spinal flexion. *J R Coll Surg* [*Edin*] 1984;29:281–4.
15. Ransford AO, Cairns D, Mooney V. The pain drawing as an aid to the psychologic evaluation of patients with low-back pain. *Spine* 1976;1:127–34.
16. Stauffer RN, Coventry MB. Posterolateral lumbar-spine fusion. *J Bone Joint Surg* [*Am*] 1972;54-A: 1195–204.
17. Turner JA, Ersek M, Herron L, et al. Patient outcomes after lumbar spinal fusions. *JAMA* 1992;268: 907–11.
18. Waddell G, McCulloch JA, Kummel E, Venner RM. Nonorganic physical signs in low-back pain. *Spine* 1980;5:117–25.

*Instrumented Fusion of the Degenerative Lumbar Spine: State of the Art, Questions, and Controversies,* edited by M. Szpalski, R. Gunzburg, D. M. Spengler, and A. Nachemson. Lippincott–Raven Publishers, Philadelphia © 1996.

# 6

# What Outcome Measures Are Chosen by Surgeons Who Perform Lumbar Spine Fusions?

Nicolas R. Panaro and *Margareta Nordin

*Department of Rehabilitation Medicine, Rusk Institute; and *Occupational and Industrial Orthopaedic Center, Hospital for Joint Diseases Orthopaedic Institute, New York University Medical Center, New York, New York 10014*

The role of spinal fusion is currently under scrutiny and remains controversial. Turner et al. (23,24) mention poor consensus on indications for spinal fusions and the lumbar degenerative spine disorders. Volinn et al. (24a) noted that in the United States the rates for hospitalization and surgery for low back pain varied substantially among geographical regions. Bigos et al. (5) suggest that these variations indicate a lack of agreement on surgical indications. This could potentially lead to inappropriate care and suboptimal results.

Deyo et al. (8) studied morbidity and mortality associated with surgery of the lumbar spine. They studied 18,122 hospitalizations for surgical procedures involving the lumbar spine. A total of 84% involved patients with herniated discs or spinal stenosis. The overall mortality rate was very low (0.007%). This rate increased with age but remained less than 1% even for patients more than 75 years old. Postoperative complication rates were approximately 10% and increased to 18% in the group 75 years and older. Deyo et al. (8) stress the importance of the patient's age, the diagnosis, and the type of operative procedure in determining lumbar spine surgery morbidity and mortality. Their database did not provide information on outcomes such as postoperative symptoms, functional ability, or new physical findings at eventual follow-up. The authors suggest that more detailed data on outcomes on larger populations are needed to assess the operative success related to impairment, disability, quality of life, and continued health care.

Frymoyer (9a) discusses outcome measures for success. He states, "The goal of lumbar surgery is usually to relieve pain and improve function, rather than to reduce deformity, except the subset of patients with significant post-traumatic, developmental and/or acquired postural deformities." Howe and Frymoyer (12) designed a 14-item questionnaire to measure success on patients undergoing surgery for lumbar disc excision, with or without fusion. The success rate varied, depending on the outcome measures used. In their study, the best results were associated with patient satisfaction and the least favorable results were associated with functional outcomes measured, such as return to work. Frymoyer (1991) suggests that using various outcome measures can significantly affect the interpretation of lumbar surgery results for degenerative spine diseases.

Most operative procedures of degenerative disorders of the lumbar spine are elective. A patient's decision to undergo a surgical procedure for relief of lumbar spine pain is complex and difficult. This topic has lately been given more attention. A "better informed consumer" is shown to yield a more satisfied patient in cases of nonchronic back pain (5). Patients vary in their willingness to take risks associated with any clinical, diagnostic, or surgical procedures. The patient can only decide whether he or she knows the outcomes and eventual risks (8). The surgeon is the primary source of information for the patient considering surgery. We therefore undertook this literature search to review what outcome measures spine surgeons commonly use. The aim of this review was to survey the literature of spinal fusion in patients with painful degenerative lumbar spine diseases, with special emphasis on outcome measures. The information could be used to structure patient information and be helpful in the patient/surgeon decision-making process to optimize success in the choice of spine surgery for degenerative lumbar spine disorders.

## METHOD

A Medline search was performed, including articles published from January 26, 1990 to January 27, 1995. The search was limited to the following keywords: human/spinal fusions/English/abstract. We then linked this search to treatment outcomes limited to one-stage fusion. Studies of fusion including neoplasm, pediatric disor-

**TABLE 1.** *Outcome assessment preference (refs. 6, 18, 20)*[a]

| Reference | Pavlovic (18) | Bridwell et al. (6) | Tonino and Van Der Werf (10) |
|---|---|---|---|
| Type of study | Case series | RCT | Case series |
| Date data collected | 1987–1990 | ? | 1981–1983 |
| Length follow-up | >2 years | >2 years | 10 years |
| Diagnosis | Spondylolisthesis, spondylosis | Degenerative spondylolisthesis | Spondylolysis |
| Procedure | H | F, G, H | H |
| Radiography | A, C, D | A | A, B |
| Total *n* | 17 | 43 | 12 |
| Psychological consideration | Not reported | Not reported | Not reported |
| Disability/litigation | Not reported | Not reported | Not reported |
| Age | 14–31 years | Mean 66 years | 16–39 years |
| Observers | Author | Independent | Author |
| Outcome | Functional scale | Ability to walk | Pain, return to work |
| Duration conservative preoperative treatment | ? | ? | ? |
| Number of surgeons | One | One | ? |
| Population identified | No | Yes | No |
| Duration of preoperative symptoms | ? | ? | ? |
| Exclusion/inclusion criteria | ? | Yes | ? |
| Complications listed | Yes | Yes | Yes |
| Grading of fusion | Yes | Yes | Yes |

[a] A, radiographs; B, discograms; C, myelography; D, CT; E, MRI; F, fusion, no instrumentation; G, no fusion; H, fusion with instrumentation.

**TABLE 2.** *Outcome assessment preference (refs. 9, 13, 24)[a]*

| Reference | Virta and Osterman (24) | Knox and Chapman (13) | Dhar and Porter (9) |
|---|---|---|---|
| Type of study | Cohort | Case series | Cohort |
| Date data collected | ? | ? | 1980–1984 |
| Length follow-up | Mean 17 years | ? | 1 year |
| Diagnosis | Spondylolisthesis | Degenerative disc disease | Multiple, not listed |
| Procedure | Fusion, conservative management | Fusion, retrospective | Fusion, discectomy, decompression |
| Radiography | A | A, B | A, C, D, and EMG |
| Total *n* | 148 | 30 | 160 |
| Psychological consideration | Not reported | Depression scale | MMPI |
| Disability/litigation | Not reported | Yes | ? |
| Age | 20–50 years | 25–54 years | 27–69 years |
| Observers | Independent | Authors | Authors |
| Outcome | ADL index, return to work, pain | Disability index, pain | Pain, return to work, patient satisfaction |
| Duration conservative preoperative treatment | ? | ? | ? |
| Number of surgeons | ? | One | ? |
| Population identified | Yes | No | ? |
| Duration of preoperative symptoms | ? | ? | ? |
| Exclusion /inclusion criteria | Incomplete | Incomplete | ? |
| Complications listed | Yes | No | No |
| Grading of fusion | No | Yes | Incomplete |

[a] A, radiographs; B, discograms; C, myelography; D, CT; E, MRI; F, fusion, no instrumentation; G, no fusion; H, fusion with instrumentation.

ders, trauma, and systemic diseases were excluded. This review considered only original articles. Meta-analysis and review articles by invitation were not included. The studies meeting these criteria were evaluated according to the McGill critical appraisal form (19). The form rates studies for admissibility of study design and outcome measures. To be included in this review we arbitrarily decided (a) to include studies that complied at least with 30% (four of 12 questions were answered with a yes) of the first part of the appraisal form and (b) that the study had to be published by a peer-reviewed journal. The following criteria were considered: Was a hypothesis clearly stated? Was a source population identified? Were inclusion and exclusion criteria stated and appropriate? Were withdrawals, refusals, and number excluded reported and were reasons stated? Was sample size large enough for adequate statistical power? Was an independent evaluator used? Were results verifiable from the raw data? Was the study a retrospective or a prospective cohort, a randomized control trial (RCT) or a case series? We then listed the outcome measures of the selected studies in a table format to display the preferred variables and/or outcome measures selected by the authors. We included no quality assessment of the outcome measures.

## RESULTS

A total of 1,318 articles were retrieved from the initial search, including fusions. When the search was linked to studies including patient treatment and outcomes, 864

**TABLE 3.** *Outcome assessment preference (refs. 11, 15, 28)[a]*

| Reference | Zuckerman et al. (28) | Grubb and Lispcomb (11) | Matsunaga et al. (15) |
| --- | --- | --- | --- |
| Type of study | Cohort | Cohort | Cohort |
| Date data collected | 1978–1986 | ? | ? |
| Length follow-up | 1–4.5 years | 2–5 years | 2–7 years |
| Diagnosis | Herniated disc with instability | Degenerative disc disease | Herniated disc |
| Procedure | F, H | F, H | F, G |
| Radiography | A | A, B, C | A |
| Total *n* | 126 | 101 | 110 |
| Psychological consideration | Yes | Yes | ? |
| Disability/litigation | ? | Yes | Not reported |
| Age | Mean 44.5 years | 20–50 years | 15–62 years |
| Observers | Independent | Authors | Authors |
| Outcome | Analgesic use, return to work | Pain, work status | Return to work, sports activities |
| Duration conservative preoperative treatment | ? | ? | ? |
| Number of surgeons | ? | ? | ? |
| Population identified | No | Yes | Yes |
| Duration of preoperative symptoms | ? | Yes | Yes |
| Exclusion/inclusion criteria | Yes | No | Yes |
| Complications listed | No | No | No |
| Grading of fusion | Yes | Yes | No |

[a] A, radiographs; B, discograms; C, myelography; D, CT; E, MRI; F, fusion, no instrumentation; G, no fusion; H, fusion with instrumentation.

studies remained. Fifty-eight studies involved fusions in patients with lumbar spine degenerative diseases. Fourteen studies met the criteria of inclusion. Tables 1–5 display the type of study, data collected, and outcome measures. The authors favored the following outcome measures in these studies: subjective pain rating by the patient (7 of 14), use of analgesics (5 of 14), and some activity level, most including return to work (12 of 14). Lumbar mobility was measured in one study. Patient satisfaction was measured in one study. Grading of fusion by radiography or imaging was indicated in seven studies. Only half of the studies used an independent evaluator (7 of 14). Duration of symptoms before surgery was mentioned in six studies, and psychological profile was used in five studies. Follow-up time was reported in 13 of 14 studies and was generally reported for more than 1 year.

## DISCUSSION

This literature review was not undertaken to evaluate lumbar spine fusion success rates. It was undertaken as a review to determine what outcome measures are favored by the surgeon performing spine surgery. Furthermore, it is of interest to discuss what outcomes are of interest to inform the patient before surgery. No study, to our knowledge, has used a systematic approach to investigate what information the patient wants to know. Little evidence exists that patients who select surgery and

**TABLE 4.** *Outcome assessment preference (refs. 17, 25, 27)[a]*

| Reference | White et al. (27) | Weber (25) | Newman and Grinstead (17) |
|---|---|---|---|
| Type of study | Case series | RCT | Case series |
| Date data collected | ? | 1970–1971 | ? |
| Length follow-up | Mean 3 years | 10 years | >4 months |
| Diagnosis | Herniated disc | Herniated disc | Degenerative disc disease |
| Procedure | G, H | G, conservative treatment | F |
| Radiography | C, D and EMG | A, C | B, E |
| Total *n* | 69 | 280 | 36 |
| Psychological consideration | Not reported | Yes | Yes |
| Disability/litigation | Not reported | Not reported | Yes |
| Age | 37–76 years | 25–55 years | 26–58 years |
| Observers | Independent | Author | Independent |
| Outcome | Activity level, analgesic use | Activity level, analgesic use | Analgesic use, ADL, return to work |
| Duration conservative preoperative treatment | 3 months | ? | ? |
| Number of surgeons | One | ? | One |
| Population identified | Yes | Yes | Yes |
| Duration of preoperative symptoms | ? | Up to 10 years | Mean 3.6 years |
| Exclusion/inclusion criteria | Yes | Yes | No |
| Complications listed | Yes | Yes | Yes |
| Grading of fusion | ? | Yes | No |

[a] A, radiographs; B, discograms; C, myelography; D, CT; E, MRI; F, fusion; G, no fusion; H, fusion with instrumentation.

fusion of the lumbar spine for degenerative spine disease will return to their previous functional level. The option to obtain pain relief may be a satisfactory outcome for the patient, provided that this is understood before surgery is performed. Pain relief was usually measured as a global measure with a questionnaire, a visual analogue scale (4) and/or the McGill pain questionnaire (16). Most common was the measure of analgesic intake, which is an indirect measure of pain relief. Pain relief is an important outcome for the patient and can be evaluated only subjectively. Nevertheless, the perceived rating can distinguish between pain at rest, pain during activity, and duration of pain.

Few studies have looked at functional outcomes in more detail. Broad categories such as return to work are mentioned in some studies (9,11,15,20,24,28). It is unclear from these studies what level of work the patients returned to. Did the patient return to previous work, restricted duty, or partial disability? One study (1) used range of motion of the lumbar spine. Range of motion or flexibility of the trunk is highly influenced by age, gender, and anthropometric factors (3). This may also be true for the patient with a lumbar spine fusion. Functional motion, including pain-free trunk motion, would be a better measure to determine success or failure for the patient considering spinal fusion. Activities of daily living, functional scales, and/or disability scales were used by several authors (13,17,25,27). One study (6) used ability to walk in an older patient population with a mean age of 66 years. Another study (15) used level of sports activity. The choice of functional scales for evaluation is be-

**TABLE 5.** *Outcome assessment preferences (refs. 1, 26)[a]*

| Reference | Axelson et al. (1) | Wetzel et al. (26) |
| --- | --- | --- |
| Type of study | Case series | Case series |
| Date data collected | 1984–1989 | 1983–1987 |
| Length follow-up | >2 years | 2 years |
| Diagnosis | Spondylolisthesis, pain post laminectomy | Degenerative disc disease |
| Procedure | F | F, H |
| Radiography | A | B, D, E, EMG, and bone scan |
| Total *n* | 61 | 48 |
| Psychological consideration | Not reported | Not reported |
| Disability/litigation | Not reported | Yes |
| Age | 11–67 years | 17–58 years |
| Observers | ? | ? |
| Outcome | Lumbar mobility, pain | Analgesic use, pain, functional scale |
| Duration conservation preoperative treatment | ? | >3 months |
| Number of surgeons | Five | ? |
| Population identified | No | No |
| Duration of preoperative symptoms | >1 year | >3 months |
| Exclusion/inclusion criteria | Incomplete | No |
| Complications listed | No | Yes |
| Grading of fusion | No | No |

[a] A, radiographs; B, discograms; C, myelography; D, CT; E, MRI; F, fusion, no instrumentation; G, no fusion; H, fusion with instrumentation.

coming more difficult, as these scales are popular. The success or failure of a functional scale used in patient evaluation must be seriously considered. It is wise to contact a clinical epidemiologist to better understand the limitations and strengths of the choice of instrument and study design. If this is not possible, we refer the clinician to publications by Troidl et al. (21) and Bellamy (4). Table 1 was prepared to show the variability of criteria in studies concerning fusion of the lumbar spine for degenerative spine diseases and outcome. Few papers provided enough data to examine more than a few variables.

A meta-analysis of lumbar spine fusions for spinal stenosis was published in 1992 to examine the efficacy of this procedure (22). The results included the following variables: type of surgery, study design, definition of outcome, and method of analysis. These authors found that the overall rate of surgical success averaged 64% and at that time no randomized trials concerning surgical vs. nonsurgical care were available. No significant relationship was found among age, gender, previous back surgery, pseudo-claudication, and number of levels of laminectomy. At the time of this review, too few papers existed to compare retrospective vs. prospective studies or independent examiner vs. author's rating. We therefore direct the reader to the meta-analysis published in Chap. 24. Prior analysis of the literature has also shown considerable variability in fusion outcomes, ranging from 16 to 95% with various diagnoses (5,22,23).

We prepared a list of suggested factors that can affect outcome measure (Table 6). These criteria can be used for discussion of study design or as structured information to be provided to the patient. The proposed list is meant as a guide and is not exhaustive.

Defined outcome criteria are essential for the patient, the surgeon, and the clinical

**TABLE 6.** *Factors affecting outcome measure*

Demographic data
  Age
  Gender
  Body build (height, weight)
  Familial aggregation
Clinical information
  Diagnosis (ICD code)
  Preoperative duration of lumbar pain (months)
  Frequency of attacks per time unit (attacks per month)
  Preoperative duration of leg pain (months)
  Degree of need for analgesics (pre- and postsurgery, type)
  Lumbar/trunk mobility or flexibility (measured or estimated)
  Pre/postoperative straight leg raising test (measured or estimated)
  Preexisting medical problems (trauma, systemic disease, other)
  Previous hospitalization for back pain (number and length)
  Previous surgery (number and time)
Diagnostics
  Preoperative disc degeneration (technique and classification by preference)
  Degree of vertebral slippage (pre/postoperatively, technique, and classification by preference)
  Degree of herniation (classification by preference)
  Solid fusion healing vs. pseudarthrosis (technique and classification by preference)
  EMG
Surgery
  Type of fusion (anterior, posterolateral, instrumented)
  Number of levels fused
Complications
  Morbidity
  Mortality
  Infections
  Implant failure
Lifestyle
  Level of activity (sedentary, activities of daily living, level of sports activity)
  Smoking (prior, current, and amount)
  Drug/alcohol intake (amount)
  Driving time (daily exposure to vibration)
  Sleeping time (amount and quality)
  Fitness level (measured or estimated)
  Sexual activity
Psychological status
  Psychological illness
  Depression
  Hysteria/hypochondria
  Health beliefs
Socioeconomic status
  Economic status
  Education level
  Pending litigation
  Disability/pension
Occupation
  Type of occupation (sedentary or physically demanding, i.e., exposure to lifting, awkward
    posture, and/or whole body vibration)
  Level of return to occupation (same, modified, disability)
  Degree of job satisfaction
Patient satisfaction
  Resolution of symptoms
  Activity level
  Quality of life

team. If the patient is provided the same message by all involved, any potential for ambiguity is decreased, and the patient can make an informed decision. Patient education is important and, in other chronic disease, has been shown to be cost-effective for osteoarthritis and chronic pain (2). Perhaps the patient who is a candidate for lumbar spine fusion surgery should first attend instructional sessions before surgery is performed. This would ensure that the information about factors affecting surgical outcomes is understood. The information can be given in a structured way and adapted to the individual patient and level of education. One center in the United States uses 1 month of preoperative fitness training, education, and smoking cessation to improve outcomes of lumbar spine fusion. No formal evaluation of this approach has yet been presented (7).

Many factors contribute to success after surgery. The factor emphasized here is the patient's level of understanding: perception, attitudes, and beliefs. Patients' beliefs and preferences can be better understood with a systematic approach and evaluation before intervention. Spine fusion is an irreversible procedure, whether successful or not. Surgical efficacy cannot be determined in isolation. Patients must not only acquire knowledge but they must also accept that the surgical result in a lifelong context may require a change in behavior and beliefs. When a fusion is successful (i.e., relief of pain) is achieved, functional gains usually follow. At present we lack the tools necessary to predict with confidence which patients will or who will not benefit from lumbar spine fusion for degenerative spine diseases. Greenough [Chap. 5] and Greenough et al. (10) state that the results obtained by lumbar spine fusion are heavily influenced by socioeconomic and psychological factors, as well as by the assessment techniques. Little and MacDonald (14) showed in a heterogenous group of 144 patients that previous surgery on the spine and low initial disability scores were significantly negative predictors at short- and long-term follow-up. Prospective, randomized, controlled trials with stringent criteria are needed to define specific methods of treatment for rigorously defined lumbar spine degenerative disorders. By utilizing a model for outcome scores and study criteria, information concerning lumbar spine fusion and postoperative long-term outcomes can be effectively pooled. Success criteria for a surgical intervention must be discussed from many different aspects, including among others the patient, the surgeon, and the cost. Finally, assessment must be done by an observer(s) demonstrably independent from the treating surgeon and the clinical team.

## REFERENCES


1. Axelsson P, Johnsson R, Stromqvist B, Arvidsson M, Herrlin K. Posterolateral lumbar fusion. *Acta Orthop Scand* 1994;65:309–14.
2. Bartlett E. Cost-benefit analysis of patient education. In: Assal JPH, Golay A, Visser APH, eds. *New trends in education. A trans cultural and inter-disease approach. International Congress Series 1076.* Amsterdam: Elsevier, 1995:87–91.
3. Battie MC, Bigos SJ, Sheehy A, Wortley MD. Spinal flexibility and individual factors that influence it. *Physical Ther* 1987;67:653–7.
4. Bellamy N. *Musculoskeletal clinical metrology.* London: Kluwer Academic Publishers, 1993.
5. Bigos S, Bowyer O, Braen G, et al. *Acute low back problems in adults.* Clinical Practice Guideline No. 14. AHCPR Publication No. 95-0642. Rockville, MD: Agency for Health Care Policy and Research, Public Health Service, US Department of Health and Human Services, 1994.
6. Bridwell KH, Sedgewick TA, O'Brien MF. The role of fusion and instrumentation in the treatment of degenerative spondylolisthesis with spinal stenosis. *J Spine Dis* 1993;6:461–72.
7. Brown MP, Seltzer DG. Perioperative care in lumbar surgery. *Orthop Clin North Am* 1991;2:353–8.
8. Deyo RA, Cherkin DC, Loeser JD, Bigos SJ, Ciol M. Morbidity and mortality in association with operations on the lumbar spine. The influence of age, diagnosis and procedure. *J Bone Joint Surg (Am)* 1992;74-A:536–43.
9. Dhar S, Porter RW. Failed lumbar spinal surgery. *Int Orthop* 1992;16:152–6.

9a. Frymoyer JW. Radiculopathies: lumbar disc herniation and recess stenosis—patient selection, predictors of success and failure and non-surgical treatment options. In: Frymoyer JW, ed. *The adult spine. Principles and practice.* Vol. 2. New York: Raven Press, 1991:1719–31.

10. Grenough CG, Taylor LJ, Fraser RD. Anterior lumbar fusion. A comparison of noncompensated patients with compensated patients. *Clinical Orthop Relat Res* 1994;300:30–7.

11. Grubb SA, Lipscomb HJ. Results of lumbar sacral fusion for degenerative disc disease with and without instrumentation: two to five year follow up. *Spine* 1992;17:349–55.

12. Howe J, Frymoyer JW. The effects of questionnaire design on the determination of end results in lumbar spine surgery. *Spine* 1985;10:804–5.

13. Knox BD, Chapman TM. Anterior lumbar interbody fusion for discogram concordant pain. *J Spinal Dis* 1993;6:242–4.

14. Little DG, MacDonald D. The use of the percentage change in Oswestry Disability Index Score as an outcome measure in lumbar spine surgery. *Spine* 1994;19:2139–43.

15. Matsunaga S, Sakou T, Taketomi E, Ijari K. Comparison of operative results of lumbar disc herniation in manual laborers and athletes. *Spine* 1993;18:2222–6.

16. Melzack R. The McGill Pain Questionnaire: major properties and scoring methods. *Pain* 1975;1:277–99.

17. Newman MH, Grinstead GL. Anterior lumbar interbody fusion for internal disc disruption. *Spine* 1992;17:831–3.

18. Pavlovic M. Surgical treatment of spondylosis and spondylolisthesis with a hook and screw. *Int Orthop* 1994;18:6–9.

19. Spitzer WO, Skovron ML, Salmi LR, et al. Scientific monograph of the Quebec Task Force on whiplash-associated disorders: redefining "whiplash" and its management. *Spine* 1995;20(suppl 8):12S–20S.

20. Tonino A, Van Der Werf G. Direct repair of lumbar spondylolysis. *Acta Orthop Scand* 1994;65:91–3.

21. Troidl H, Spitzer WO, Peek B, et al. *Principles and practice of research. Strategies for surgical investigators.* New York: Springer-Verlag, 1991.

22. Turner JA, Ersek M, Herron L, Deyo R. Surgery for lumbar spinal stenosis: attempted meta-analysis. *Spine* 1992;17:1–8.

23. Turner JA, Ersik M, Herron L, et al. Patient outcomes after lumbar spinal fusions. *JAMA* 1992;268:907–11.

24. Virta L, Osterman K. Radiographic correlations in adult symptomatic spondylolisthesis: a long term follow up study. *J Spinal Dis* 1994;7:41–8.

24a. Volinn E, Turczyn KM, Loeser JD. Theories on back pain and health care utilization. *Neurosci Clin N Am* 1991;2:739–48.

25. Weber H. Lumbar disc herniation: a controlled, prospective study with ten years of observation. *Spine* 1983;8:131–40.

26. Wetzel FT, LaRocca H, Lowery GL, Aprill CN. The treatment of lumbar spinal pain syndromes diagnosed by discography. *Spine* 1994;19:792–800.

27. White AH, Von Rogov P, Zucherman J, Heiden D. Lumbar laminectomy for herniated disc: a prospective controlled comparison with internal fixation. *Spine* 1987;12:305–7.

28. Zuckerman J, Hsu K, Picetti G, White A, Wynne G, Taylor L. Clinical efficacy of spinal instrumentation in lumbar degenerative disc disease. *Spine* 1992;17:834–7.

*Instrumented Fusion of the Degenerative
Lumbar Spine: State of the Art, Questions,
and Controversies,* edited by M. Szpalski,
R. Gunzburg, D. M. Spengler, and
A. Nachemson. Lippincott–Raven
Publishers, Philadelphia © 1996.

# 7

# The Failed Fused Back

Pieter F. van Akkerveeken

*Department of Orthopaedics, RugAdviesCentra Nederland,
3702 AD, Zeist, The Netherlands*

Joints damaged by disease or trauma are usually not functioning well. To restore function the joint can be surgically reconstructed by an endoprosthesis in a number of indications. When reconstruction of a joint is not possible, fusion is the only alternative. For joints such as the wrist and the big toe, arthrodesis is still the operation of choice, yielding a high percentage of excellent functional results.

Failure of fusion can be differentiated into clinical failure and surgical failure. Clinical failure is defined as a condition in which the patient has persisting symptoms after the operation, particularly pain. When bony ankylosis is absent, the condition is called a surgical failure.

Fusion of one or more lumbar segments may be indicated in patients with severe damage, e.g., in fractures, tumor, and infection. In view of the good results obtained in these conditions, the concept of fusion was applied to pain problems in patients without gross damage of the spines: degenerative changes with or without segmental hypermobility. Because degenerative changes are common in advancing age in people with no back pain at all, symptomatic and asymptomatic degenerative changes have to be differentiated. In theory, this can be done by provocative discography and diagnostic facet blocks. The latter has proved not to have any predictive value (2). A recent review of lumbar discography (15) concluded that "most of the current literature supports the use of discography in select situations." Four indications were presented: patients with suspected disc abnormality, patients in whom fusion is being considered to determine whether or not the proposed fusion segment is symptomatic and whether the adjacent discs are normal; patients with persisting symptoms after previous surgery; and patients in whom minimally invasive discectomy is being considered to confirm a contained disc herniation and to exclude a sequestered disc. Only one publication (17) dealt with discography in patients with persisting symptoms after a fusion. Symptom reproducibility identifying the symptomatic abnormality occurred in 21 of 24 patients. The authors considered the negative result of discography in three patients as false-positive, attributable to poor needle placement. They used discography to differentiate between symptoms at the pseudarthrosis level from those at an adjacent level. Discography was also used to identify the source of symptoms in patients with persistent symptoms but with a solid posterior anterolateral fusion (36). It can be concluded that discography as a procedure to differentiate between symptomatic and asymptomatic pseudarthrosis has not been studied sufficiently well.

Because the subject of failed fusions of the lumbar spine is complex, it is discussed here only in broad terms. This chapter presents an overview with a classification and diagnostic recommendations.


## SURGICAL FAILURE

Surgical failure or pseudarthrosis is a condition that occurs after an attempted fusion of at least one spinal segment in which no bony union occurred between the vertebrae. Pseudarthrosis may be atrophic or hypertrophic, and may be caused by infection or may occur without infection.


### Atrophic Pseudarthrosis

Atrophic pseudarthrosis is characterized by absence of bony reaction. When bone grafts are applied they are resorbed. Bone resorption is considered to be the result of stress shielding by intact facets or by rigid spinal instrumentation: Heggeness and Esses (16) observed an atrophic pseudarthrosis in 38% of patients without instrumentation, whereas in patients with instrumentation it occurred in 61% of the pseudarthroses. Atrophic nonunion is usually accompanied by implant failure caused by metal fatigue or loosening. Atrophic pseudarthrosis can occur after intertransverse fusion with facet arthrodesis and also after interbody fusion. Resorption of the interbody graft has been observed, although a pseudarthrosis after interbody fusion is usually of the hypertrophic type.

Infected pseudarthroses are usually of the atrophic type. The atrophy indicates poor biologic conditions as a result of tissue destruction by the infective process. To repair the pseudarthrosis in those patients, extensive bone grafting is usually indicated. In some patients, vascularized bone grafts must be used, but only in a small minority because of the extensive collateral blood circulation of the spine.


### Hypertrophic Pseudarthrosis

Hypertrophy indicates optimal biologic conditions but inadequate mechanics (37). Radiologically, bony sclerosis is observed. Although this may be confused with dead bone, it represents excessive bone formation with an optimal blood supply. As has been proved in animal experiments for long bones, the therapy of choice is stabilization, preferably by internal fixation and, in case of a malalignment, in combination with a correction osteotomy.

Heggeness and Esses (17) recognized two subtypes after posterolateral fusion: a "transverse" pseudarthrosis in the fusion mass and a pseudarthrosis in the form of a "shingle." These types can also occur in combination, called a "complex" pseudarthrosis. Defects in the fusion mass are often observed in patients with a transverse

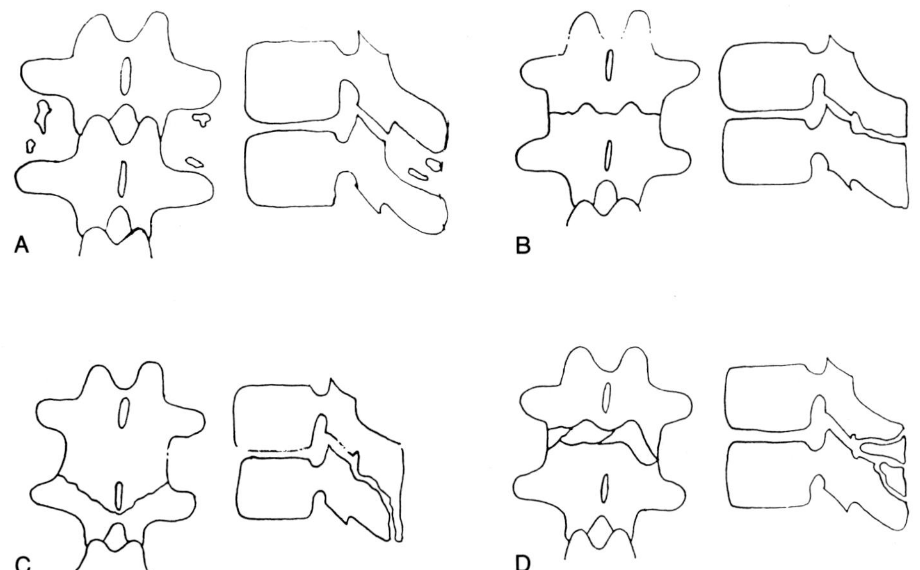

**FIG. 1.** Drawing of an atrophic **(A)**, transverse **(B)**, shingle **(C)**, and complex **(D)** pseudarthrosis. Adapted from ref. 16.

pseudarthrosis. Heggeness and Esses consider an intact facet joint one of the reasons for pseudarthrosis due to stress shielding (Fig. 1).

### Diagnosis

The condition of the lumbar spine after a fusion operation does not correlate well with symptoms as experienced by the patient. Patients with pseudarthrosis may be free of pain and perform normally in daily life. On the other hand, persistent or recurrent pain has been reported in 30 to 40% of patients (18), even in the presence of a solid fusion. Flatley and Derderian (10) reported poor clinical results in seven of 10 patients with solid fusions. Even in the 1960s, similar observations had been reported (8). However these "solid" fusions were not surgically verified, and the radiologic observations may be false-positive in the sense that the "solid" fusions were actually pseudarthroses. To assess fusion postoperatively, plain radiographs in posteroanterior and lateral projection, usually in combination with standing extension/flexion views, are commonly used (4,7,18,27,28).

As early as 1947, Ralston and Thompson (28) demonstrated that in 23 of 175 patients with a fusion on plain films, bending films demonstrated abnormal segmental motion. Brodsky and co-workers (4) compared plain radiographs, tomograms, extension/flexion views, and computed tomography (CT) with the findings at surgical exploration. A solid fusion was considered to be present when by direct manipulation at vertebrae and fusion mass no motion could be evoked and when by visualization the bone mass appeared continuous. They noted in many patients "a solid plate of bone that moved on the underlying deeper layers, indicating failure to fuse to the transverse processes." Their study demonstrated a large number of false-negatives and false-positives of the radiologic assessment before operation. In a total

**TABLE 1.** *The failed fused back: specificity, sensitivity, and predictive values*

| Preoperative radiologic modality | No. of sites | True + | True − | False + | False − | Specificity | Sensitivity | +PV | −PV |
|---|---|---|---|---|---|---|---|---|---|
| Roentgenography | 758 | 399 | 185 | 123 | 51 | 60 | 89 | 76 | 78 |
| Tomography | 240 | 74 | 107 | 20 | 39 | 84 | 65 | 79 | 73 |
| Bending films | 216 | 127 | 31 | 53 | 5 | 37 | 96 | 70 | 86 |
| CT scan | 150 | 34 | 13 | 20 | 86 | 86 | 63 | 72 | 81 |

From Brodsky et al., ref. 4.
+PV, positive predictive values; −PV, negative predictive values.

of 214 surgical explorations, 36% of plain radiographs and 43% of CT scans did not correlate with symptoms. Specificity, sensitivity, and predictive values were calculated for individual sites of fusions (Table 1). Because of their high sensitivity, extension/flexion views "are less likely to miss a solid fusion." The highest positive predictive value (79%) was from tomography; bending films, on the other hand, had the highest negative predictive value (86%).

In a recent report, Kant and co-workers (18) studied 126 levels in 75 patients who had their instrumentation removed between 1 month and 212 weeks postoperatively. During this operation the fusion mass was directly observed. The results were compared with the assessment of plain radiographs, including oblique views, by an orthopedic surgeon not involved in the surgical management. The overall agreement between the radiographs and direct observation at surgery was poor (K 0.26, 95% confidence limit 0.07–0.44).

Morris and co-workers (24) differentiated on radiographic assessment between functional and structural integrity. Functional integrity can be demonstrated by bending films. These may fail to show segmental motion in the presence of muscle action or internal fixation.

Structural integrity is assessed by plain radiography, tomography, and CT scanning, looking for a continuous bony mass. More sophisticated methods such as stereo photogrametry, first applied by Olsson et al. (25) in the 1970s, has proved to be very accurate in detecting segmental motion. However, this method has not been used systematically and studies correlating the results of this technique with direct observations at surgical exploration have not been reported.

Scintigraphy has also been reported as an assessment tool for pseudarthrosis (31). Although this modality, particularly SPECT, appears promising, no validating studies have been reported. CT with three-dimensional reconstruction and MRI also appear to be promising modalities, but no studies of their sensitivity, specificity, and predictive value have been published.

Infected pseudarthrosis can be diagnosed in the majority of patients by an elevated erythrocyte sedimentation rate (ESR) in combination with positive findings on scintigraphy. However, this can be difficult in patients with low-grade infection. Only one of seven such patients had a positive gallium scan, and two had a normal ESR. No patient had an elevated white blood cell count (30).

Pseudarthrosis of a lumbar segment can be the cause of re-occurring or persisting symptoms but can also be asymptomatic. Therefore differentiation is indicated in patients with re-occurring or persisting symptoms. Discography has been used by Johnson and MacNab (17) but has not been validated. Direct infiltration of the pseudarthrosis with bupivacaine HCl has also been used to assess whether or not the pseudarthrosis is painful. However, no studies indicating the diagnostic value of this method have been found. In conclusion, differentiation between symptomatic and asymptomatic pseudarthrosis is still very much a trial-and-error phase: not one diagnostic modality has been validated.

## CLINICAL FAILURE

Persistence or recurrence of symptoms after lumbar fusion characterizes clinical failure. The symptoms may be the result of a symptomatic pseudarthrosis. However, symptoms may persist in the presence of a solid bony ankylosis. Symptoms may be radicular or nonradicular. Radicular symptoms may be new and not present before the operation, or they were present before and persist or recur after the operation.

### Radicular Symptoms

Pain radiation with a segmental pattern in a leg indicates radicular pain. For example, radiation into the big toe indicates an L5 nerve root entrapment and in the lateral aspect of the foot an S1 entrapment. The diagnosis is certain when signs of nerve root entrapment, such as straight leg raising and the Lasegue test, are positive. The location of the entrapment must be demonstrated by imaging: magnetic resonance imaging (MRI) with gadolinium enhancement or CT with intrathecal contrast and three-dimensional reconstruction is the method of choice. However, in patients with pain radiating below the knee without a typical pain pattern and without signs of nerve root irritation, the diagnosis of nerve root entrapment is questionable. Even when imaging techniques demonstrate decreased space for the nerve root, the dorsal root ganglion, or the spinal nerve, this may be asymptomatic. To demonstrate a correlation between the radiological observations and the symptoms, nerve root sheath infiltration (1,2,6) is the method of choice, particularly in the presence of negative neurophysiologic findings. When symptomatic nerve root entrapment has been demonstrated as the cause of the symptoms, pinpoint decompression of only the entrapped nerve root by an interlaminar or lateral approach will yield a high success rate when the leg pain is predominant (1) and when other factors, as discussed below, are absent.

### *Deafferentation Pain*

Radicular pain may also be due to deafferentation. Deafferentation pain is defined as "discomfort arising in any part of the body when the flow of afferent nervous impulses has been partially or completely interrupted" (32). In the majority of patients this is caused by lesions of nerves, dorsal roots, spinal cord, brainstem, or cerebral cortex. Patients must demonstrate a loss of one or more modalities of somatosensory function with pain in the area of the sensory loss. Tasker (32) describes two groups: one group with only pain and another with pain and "hyperpathia." Hyperpathia is defined as unpleasant sensations induced by normally nonnociceptive stimulation in areas with sensory impairment. Summation of impulses appears to be a pathognomonic sign. This can be elicited by gentle tapping or continuous rubbing of the hyperpathic area. For guidelines on management of these patients, the reader is referred to the appropriate literature.

### Nonradicular Pain

Back pain radiating into the buttock and the posterolateral aspect of the thigh, and sometimes into the proximal aspect of the calf, is called referred or nonradicular pain. Signs of nerve root entrapment, such as a positive Lasegue test and straight leg raising test, must be negative. Symptoms may persist or recur in patients after a fusion in the presence or absence of a bony ankylosis.

### *Bony Ankylosis*

When symptoms persist despite a bony ankylosis, in theory the selection of the patient for lumbar fusion has been incorrect. One can assume that the observed pathology was not the cause of the symptoms. The pain pattern of these patients will not significantly be changed by the operation. The course of symptoms may have predictive value, although this has thus far not been studied.

Symptoms and signs may change after the operation. Symptoms may disappear completely and recur, or the pattern and other characteristics of pain may change during the postoperative period. In such cases, again, the selection was incorrect, but this time due to an incomplete diagnosis. In theory, it is possible that the observed pathology was indeed symptomatic but was not the only contributing factor. This diagnostic enigma can be solved by a multifactorial paradigm that considers not only the pathology of the lumbar spine but also other factors (3,33,34); the back pain is multifactorial.

### Multifactorial Chronic Back Pain

Chronic low back pain is often divided into two subgroups, "specific" and "aspecific." The term "specific" refers to the relation of symptoms to specific somatic pathology. However, somatic pathology such as stenosis, disc protrusion, and degenerative changes has been described in patients with symptoms as well as in patients without symptoms. Moreover, in patients with symptoms the amount of pain varies widely in the presence of identical pathology. A dichotomous model differentiating between pathology or lack thereof cannot explain this. It is, however, understandable in view of current pain theories: tissue damage results in nociceptive impulses, and when these impulses arrive in the brain they may evoke a pain experience. Arousal, anxiety, and attention sensitize this system, and the patient experiences an increase in pain. This implies that even in patients with clear-cut somatic pathology, psychological variables must be taken into account. Pain, both acute and chronic, is therefore multifactorial by definition.

For back pain, the following factors and processes have been recognized.

### *Physical Condition in Terms of $VO2_{max}$*

Over 20 years ago, Cady et al. (5) demonstrated in an occupational setting the correlation between $VO2_{max}$ and back pain. People with a poor aerobic capacity had more episodes of back pain and absenteeism of a longer duration compared to people with an average capacity. This implies that poor physical condition increases morbidity in patients with back pain, although it is probably not a causative factor.

### Trunk Muscle Performance

In theory, good muscle performance is needed to protect a joint from overload under physiological conditions. Overload ("sprain") may become manifest as joint pain with or without muscle spasm. It may be acute, e.g., a lifting incident, or may build up gradually. This is particularly the case in patients with poor trunk muscle performance. Their capacity to sustain physiologic loads is not sufficient and therefore they are continuously overloading their spine.

Indeed, trunk muscle endurance is a significant factor in back pain (26). Information on strength, coordination and endurance of abdominal and erector spinae muscles is essential in the management of patients with chronic back pain. Clinically, a sit-up test is used to obtain an impression of abdominal muscle function. However, this test is not validated, and a suitable test for back muscles is not available. To obtain reliable data one must use computer-assisted dynamometers (23).

Mayer and Gatchel (23) use the term "deconditioning syndrome" for patients with poor aerobic capacity and poor trunk muscle performance. Those patients display usually inadequate pain behavior. This pain behavior can be assessed by symptoms and signs according to Waddell et al. (35). The poor physical condition is the result of pain avoidance behavior, leading to a decrease in daily activities. Poor physical condition reinforces back pain, and patients may respond to it with increased inadequate pain behavior. They enter a circle that cannot be escaped without professional intervention. Meanwhile, patients experience loss of perspective, which may result in a depressed state. This is a stressor that may increase back pain.

### The Process of Somatization

Somatization is defined (19) as a condition indicated by one or more physical complaints such as fatigue, gastrointestinal or urinary complaints, headache, and neck or back pain. Appropriate evaluation uncovers no organic pathology or pathophysiologic mechanism or, in the case of related organic pathology, physical complaints or resulting social or occupational impairment are grossly in excess of what would be expected from the physical findings. In this process, psychophysiologic reactions under conditions of emotional and mental load appear to play a major role.

In patients with neck and/or back pain, the pain is hypothetically related to abnormal muscle activity in back and/or neck, particularly during disturbed sleep, as an unconscious reaction to mental and emotional load leading to exhaustion of muscle and subsequently to a decrease in condition while muscle tenderness increases. Indications for this mechanism are the observation of increased muscle activity as measured by EMG during experimental stress. Further more, EMG levels are higher in anxious patients compared to controls (14,21). Particularly in patients with occipital and neck pain, EMG activity is higher in neck muscles during experimental stress compared to other people (20). In addition, when patients have pain, some of them react with reflex muscle contraction. Patients suffering from headache and neck pain show higher EMG activity than controls when pain is experimentally inflicted on the forearm (22). Some patients with low back pain have higher paravertabral muscle activity measured on EMG (9), particularly when they are under emotional stress (12,21).

### Operant Conditioning

Pain experience may be the consequence of nociception, i.e., tissue damage. Pain has cognitive and emotional aspects and may result in pain behavior, which is defined as the interaction between the patient and the environment. It is a way of communication. Fordyce (13) proposed the application of theories of behavior to patients with pain. In other words, pain, particularly chronic pain, is studied as a form of behavior. It can be assessed and modified by application of the principles of "learning." Three modes of learning have been described: respondent conditioning as described by Pavlov, which appears to be an important mechanism in the process of somatization, and operant conditioning as described by Skinner, who indicated three types of reinforcing factors:

1. A positive reinforcer: after the experienced pain a positive experience occurs systematically, e.g., empathy and care by a relative.
2. A negative reinforcer: e.g., conflicts at work due to problems with the supervisor. The patient tries to avoid this negative impulse ("pain avoidance behavior").
3. Healthy behavior is no longer reinforced: e.g., the patient stays in bed because he or she does not feel well enough to get up.

The third mode of learning is modeling: children imitate the behavior of their parents. For example, if a father used to stay home in the presence of work pressure, children tend to display similar behavior when they are adults.

Chronic back pain can be considered as caused by operant processes and is not merely acute pain that lasts longer. This is why most patients think that "the real cause has not been found" and "maybe another investigation is needed."

Applying a multifactorial concept to a patient with persisting "nonspecific" symptoms after fusion means, in daily practice, ergometry to define $VO2_{max}$, assessment of trunk muscle performance, preferably with computerized dynamometry, and psychological assessment to answer the question of whether or not somatization and operant conditioning play a role and, if so, which factors are involved in these processes.

These factors and processes are not rare in patients with failed back surgery syndrome! In about two-thirds of patients referred to me, these factors were found on multifactorial assessment. Subsequent cognitive behavioral training was successful in 78% of these patients. This is compatible with the results of a meta-analysis by Flor et al. (11), who found better results of a multifactorial management program compared to "no treatment," "unifactorial treatment," and "conventional physiotherapy." These positive effects were consistent over time. The rate of return to work was found to be twice as large, and similar figures were found for medical handling after treatment. A drawback to these cognitive behavioral programs is their costs. They are also very time-consuming and require a team of professionals working closely together. Therefore, one has to look for prevention of the chronic state. I strongly suggest use of this multifactorial concept in patients with radiologically observed pathology that correlates only weakly with symptoms such as degenerative changes, lytic spondylolisthesis, L5–S1 grade 1, and enchondrotic changes without deformity.

## MANAGEMENT OF FAILED FUSION PATIENTS

### Diagnosis

A team approach is mandatory: not only must a spinal surgeon assess the patient but other disciplines must also be involved.

1. $VO2_{max}$ by ergometry (kinesiologist or physiotherapist).
2. Trunk muscle performance by computerized dynamometry (kinesiologist or physiotherapist).
3. Pain behavior assessment according to the symptoms and signs of Waddell et al. (35) and the pain drawing of Ransford et al. (29) (spinal specialist or surgeon).
4. Symptomatic pathology (spinal specialist or surgeon) (see below).
5. Operant conditioning: Which positive and negative reinforcing factors are significant (psychologist by structured interview and MMPI 2 or other psychometric assessment).
6. Somatization: If present, which stressors are provoking the somatization reaction (psychologist by structured interview and MMPI 2 or other psychometric assessment).
7. Cognition: Information about the belief system of the patient in relation to the symptoms. Does the patient believe that he has a serious disease which cannot be cured?

### Symptomatic Pathology

When pathology has been observed, the question arises of whether the pathology is symptomatic or asymptomatic. As a coincidental finding it may have no relation to the symptoms.

In the case of pain radiating into a leg, differentiation must be made between radicular and referred pain. Radicular pain is indicated by a segmental pain pattern, signs of nerve root entrapment (e.g., positive straight leg raising and Lasegue test, signs of neurological deficit, imaging (CT or MRI), and nerve root sheath infiltration (6) in the case of an atypical clinical presentation or multilevel pathology at imaging.

A radicular syndrome may be caused by nerve root entrapment or by deafferentation pain. Deafferentation pain is characterized by pain in a typical segmental pattern, dysesthesia in a hypo- or anaesthetic skin area, and summation of impulses in those areas as demonstrated by an increased pain experience evoked by gentle rubbing or tapping of the skin. The sensory deficit can be also demonstrated by neurophysiologic assessment, including sensory evoked potentials. Referred pain (nonradicular) may relate to symptomatic pathology such as pseudarthrosis or degenerative changes at an adjacent level.

In symptomatic pseudarthrosis, the continuity of the fusion bone mass must be demonstrated by CT or MRI, segmental motion by extension/flexion films, and an increase in biologic activity, indicating a pseudarthrosis, by scintigraphy. Infiltration of the pseudarthrosis with bupivacaine HCl must have a positive result, whereas injecting bupivacaine into a facet joint at a different level should not decrease symptoms.

For a symptomatic segment at an adjacent level, assessment of symptomatology by provocative discography after degenerative changes should be demonstrated by

MRI. The validity of discography has not been well confirmed. The clinician must be aware of the possibility of deconditioning syndrome, and multifactorial assessment (see above) is definitely indicated. For symptomatic disc degeneration at the level of a posterolateral fusion (36), the only mode of assessment is provocative discography.

## Treatment

Patients with a radicular syndrome due to nerve root entrapment required surgical treatment when conservative management fails. Other factors and processes as described above should be addressed by physical training only or in combination with cognitive behavioral modification. Deafferentation pain is difficult to treat. Repeated nerve root infiltration in combination with cognitive behavioral training has been employed. Symptomatic pseudarthrosis without nerve root involvement is an indication for revision surgery to obtain a solid bony ankylosis. When other factors and processes are also present, these should be addressed by cognitive behavioral modification and functional restoration (13,23).

## CONCLUSION

Prevention of failed fusion starts with proper selection of patients. In view of our present scientific knowledge, a multifactorial model of pain must be used. When operant conditioning resulting in poor physical performance and somatization has been ruled out and symptomatic pathology, preferable only at one segment, has been demonstrated, fusion will cure the majority of patients. However, attempted fusion in patients who demonstrate poor physical performance in the presence of psychological processes such as operant conditioning and somatization has a low success rate, even in the case of symptomatic pathology. Therefore, an important consideration *in dubio abstinens*. Do not operate when in doubt!

## REFERENCES


1. Akkerveeken PF van. *Lateral stenosis of the lumbar spine*. Thesis, Rijksuniversiteit Utrecht, The Netherlands, 1989.
2. Akkerveeken PF van. Diagnostic injections: an overview of discography, facet arthrography and nerve root infiltration. In: Frymoyer JW, ed. *The adult spine, principles and practice*. 2nd ed. Philadelphia: Lippincott Raven, 1996 [*in press*].
3. Allan DB, Waddell G. An historical perspective on low back pain and disability. *Acta Orthop Scand* 1989;234(suppl).
4. Brodsky AE, Kovalsky ES, Khalil MA. Correlation of radiologic assessment of lumbar spine fusions with surgical exploration. *Spine* 1991;16:S261–5.
5. Cady LD, Bischoff DP, O'Connel ER. Strength and fitness and subsequent back injuries in firefighters. *Occup Med* 1979;4:269–72.
6. Castro WHM, Akkerveeken PF van. Der diagnostische Wert der selektiven lumbalen Nervenwurzelblockade. *Z Orthop* 1991;129:374–9.
7. Dawson EG, Clader TJ, Bassett LW. A comparison of different methods used to diagnose pseudarthrosis following posterior spinal fusion for scoliosis. *J Bone Joint Surg* 1985;67A:1153–9.
8. De Palma AF, Rothman RH. The nature of pseudarthrosis. *Clin Orthop Relat Res* 1968;59:113–8.
9. Dolce JJ, Raczynski JM. Neuromuscular activity and electromyography in painful backs: psychological and biomechanical models in assessment and treatment. *Psychol Bull* 1985;97:502–20.
10. Flatley TJ, Derderian H. Closed loop instrumentation of the lumbar spine. *Clin Orthop Relat Res* 1985;196:273–8.
11. Flor HC, Fydrich TH, Turk DC. Efficacy of multidisciplinary pain treatment centers: a meta-analytic review. *Pain* 1992;49:221–30.

12. Flor HC, Turk DC, Birbaumer N. Assessment of stress-related psychophysiological reactions in chronic back pain patients. *J Consult Clin Psychol* 1985;53:3654–64.
13. Fordyce WE. *Behavioral methods for chronic pain and illness.* St. Louis: CV Mosby, 1976.
14. Goldstein EB. Physiological responses in anxious women patients: a study of autonomic activity and muscle tension. *Arch Gen Psychiatry* 1964;10:382–8.
15. Guyer RD, Ohnmeiss DD. Lumbar discography. Contemporary concepts in spine care. *Spine* 1995; 20:2048–59.
16. Heggeness MH, Esses SI. Classification of pseudarthrosis of the lumbar spine. *Spine* 1991;16: S449–54.
17. Johnson RG, MacNab I. Localization of symptomatic lumbar pseudarthrosis by use of discography. *Clin Orthop Relat Res* 1985;197:164–70.
18. Kant AP, Daum WJ, Dean SM, Uchida T. Evaluation of lumbar spine fusion. *Spine* 1995;20:2313–7.
19. Kellner R. Psychosomatic syndromes, somatization and somatoform disorders. *Psychother Psychosom* 1994;61:4–24.
20. Malmo RB, Schagass C. Physiologic study of symptom mechanism in psychiatric patients under stress. *Psychosom Med* 1949;11:25–9.
21. Malmo RB, Shagass C, Davis JF. A method for the investigation of somatic response mechanisms in psychoneurosis. *Science* 1950;112:325–8.
22. Malmo RB, Wallerstein H, Schagass C. Headache proneness and mechanisms of motor conflict in psychiatric patients. *J Pers* 1953;22:163–87.
23. Mayer TG, Gatchel RJ. *Functional restoration for spinal disorders.* Philadelphia: Lea & Febiger, 1988.
24. Morris J, Chafetz N, Baumrind S, Genant H, Korn EL. Stereophotogrammetry of the lumbar spine: a technique for the detection of pseudarthrosis. *Spine* 1985;10:368–75.
25. Olsson TH, Selvik G, Willner S. Mobility in the lumbosacral spine after fusion studied with the aid of röntgen stereo-photogrammetry. *Clin Orthop Relat Res* 1977;129:181–90.
26. Parnianpour M, Nordin M, Kahanovitz N, Frankel V. The tri axial coupling of torque generation and trunk muscles during isometric exertions and the effects of fatiguing iso inertial movements on the motor output and movement patterns. *Spine* 1988;13:982–92.
27. Pearcy M, Burrough S. Assessment of bony union after interbody fusion of the lumbar spine using a biplanar radiographic technique. *J Bone Joint Surg* 1982;64B:228–32.
28. Ralston EL, Thompson WAL. The diagnosis and repair of pseudarthrosis of the spine. *Surg Gynecol Obstet* 1947;89:37–42.
29. Ransford AO, Cairns D, Mooney V. The pain drawing as an aid to the psychologic evaluation of patients with low back pain. *Spine* 1976;1:127–34.
30. Schofferman L, Zucherman J, Schofferman J, et al. Diphtheroids and associated infections as a cause of failed instrument stabilization procedures in the lumbar spine. *Spine* 1991;16:356–8.
31. Slizofski WJ, Collier BD, Flatley TJ, Carrera GF, Hellman RS, Isitman AT. Painful pseudarthrosis following lumbar spinal fusion: detection by combined SPECT and planar bone scintigraphy. *Skel Radiol* 1987;16:136–41.
32. Tasker RR. Deafferentation. In: Wall PD, Melzack R, eds. *Textbook of pain.* Edinburgh: Churchill Livingstone, 1984:119–32.
33. Waddell G. A new clinical model for the treatment of low back pain. *Spine* 1987;12:632–44.
34. Waddell G. In: Weinstein JN, Wiesel SW, eds. *The lumbar spine.* Philadelphia: WB Saunders, 1990:43–8.
35. Waddell G, McCulloch JA, Kummel E, Venner RM. Non organic signs in low back pain. *Spine* 1980;5:117–25.
36. Weatherley CR, Prickett CF, O'Brien JP. Discogenic pain persisting despite solid posterior fusion. *J Bone Joint Surg* 1986;68B:142–3.
37. Weber BG, Cech O. *Pseudarthrosis. Pathophysiology, biomechanics, therapy, results.* Bern: Huber, 1976.

*Instrumented Fusion of the Degenerative
Lumbar Spine: State of the Art, Questions,
and Controversies,* edited by M. Szpalski,
R. Gunzburg, D. M. Spengler, and
A. Nachemson. Lippincott–Raven
Publishers, Philadelphia © 1996.

# 8

# Biomechanics and Clinical Results of the SOCON Spinal System

R. H. Wittenberg, R. Steffen, R. E. Willburger, and *L. P. Nolte

*Department of Orthopaedic Surgery, St. Josef Hospital, Ruhr University,
44791 Bochum, Germany; and *Maurice Mueller Institute of Biomechanics,
3010 Bern, Switzerland*

Development of spinal fixation devices has focused on intrapedicular systems with a constrained screw–rod connection. Various systems have been introduced during the recent years, but the biomechanical principle is basically the same. The major difference is the versatility that these devices allow for short- or multisegmental fusion. Even though there is an advantage of an universal system, most fusions are performed as single- or double-level fixation.

There are a number of indications for short segmental lumbar fusion in orthopedic surgery, and the number of fusions is increasing rapidly. Lehmann et al. (21) reported that the incidence of lower lumbar fusions for degenerative diseases in the United States doubled between 1979 and 1983. In spinal trauma surgery, various authors (5,6,14) have described an advantage of the operative treatment of compression and burst fractures over nonoperative treatment. The considerations as to whether an internal fixation device is necessary differ, depending on the severity of the trauma. The operative treatment of thoracolumbar fractures requires internal stabilization to maintain the reposition and reduce the load on the anterior and middle column of the spine until the fracture has healed, irrespective of the necessity of simultaneous anterior or posterolateral fusion (14). Lower lumbar or lumbosacral fusions in degenerative spine diseases are usually performed as an in situ fusion except in cases of spondylolisthesis, for which some authors recommend repositioning. Without repositioning, noninstrumented fusion can also be considered as a possible and easy technique.

The advantage of instrumented over noninstrumented fusion is the significantly reduced rate of pseudarthrosis. The main problem of lumbar fusion was the considerably high rate of pseudarthrosis, between 18 and 49% (18) depending on the number of fused segments and the kind of fusions (posterolateral or interbody). Various authors have shown that the rate of pseudarthrosis can be reduced by use of an internal fixation device (18). This might be explained by the high amount of stability provided by an internal fixation compared to the effect of external bracing.

Animal studies have shown that the stability of bony fusion can be improved by the use of an implant (16,23). A reduced initial strain rate has also been shown in an animal model to correlate with a successful fusion (24). Therefore, the main reason for the use of an internal fixation device in orthopedic cases is the internal stability provided. In addition, the implant allows compression of the anterior bone graft in combined anterior and posterior fusions (19). These requirements are met by the so-called fixateur interne first described by Dick (6). The clinical success of this system led to the development of a number of devices along the same constructive principle, differing only in pedicle screw design, type of distraction rod, and the connection mechanism of the two, as well as in handling factors.

## IMPLANT REQUIREMENTS

For selection of an implant, certain factors must be considered. Initially, the main indications and the fusion levels should be defined. The implants that meet these requirements should then be compared concerning their biomechanical characteristics. Because of the larger experience and the learning curve from the early period, most implants are biomechanically more or less the same in strength and flexibility. They might vary, however, in their fatigue life. The next thing, and most important for the surgeon, is the simplicity and effectivity with respect to intraoperative handling and instruments available for corrective procedures. Finally, the costs and service provided by the manufacturer must be considered. The two systems most commonly used at present are implants with a constrained screw–rod connection that allow short single and double (fixateur interne) or multisegmental fixation (universal spine systems).

Even though pedicle screw fixation can be performed in the thoracic and lumbar spine as well as on the sacrum, most of these procedures are carried out on the lumbar spine. The majority of fusions are performed as single- or double-level fixation. The indications are trauma, tumors, or degenerative spine diseases such as spondylolisthesis or failed back surgery. The main indications for long segmental fusions are scoliosis and tumors. Multisegmental fusions in degenerative lumbar spine diseases have shown a considerable high complication rate and disappointing clinical results (30). Because about 90% of all thoracic and lumbar fusions are performed as single- or double-level fixations, these indications should determine the implant selection. The internal spine fixateur, a device that is specifically designed for short segmental fusion, therefore appears to be the first choice if an implant is selected for the spine, even though there is now a trend in the development of spinal fixation devices toward more universal instrumentation systems. These have the theoretical advantage of the greatest span of indication, but the option for long fusion result in more complicated handling because of the increased number of instruments and implants. Therefore, one is working most of the time with a suboptimal device. We therefore prefer a system that is designed for short segmental fusion, with the option to treat several levels but without the possibility to correct scoliotic deformities.

## BIOMECHANICS

In a biomechanical study, the SOCON spinal system (Aesculap AG, Germany) was compared to two other fixateur interne system (AO-Synthes, Kluger-Endotec,

Germany). All the systems are described as constrained and thereby fulfill the demands of Wörsdörfer (35) for the treatment of thoracolumbar fractures. Each system consisted of pedicle screws and adjusted distraction rods that could be fastened to one another at different angulations. Eighteen fresh human cadaveric spines from the L3–L5 level were harvested from donors with a mean age of 43 years. After the standardized preparation, determination of the bone mineral density, and biomechanical testing of the intact specimens, they were tested in three comparable groups. On each specimen in a group, one of the fixateur interne systems was attached. The following conservative loads were applied incrementally in combination with a small stabilizing preload of 40 N: (a) axial compression ($-Fy = 0$–1,000N); (b) flexion–extension ($\pm Mx = 0$–7.5 Nm); (c) lateral bending ($\pm Mz = 0$–7.5 Nm); and (d) axial torsion ($\pm My = 0$–10 Nm). Special care was taken to minimize viscoelastic effects during the experiment. The following clinically relevant parameters have been studied: (a) range of motion (ROM); (b) neutral zone (NZ), both according to the definition by Panjabi et al. (27); (c) strain energy; and (d) the center of rotation. The specimens were investigated in the following steps: intact, intact with one of the internal fixateurs applied, and after corpectomy with the SOCON.

### Results

The typical load displacement curves of a single specimen are shown in Fig. 1. The loads are marked on the horizontal axis and the resulting dominant deformations are marked on the vertical axis. The shape of the path clearly demonstrates the stabilizing effect of the SOCON spinal system. In all three dimensions of movement, the intact specimens demonstrated a nonlinear-shaped path with decreasing deformation under increasing load. In contrast to this, after application of the spinal fixation device the path became linear, i.e., the deformation showed a constant correlation to the applied load. Under smaller loads the intersegmental stiffness of the specimens with applied devices was 15 to 50 times higher than that of the noninstrumented specimens. Under maximal loading there was no great divergence in the degree of stiffness. Assuming a nonlinear behavior of the enclosed intervertebral discs and the ligamentous structures, the results suggested that the deformation after instrumentation was due to a certain deformation in the interface between pedicle screw and bone, on the one hand, and in the implant itself.

Of clinical interest is the deformation energy, i.e., the energy that is necessary to produce an equal deformation with and without instrumentation. The increase of the deformation energy after application of an internal fixateur was at most 13 times higher in flexion–extension and lateral bending and three times higher under axial torsion (Fig. 2).

After application of the various internal fixateurs, a similar reduction of flexibility, expressed as SUMROM for the different dimensions of movement, was recorded (Fig. 3). The results demonstrated for the investigated fixation devices almost the same decrease of SUMROM flexion–extension and lateral bending from 20° to 4°. The effectiveness of instrumentation was considerably lower under axial torsion, with a decrease from 10° to 5°.

Further investigation of the clinical effectiveness of the internal fixation devices in the treatment of thoracolumbar fractures was carried out with the SOCON spinal

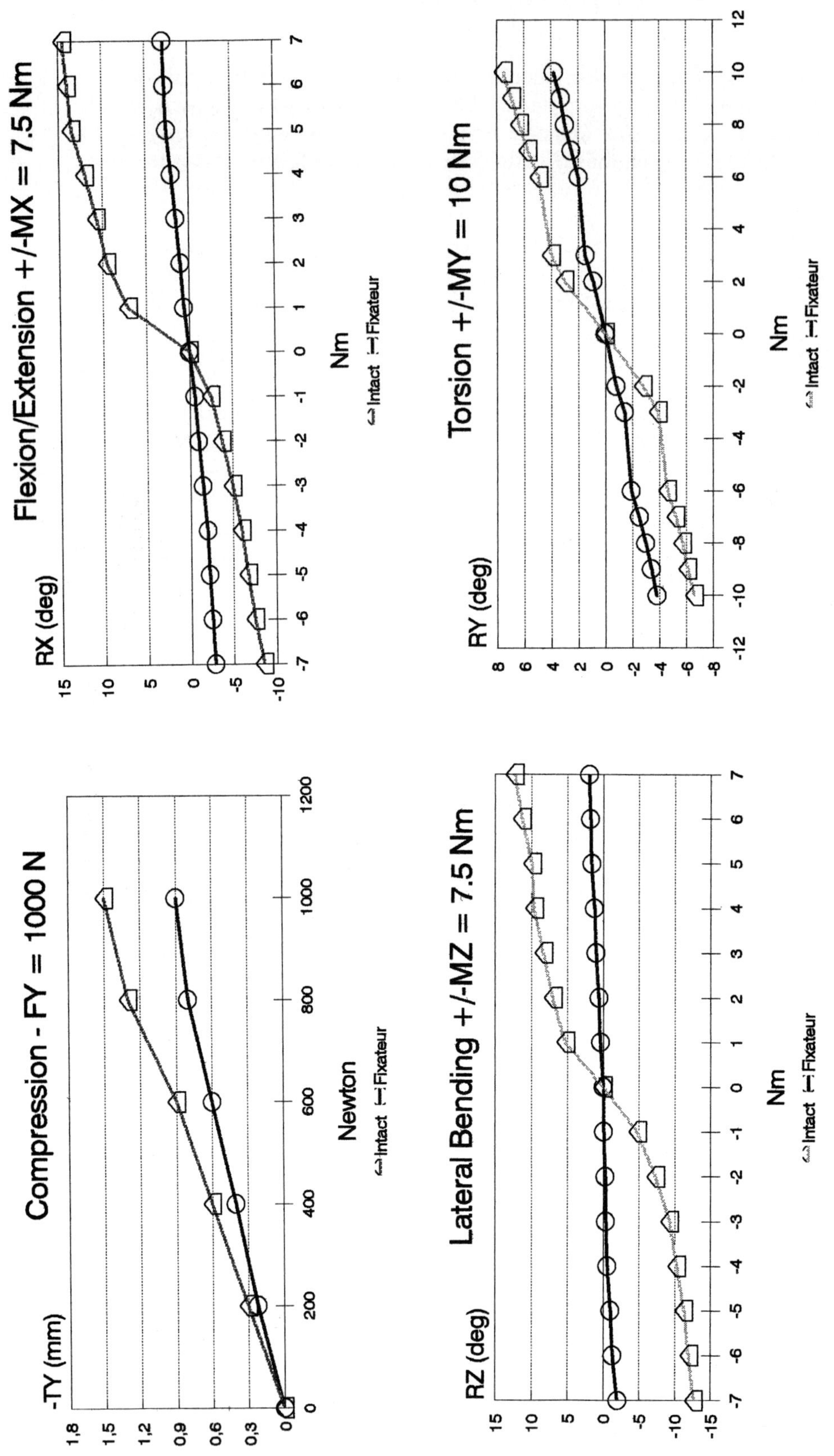


**FIG. 1.** Load displacement curves of a single specimen L3–L5 with and without instrumentation (SOCON). Applied loads: FY, force on y-axis; MX, moment on x-axis; MY, moment on y-axis; MZ, moment on z-axis. Resulting deformation: TY, axial compression; RX, flexion/extension; RZ, lateral bending; RY, axial rotation.

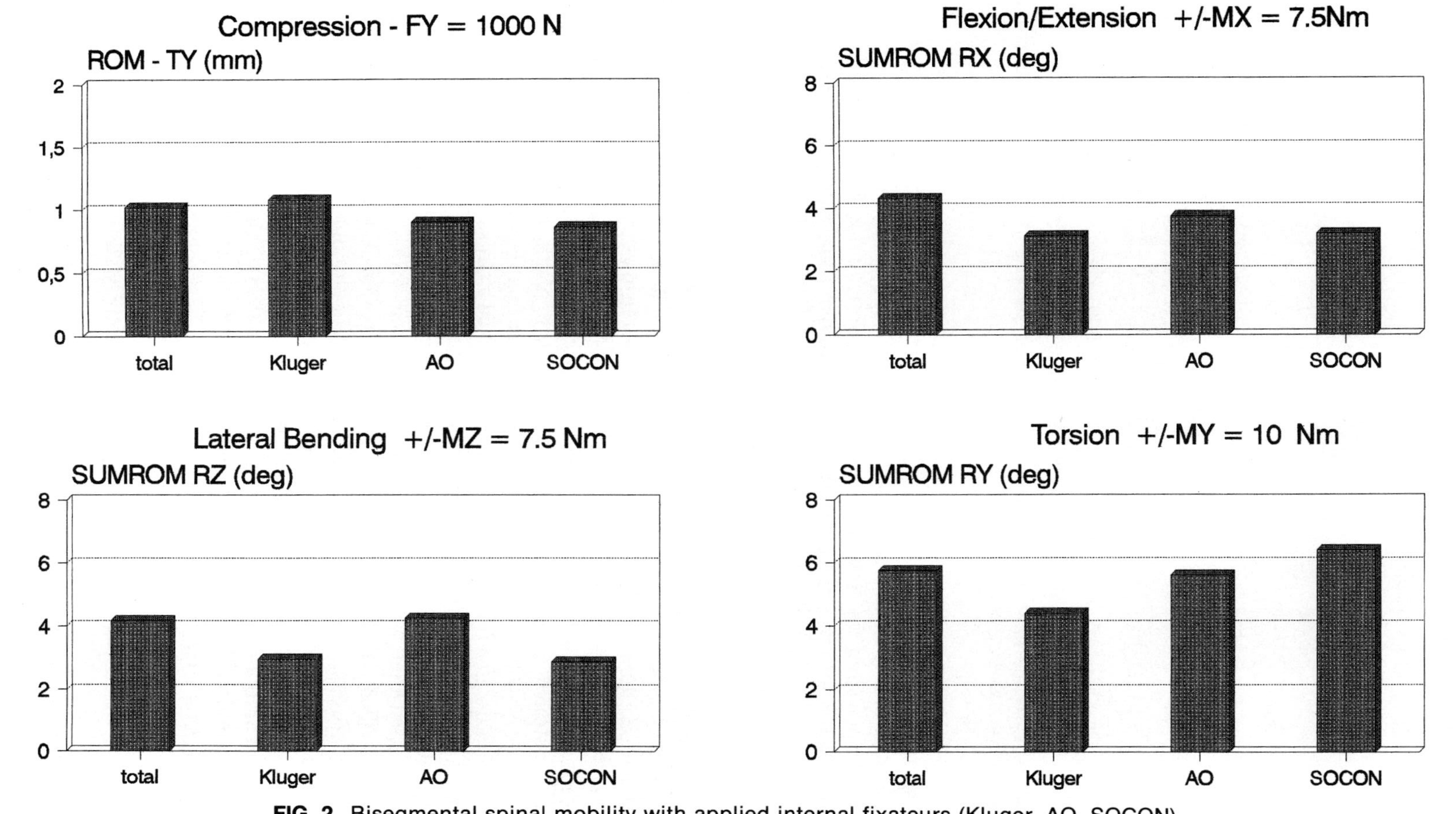


**FIG. 2.** Bisegmental spinal mobility with applied internal fixateurs (Kluger, AO, SOCON).

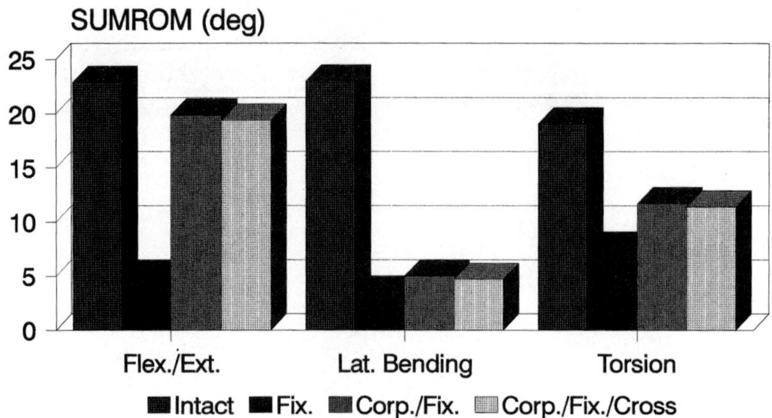


**FIG. 3.** Bisegmental spinal mobility with applied SOCON (*n* = 3) after corpectomy (L4) and influence of crossloading.

system on a corpectomy model. The corpectomy simulated a severe instability in the anterior and middle columns of the spine. This severe instability was sufficiently compensated by instrumentation, and the resulting flexibility expressed in SUMROM did not exceed the values of the intact, noninstrumented segments.

## Discussion

Biomechanical investigation of the three different devices showed that all of the systems provided almost the same degree of stabilization, with a distinct weakness under axial torsion. The corpectomy model confirms the stabilizing capacity of the investigated SOCON spinal system in the treatment of highly unstable thoracolumbar fractures. However, the results of testing procedures under cyclic loads (34) have demonstrated a certain failure rate of spinal implants by screw or rod breakage between 60,000 and 90,000 load cycles. Another failure mode is described by Goel et al. (11) who, in a finite element model, established a stress shielding along the pedicle screw in the vertebral body and deduced a risk for screw loosening. These investigations suggest an implant failure after a certain period of time and lead to the conclusion that we have to protect the internal fixation device in patients from uncontrolled strain and movement during the period of fracture healing or consolidation of spinal fusion. On particular consideration of our findings, it becomes clear that extensive loads for compression and axial torsion conceal the highest risk for implant failure. For further clinical use of an internal fixateur for posterior fixation without anterior stabilization, we still recognize the necessity to apply a brace for the first 4 months after surgery if the patient is unreliable and does not fully comply with the surgeon's recommendations.

## CLINICAL EXPERIENCE

Clinically, the success of a device should be determined by the bony fusion, intraoperative handling, implant failure rate, and functional outcome. Of an early series of SOCON instrumentations, 100 patients have thus far been followed up by clinical investigation and x-ray evaluation. These patients underwent fusion for the following diagnoses: spondylolisthesis, lumbar instability, and failed back syndrome. The largest group consisted of 61 patients with failed back syndrome. This is also, according to Frymoyer et al. (9) as well as Caldwell and Sheppard (3), unfortunately the main indication for lumbar fusion.

## Materials and Methods

A total of 61 patients who had undergone previous back surgery were treated by lumbar and lumbosacral fusion for intractable back and/or leg pain. Before surgery, all patients underwent conservative treatment for a minimum of 3 or more months, including a 2-week stay in our institution. This treatment included a number of nerve root blocks, epidural injections, and radiculography for diagnostic purposes and with a steroid as a treatment modality. All patients received a full diagnostic work-up, including MRI studies with gadolineum, as well as a neurologic investigation with EMG and motor evoked potentials. After the inpatient period, they had to continue the rehabilitation program for another 6 weeks on an outpatient basis. After failure of the conservative treatment only those patients were scheduled for surgery who responded to bracing and to facet or nerve root blocks. Patients whose psychological impairment was obvious were excluded from surgery.

Surgery was performed on the delordoting Wilson frame (Zimmer) in a prone position. The patient and the image intensifier were draped steril and then posterior lumbar fusion was performed with ($n = 26$) or without ($n = 35$) decompression of the

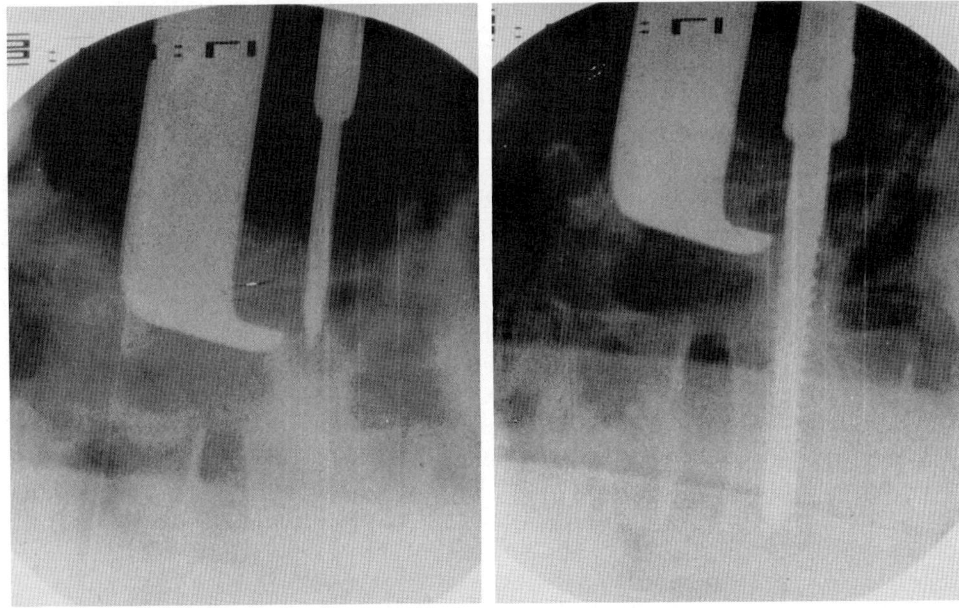

**A**  **B**

**FIG. 4.** Intraoperative image intensifier picture of the pedicle screw insertion. First the pedicle is penetrated by a graduated Steinmann Pin **(A)** and then the screw is inserted along this path **(B)**.

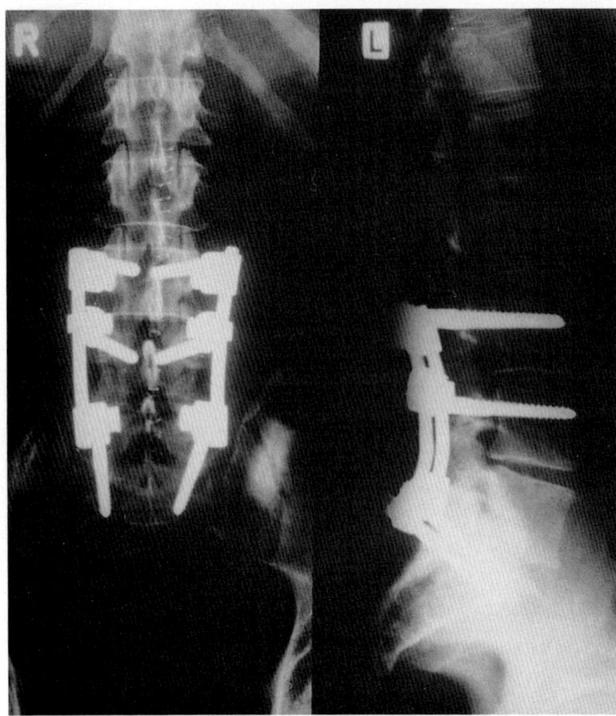

**FIG. 5.** Three-level SOCON fixateur interne fusion with pedicle screws in S1, L4, and L3.

involved nerve root. To avoid postoperative spinal instability due to the laminectomy (16) and graded facetectomy (1), a fusion was always added to the decompression. The fusion was supported by an internal fixation system (SOCON) and was always performed with autologous bone grafts from the posterior iliac crest. After preparation from a midline approach, the facet joints and transverse processes were exposed. The bone bed for the fusion was prepared by decortication of the transverse processes L4 and L5, the base of the sacrum, and the facet joints L4–L5 and L5–S1. Pedicle screws were introduced from the lateral approach described by Magerl (22). Under fluoroscopic control, all four in patients with a two-level fusion or six pedicle screws in patients with three-level fusion were inserted (Fig. 4). All screws were advanced to the anterior cortex, and in patients with decreased bone density slightly through the anterior cortex. Thereafter, the clamp, together with the longitudinal rod, was attached to the pedicle screws and tightened. Finally, bone grafts were carefully placed in the decorticated areas (Fig. 5).

All patients were mobilized the day after surgery in the preoperatively applied brace. A mobilization program was performed that allowed only limited spine motion and activities for 4 months. Regular x-ray controls were performed after 8 and 16 weeks and the brace treatment was terminated with respect to the assumed consolidation of the bone fusion mass (Fig. 6). After 4 months a second rehabilitation program focused on muscle strengthening and daily living activities. If patients had difficulties in completing this on an outpatient basis, they were referred to rehabilitation centers for a period of 4–6 weeks to get back to full activity. This should take place around the sixth month. Follow-up investigations were carried out routinely after 2, 4, and 6 months and after 1 year. Implant removal was recommended after 1 year. After 2 years the final clinical results were evaluated by an independent

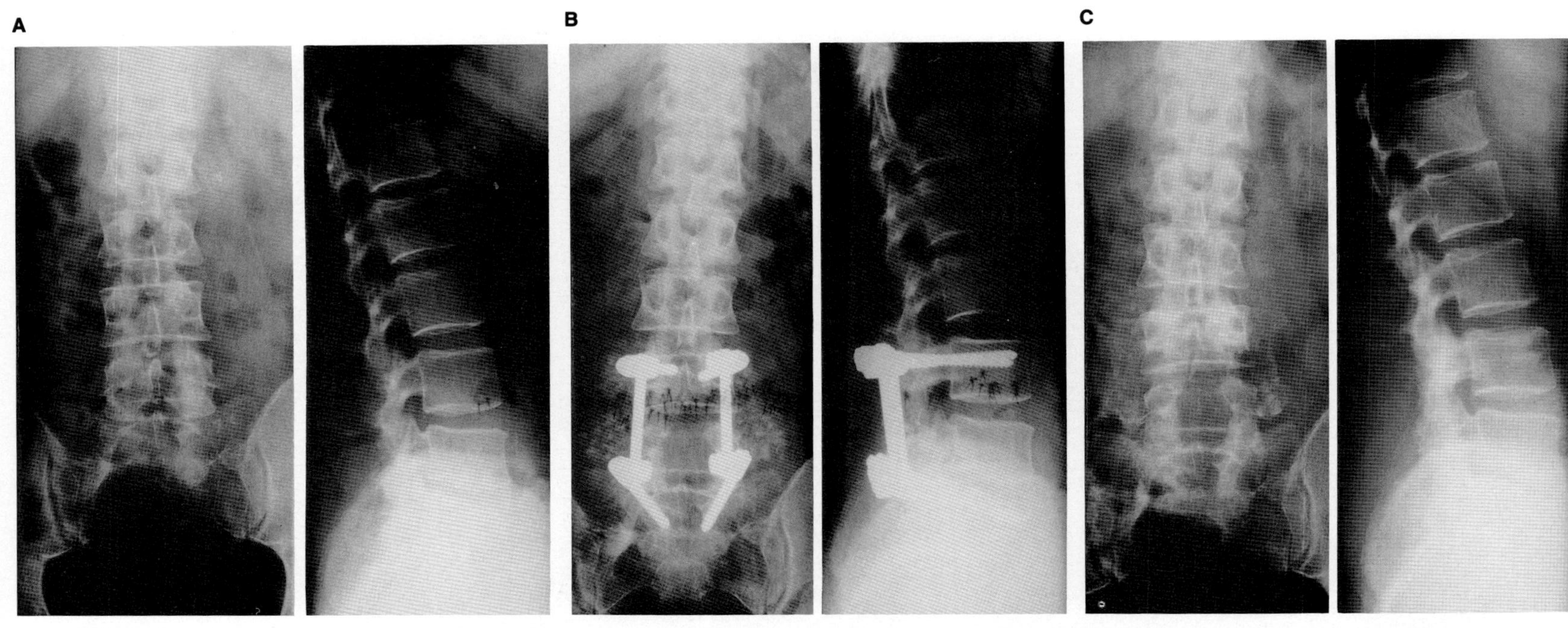

**FIG. 6.** Roentgenograms before **(A)** and after **(B)** surgery as well as after 1 year and after implant removal **(C)** (36-year-old patient with L4–S1 fixation). Solid fusion with no loss of disc height.

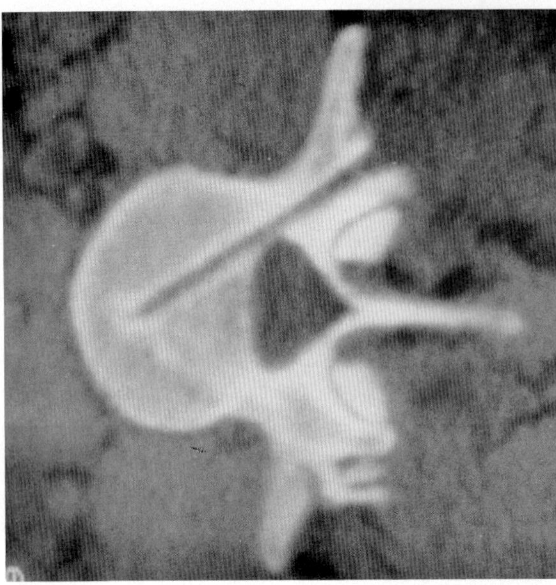

**FIG. 7.** CT after implant removal shows the screw path in the pedicle and the screw tip.

observer. Routine preoperative anterior-posterior and lateral films were used in addition to the intraoperative evaluation during implant removal to assess the fusion mass after implant removal. After implant removal the screw path and position were controlled on CT images (Fig. 7). Objective quantification of the disability was achieved by the Oswestry Low Back Pain Disability Questionnaire (7). In addition, pain was scored on an analogue scale from 0 to 10.

## Results

In 100 patients, three cases of hardware failure occurred, accompanied by a pseudoarthrosis. These were seen in patients with spondylolisthesis reduction without anterior fusion (Fig. 8). The implant failed with a breakage of the pedicle screw in the entrance area of the pedicle. Two additional cases of pseudoarthrosis were associated with severe pedicle screw loosening and three with no obvious radiologic finding. The fusion rate, as evaluated by plain x-rays and by surgical exploration of the fusion mass at the time of implant removal, was 92%.

The 2-year clinical outcome of 61 patients with a failed back syndrome is reported. On the basis of self-rating, 74% of the patients described significant pain reduction and 20% slight improvement, whereas in 6% the degree of pain increased. Disability, as assessed by the Oswestry Low Back Pain Disability Questionnaire, improved significantly in 66% and worsened in 25%. There was a slight tendency of the group without decompression compared to the patients who underwent decompression and fusion towards a better disability improvement. The walking capacity was restricted to less than 1 km in 72% preoperatively and improved in 53%. In particular, the decompression led to an improvement of a preexisting paresis (maximal grade 3) in 64%, whereas a worsening was seen in 15%. The use of pain medication could also be reduced in 54% of the patients. Surprisingly, 72% of the patients were retired at

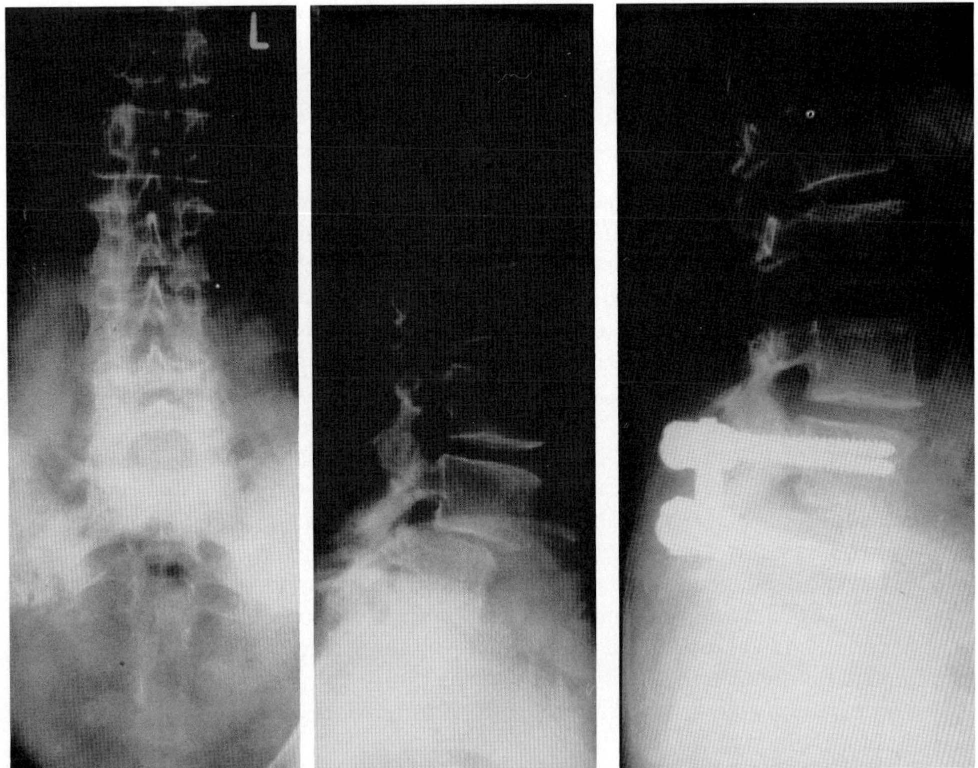


**FIG. 8.** Monosegmental SOCON fixation. Spondylolisthesis L5–S1 **(A)** with complete correction of the listhetic slip and anterior fusion **(B)**.

the time of follow-up. Only 28% returned to work. This disappointing figure appeared to be influenced mainly by the length of working disability preoperatively (average period 19 months) and the residual pretension of sick pay.

There was a considerably low postoperative complication rate of 12%, including one pulmonary embolism, one deep vein thrombosis, and the three implant failures mentioned above. In addition, we found 18 uncomplicated hematomas, mainly at the bone grafting site. One infection healed after operative revision without implant removal. There was no death or nerve root irritation due to the pedicle screw placement.

A prospective clinical investigation by Brunon and co-authors (2) was performed to compare the titanium and stainless steel version of the SOCON spinal system (19 fractures, two tumors, two spondylolistheses, one instability). This study showed an extraordinarily high number of nonimplant-related complications, with three cases of infection and two cases requiring extension of the fusion. However, there was no loss of correction, no implant failure, and no difference between the titanium and steel SOCON for the fixation. The titanium patients, however, could be investigated by MRI postoperatively.

In a separate study we investigated the pedicle screw placements in SOCON fixations (12). A total of 144 screws were positioned in 36 patients. Nine screws perforated the pedicle laterally and six screws medially (10.6%). There was no perforation greater than 3–4 mm. In none of these patients was a nerve root irritation observed.

### Discussion

The use of pedicle screws was introduced to achieve a higher fusion rate. In addition, Whitecloud and co-authors (33), among other authors, described a considerably high rate of implant-related complications for a spinal plating system (VSP), such as screw breakage (17.5%), increased blood loss, and increased operative time, with a consequently increased infection rate (7.5%). In addition, they described an impingement of the plate on the inferior facet of the vertebral body above the system, due to the size of the plate, and skin irritation in the sacral region in thin patients due to the bulkiness of the system. Unlike Whitecloud and co-authors (33), our second clinical series with the SOCON system in 100 patients showed a considerably low rate of implant-related complications. Because of the design of the internal fixateur and the chosen lateral approach to the pedicle, there was no irritation of the facet joints above or below the applied system. The initially higher rate of implant failure (7.5%) could be reduced to 3% by a further strengthening of the screw in the entrance area to the pedicle when the minor screw diameter was changed to a conical form. The patients' clinical results did not correlate with their radiologic outcome and were fundamentally determined by the patient selection.

In some patients the complaints were not absolutely clear before surgery, and after fusion their main problem or a new one became obvious. Weatherly and co-authors (31) described discogenic pain as a reason for failure of a posterior or posterolateral fusion. Discogenic pain is strongly correlated to a so-called inflammation of the disc space (15). Disc degeneration comparable to osteoarthritis can lead to an increased release of neurochemical transmitters, such as substance P or vasoactive intestinal peptide (32), and can produce pain by irritating the free nerve ending in the outer annulus (22). According to Simmons et al. (29), the symptomatic level of discogenic pain can be localized by discography. A further refinement of discography was introduced by Sachs et al. (28) with the Dallas Discogram Description. Annular discruptures are identified by additional CT investigation and correlated to pain reproduction during discography. Even after posterior fusion and instrumentation, the main part of the axial load is still transferred through the disc (25) and is therefore a persistent provocation for back pain. In two cases of our study we could identify the discogenic pain within the fused segment as the reason for disabling back pain. Both patients responded to additional interbody fusion.

The main reason for clinical failure of the operative procedures was linked to the socioeconomic situation of the patient at the time of surgery and during the recovery period. The German health care system guarantees sick pay over a period of 18 months. Afterwards, the patient is thought to be "unable to do regular work" and is encouraged to ask for an early retirement, and any further financial support is cut off. Therefore, the time the patients were off work preoperatively had the most significant influence on the final outcome. When degenerative spine diseases are treated with fusion, the indication as well as the treatment goals become complicated, especially with the lack of prospective trials from which one can evaluate the efficacy of lower lumbar fusion compared to the natural history of patients with disabling pain. In most degenerative spine diseases, the major indication for surgery is disabling pain that cannot be controlled by conservative treatment only based on clinical experience (4,10,13). The indication for any invasive treatment must therefore be considered very carefully and only after a well-structured nonoperative treatment protocol has not been successful in reducing the patient's complaints.

## REFERENCES


1. Abumi K, Panjabi MM, Duranceau J. Biomechanical evaluation of spinal fixation devices. Part III. Stability provided by six spinal fixation devices and interbody bone graft. *Spine* 1989;14:1249.
2. Brunon J, Duthel R, Potso MJ, et al. Comparative study of Socon steel/Socon titanium instrumentation in osteosynthesis of the dorsolumbar rachis (preliminary results). Company report, 1995.
3. Caldwell GA, Shepard WB. Criteria for spine fusion following removal of lumbar nucleus pulposus. *J Bone Joint Surg* 1948;30A:97.
4. Crock HV. Observations on the management of failed spinal operations. *J Bone Joint Surg* 1976;58B:193.
5. Denis F. The three column spine and its significance in the classification of acute thoracolumbar spinal injuries. *Spine* 1983;8:817.
6. Dick W. *Innere Fixation von Brust- und Lendenwirbelfrakturen. Aktuelle Probleme in Chirurgie und Orthopädie*. Vol. 28. Bern, Stuttgart, Toronto: Huber, 1984.
7. Fairbank JCT, Cooper J, Davis JO, O'Brien JP. The Oswestry Low-Back Pain Disability Questionnaire. *Physiotherapy* 1980;66:271.
8. Ferguson RL, Tencer AF, Woodard P, Allen BL. Biomechanical comparisons of spinal fracture models and stabilizing effects of posterior instrumentations. *Spine* 1988;13:453.
9. Frymoyer JW, Metteri E, Hanley EN, Kuhlmann D, Howe J. Failed lumbar disc surgery requiring a second operation: long term follow up study. *Spine* 1978;3:7.
10. Frymoyer JW, Selby DK. Segmental instability: rationale for treatment. *Spine* 1985;10:280.
11. Goel VK, Nye TA, Clark CR, Nishiyama K, Weinstein JN. A technique to evaluate an internal device by use of the selspot system. *Spine* 1987;12:150.
12. Haaker R, Kielich T, Steffen R, Krämer J. Verification of position of pedicle screws in dorsal lumbar spinal fusion. 6th European Spine Society Meeting, Noordwijk, 1995.
13. Hoover NV. Indications for fusion at time of removal of intervertebral disc. *J Bone Joint Surg* 1968;50A:189.
14. Jacobs RR, Casey MP. Surgical management of thoracolumbar spinal injuries. *Clin Orthop* 1984;189:22.
15. Jaffray D, O'Brien JP. Isolated intervertebral disc resorption. A source of mechanical and inflammatory back pain. *Spine* 1986;11:397.
16. Johnsson K, Willner S. Postoperative instability after decompression for lumbar spinal stenosis. *Spine* 1986;11:107.
17. Johnston CE, Ashmann RB, Baird AM, et al. Effect of spinal construct stiffness on early fusion mass incorporation. *Experimental study. Spine* 1990;15:908.
18. Kozak JA, O'Brien JP. Simultaneous combined anterior and posterior interbody fusion. *Spine* 1990;15:322.
19. Krödel A, Refior H, Plitz W. Biomechanical basis of compressive ventral interbody fusion [Abstract]. *Abstracts of the 18th Annual Meeting ISSLS*, Heidelberg, 1991;29.
20. Lehmann TR, Spratt KF, Tozzi JE, et al. Long term follow up of lower lumbar fusion patients. *Spine* 1987;12:97.
21. Magerl FP. Stabilization of the lower thoracic and the lumbar spine with external skeletal fixation. *Clin Orthop* 1984;189:125.
22. Malinski J. The ontogenetic development of nerve terminations in the intervertebral discs of man. *Acta Anat [Basel]* 1959;38:906.
23. McAffee PC, Farey ID, Sutterlin CE, Gurr KR, Warden KE, Cunningham BW. The effect of spinal implant rigidity on vertebral bone density: a canine model. *Spine* 1991;16:190.
24. Nagel DA, Kramers PC, Rahn BA, Cordey J, Perren SM. A paradigm of delayed union and non-union in the lumbosacral joint: a study of motion and bone grafting of the lumbosacral spine in sheep. *Spine* 1991;16:553.
25. Nolte L-P. Biomechanics of spinal implants. In: Wittenberg RH, ed. *Biomechanics of spinal implants in instrumented spinal fusion*. Stuttgart: Thieme, 1994:15.
26. Panjabi MM. Biomechanical evaluation of spinal fixation devices: I. A conceptual framework. *Spine* 1988;13:1129.
27. Panjabi MM, Abumi K, Duranceau J, Crisco JJ. Biomechanical evaluation of spinal fixation devices: II. Stability provided by eight internal fixation devices. *Spine* 1988;13:1135.

28. Sachs BL, Vanharanta H, Spivey MA, et al. Dallas discogram description. A classification of CT/ discography in low-back disorders. *Spine* 1987;12:287.
29. Simmons JW, Aprill CN, Dwyer AP, Brodsky AE. A reassessment of Holts's data on: "The question of lumbar discography." *Clin Orthop* 1988;237:120.
30. Stoll TM, Dick W. The problem of the thoracolumbar junctions following a polysegmental lumbar fusion. 5th European Spine Society Meeting Madrid.
31. Weatherley CR, O'Brien P. Discogenetic pain persisting despite solid posterior fusion. *J Bone Joint Surg* 1986;68B:142.
32. Weinstein JN, Claverie W, Gibson S. The pain of discography. *Spine* 1988;13:1344.
33. Whitecloud TS III, Butler JC, Cohen JL, Candelora PD. Complications with the variable spine plating system. *Spine* 1989;14:472.
34. Wittenberg RH, Coffee MS, Edwards WT, White AA. Zyklische Belastungstests verschiedener Wirbelsäulenimplantate. *Hefte Unfallheilk* 1990;212:528.
35. Wörsdörfer O. Operative Stabilisierung der thorako-lumbalen und lumbalen Wirbelsäule: Vergleichende biomechanische Untersuchungen zur Stabilität und Steifigkeit verschiedener dorsaler Fixationssysteme. Thesis, Klinisch-Medizinische Fakultät, Ulm, 1981.

*Instrumented Fusion of the Degenerative Lumbar Spine: State of the Art, Questions, and Controversies,* edited by M. Šzpalski, R. Gunzburg, D. M. Spengler, and A. Nachemson. Lippincott–Raven Publishers, Philadelphia © 1996.

# 9

# New Orleans Spinal System in Degenerative Lumbar Disorders (Semi-Rigid Instrumentation)

R. Cavagna

*Clinique du Ter, 56270 Lorient, France*

Indication of an arthrodesis in the treatment of degenerative diseases of the spine is a subject of gripping controversy. Many authors consider arthrodesis a technique that is rarely indicated in the degenerative spine. Their arguments are clear and perfectly acceptable: the degenerative spine is arthrotic and hence rigid, and the measures necessary for a decompression do not destabilize the spine. The other argument is based on the technical laboriousness of instrumentation in these patients, who are often fragile (18).

These ideas are quite correct in a certain number of cases. It is true that the clinical picture is at first sight often constituted by neurogenic claudication (limp), treatment of which suffices to give relief to the patient. It is also true that instrumentation prolongs the operative time and the potential morbidity of this type of surgical intervention. Nevertheless, the steady increase in lifespan and especially the maintenance of the quality of life have considerably increased the demand for this type of surgery and have imposed a quality of both neurologic and functional results that has previously been unusual.

This new information undoubtedly modifies our approach to the treatment of the degenerative spine; the indications most often apply to relatively elderly patients whose spine is not only arthrotic but is also deformed. The quality of the result depends increasingly on definite improvement and even on total disappearance of the lumbalgias (9) (in addition to cure of the neurologic disorders).

This genuine development of the indications demands a search for technical solutions directly adapted to surgery of the degenerative spine, and no longer just a modification of techniques or materials created for other uses. In this respect semi-rigid instrumentation is one possible answer to this very special surgery.

## INDICATIONS FOR ARTHRODESIS IN THE DEGENERATIVE SPINE

The indication for an arthrodesis is a frequently discussed topic. It is difficult to apply formal criteria to its execution, as every author has had different experiences with it. These divergent ideas probably arise from the diversity of the patients who undergo surgery for these types of diseases. Proposition of an arthrodesis depends on local and general factors:

Local conditions: quality of the bone (osteoporosis), the articular processes, necessity for an extensive decompression (arthrectomy), surgical history
Regional conditions: frontal and/or sagittal deformation, spondylolisthesis, sagging of the body, instability
General conditions: sex, age, activity, osteoporosis

These various parameters usually permit arrival at a logical indication of arthrodesis.

The situation is sometimes simple: Indication for decompression without arthrodesis is perfectly logical in a man whose spine lies on the normal axis, is stable, and is of correct bone density (Fig. 1). Moreover, indication for an arthrodesis is perfectly legitimate in a woman whose skeleton is osteoporotic, with sagging fractures and frontal and sagittal deviation (14,18) (Fig. 2A,B).

The difficulty lies in the treatment of all the intermediate forms, in which the surgeon must consider not only the above-mentioned criteria but also personal ex-

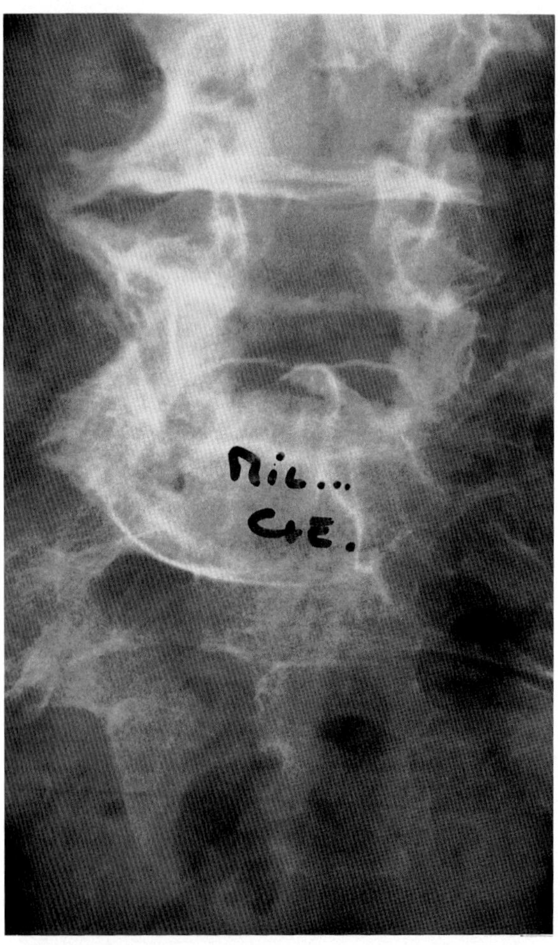

**FIG. 1.** Laminectomy without instrumentation.

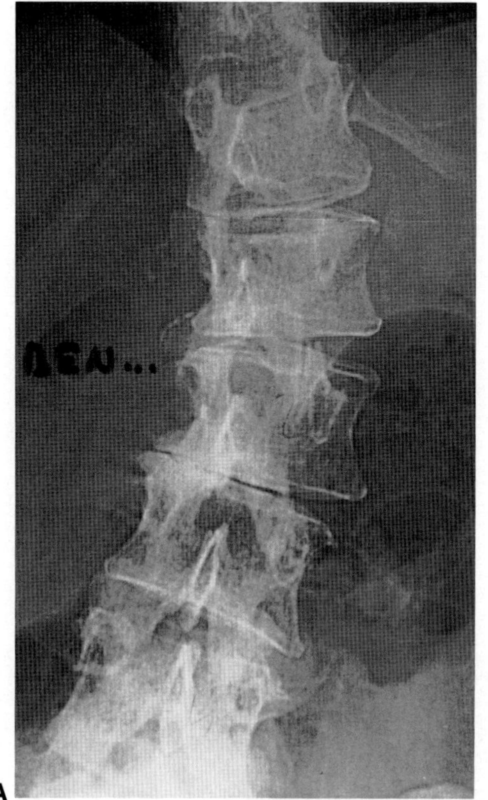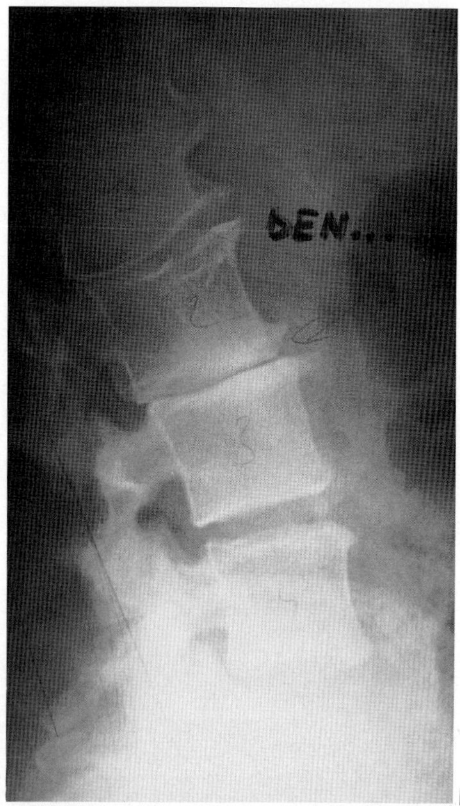

**FIG. 2. A, B:** A 71-year-old woman, osteoporosis, frontal deviation.

perience and the capacity of the patient to tolerate more prolonged surgery. In my experience, three principal criteria dictate the decision to perform an arthrodesis:

1. The presence of a frontal and/or sagittal deformation. In adults, restoration of correct equilibrium of face and profile rather than complete or partial reduction is a determining element in the quality and permanence of the final result (3,6) (Fig. 3A–C).
2. The existence of degenerative spondylolisthesis is a criterion for arthrodesis (14) (Fig. 4A,B).
3. The presence of a rotatory dislocation, even without substantial deformation, is also a criterion, as it always advances towards clinical and radiologic exacerbation.

Analysis of these three parameters clearly shows the importance of osteoporosis, which provokes (by microfracture) or aggravates these various deformations. The other criteria are less formal, except for perhaps extensive surgery (laminoarthrectomy) or previous surgery in the treated area.

Most authors have emphasized the difficulty of successfully performing an arthrodesis without instrumentation. Various studies show the considerable advantage of instrumentation in fusion of the graft (4,8,10,13,16,20,21). It is logical to propose instrumentation in surgery of the degenerative spine, especially because angular correction is sometimes required.

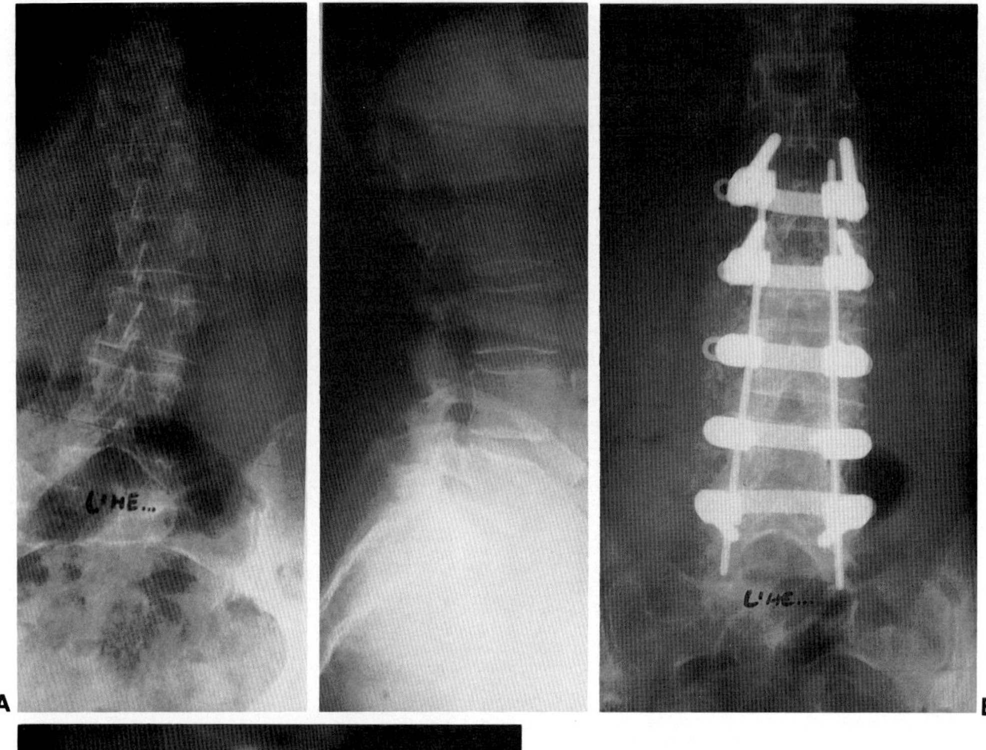

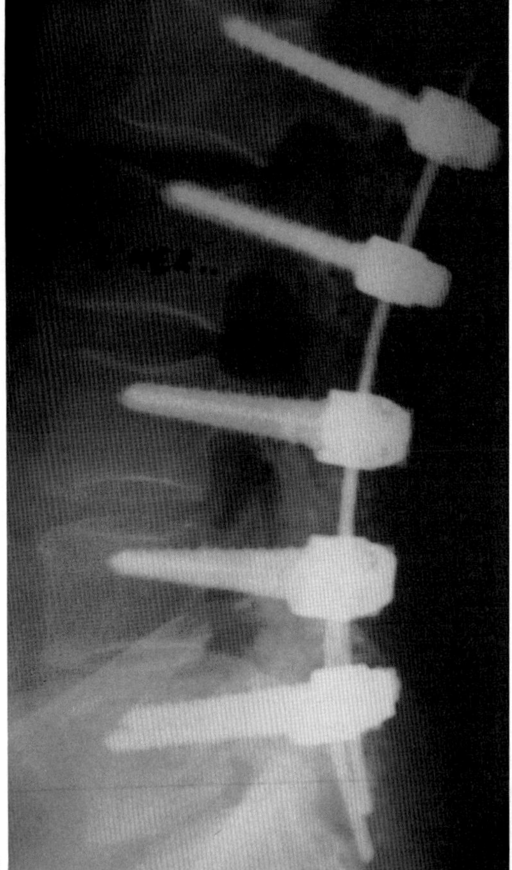

**FIG. 3. A:** A 52-year-old woman, preoperative radiograph. **B:** Postoperative frontal radiograph: good frontal re-equilibration. **C:** Anatomic lordosis.

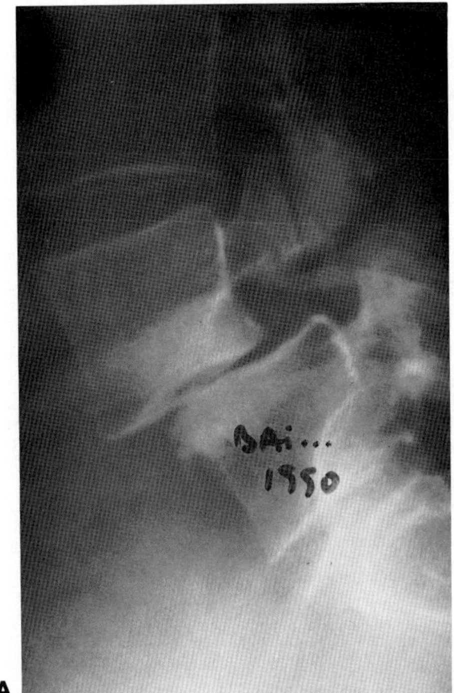
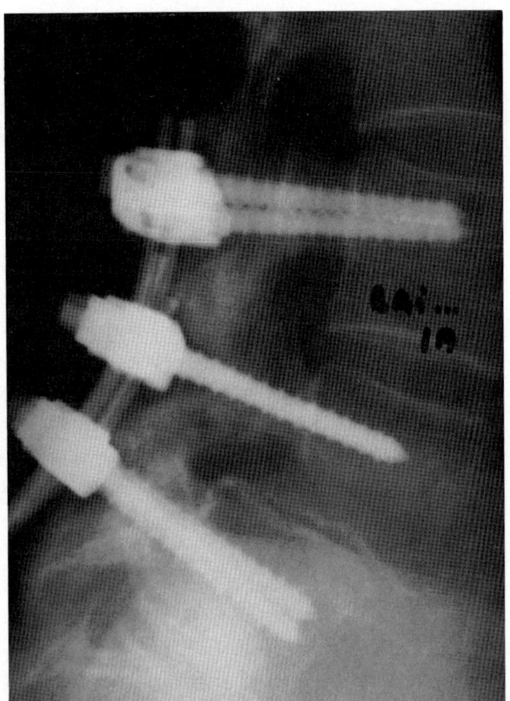

**FIG. 4. A:** Degenerative spondylolisthesis. **B:** Check after 1 year.

## CHOICE OF INSTRUMENTATION

The choice of instrumentation is necessarily dictated by the desired objective. It is illusory to imagine that there exists at present some universal instrumentation responding to all indications. In surgery of the degenerative spine, the instrumentation must certainly permit fusion of the arthrodesis but must also be tolerated by a bone that is often fragile. Finally, it must be capable of at least partially reducing deformations.

1. Fusion of the arthrodesis. According to White and Panjabi (19), an ideal instrumentation is at first rigid to protect the neovascularization of the graft, then dynamic to ensure its corticalization. No such instrumentation exists as yet, but various studies are aimed at finding an acceptable compromise (5,12,15).
2. Tolerance. The degenerative spine is often fragile, both in its bone structure and in its disc or articular components. Certain experimental or clinical studies show the influence of the rigidity of the instrumentation on the instrumented segment (stress shielding) (1,2,13), on the adjacent segments (discopathies) (11,17), and on anchorage of implants (2,7). Although not all authors agree about the extent of the fairly harmful effects of an instrumentation, the latter nevertheless cannot be denied.
3. Reduction of deformations. The material used must be capable of correcting the deformations and permit the reequilibration of the spine. This correction is not brought about in an identical manner in deformations of the young spine (derotation) and in deformations of the degenerative spine (reduction step by step) (3).

All of these considerations together lead us toward specifications specific for surgery of the degenerative spine. This explains the deliberately chosen option of a semi-rigid instrumentation such as the New Orleans system.

## SURGICAL MATERIAL AND TECHNIQUE

### Material

The New Orleans material consists of pedicle screws, fastening plates, rods, and crossplates. The complete implant is made of anodized (electrolytically plated) titanium, which enables it to occupy less space and permits postoperative exploration by scanner or magnetic resonance imaging (MRI). The anodization to a great extent prevents release of metallic particles. The principle of fastening is based on the pedicle screw, which corresponds to an optimization of the anchorage, especially on a fragile bone and on a spine where a laminectomy is usually carried out together with the arthrodesis. The shape of the screw enables it to fit into a cavity in a porotic bone. A platen is fitted onto the screw.

This basic assembly makes it possible to use ancillary material. The latter consists principally of reduction tubes screwed onto the platens. All the necessary reduction manipulations—compression, distraction, and derotation—can thus be effected. These manipulations are effected step by step under the control of the surgeon to prevent any lesion at the points of anchorage. The rods, 3 mm in diameter, are inserted into the platens, progressively determining the anticipated alignment of the instrumented segment of the spine. The modular nature of the system permits doubling of the rods over one or more stages according to local conditions. Finally the crossplates are put into position; these partly rigidify the assembly by neutralizing the forces of rotation, and they reinforce the pedicular anchorage points on the same vertebra.

The design and the dimensions of the material have been studied experimentally to ensure an acceptable compromise between the rigidity necessary for fusion of the graft and a pliability sufficient to reduce the side effects of instrumentation. The semi-rigid option of instrumentation arises from the desire not to exacerbate the already harmful effects of an arthrodesis without instrumentation, yet at the same time to optimize the success of the fusion.

### Surgical Technique

The technique can be varied according to the individual case. The preoperative balance depends on the symptomatology and on the results of standard radiography. Computed tomography (CT) scanning and/or MRI examination are usually supplemented by dynamic saccoradiculography. The latter examination is indispensable for evaluation of the lumbar stenosis in the various positions. It is thus possible to determine the stage (vertebral disc) number to be decompressed, aided by the clinical signs, and in certain cases (e.g., dynamic stenoses) a simple reduction of the deformation can be planned preoperatively without opening the spinal canal. Scanning is a particularly useful examination when the rotation of the vertebrae is substantial, as it aids the centering of the pedicle screw.

The patient lies face down on a remote-controlled operating table, with the lumbar region exposed in kyphosis. The start of the operation and the decompression do not present any particular problems. The pedicle screws and the platens are put into place, their position being checked radiologically. Remote control of the operating table permits alteration of the patient's position according to the desired reduction, the lumbar region of the spine usually being placed in a neutral position or, more rarely, in the lordosis position. This modification of the position on the operating table facilitates reduction of the deformations and positioning of the material.

The rods are moulded and then inserted stage by stage with the aid of reduction tubes. In certain cases the rod is doubled to permit stiffening of all or part of the instrumented segment. Finally, the transverse plates are fixed. The patient is able to get up the next day without any difficulty and usually begins rehabilitation activities about 6 or 7 days later.

## MATERIALS AND METHODS

The study was made on a first group of patients who underwent surgery between August of 1992 and October of 1994. The follow-up was between 12 and 38 months (average 23 months). The group was composed of 33 women and 34 men, with a mean age of 61 years (range 34 to 80 years).

The etiologies were as follows: degenerative scolioses 20 (11 of these also had lumbar stenosis); lumbar stenosis 23; degenerative kyphosis 5; and degenerative spondylolisthesis 19.

Surgical techniques used included 48 laminectomies, eight laminoarthrectomies, and 11 extracanalar approaches.

The number of levels instrumented [number of patients] were: two levels [nine]; three levels [31]; four levels [16]; five levels [7]; seven levels [2]; and eight levels [2]. No correction of deformation was performed in 21 patients, partial correction in 24, and complete correction in 22. Simple rods were used in 61 patients and double rods (at one or more levels) in six.

Posterior grafts were performed in 10 patients, posterolateral grafts in 13, and articular grafts in 44. None of the grafts in the first group was composed of bone from the iliac crest. All were composed of a mixture of spinal resection and laminectomy material and a bone substitute.

## RESULTS

### Clinical Results

All of the patients were analyzed according to the Beaujon classification (Table 1). This classification gives a useful idea of the neurologic signs and also of the lumbalgias and the lifestyle. All of the patients were seen again. The mean preoperative score was 9.4; the mean postoperative score was 17.6; and the mean score gain was 8.2. No patients suffered postoperative exacerbation of the condition (Fig. 5).

As to the incidence of complications, 65 patients had no complication whatever, one patient developed a meningocele, which healed spontaneously; and one hematoma had to be evacuated surgically.

In this group of patients there were no fatalities, nor were there any thromboembolic or postoperative neurologic complications.

**TABLE 1.** *The Beaujon classification*

| | 0 | 1 | 2 | 3 | 4 | Maximum |
|---|---|---|---|---|---|---|
| Claudication (limp) | 100 m | 100–500 m | 500 m | Unlimited | | −3 |
| Resting radiculopathy | Permanent | Crisis | Moderate | Absent | | −3 |
| Effort radiculopathy | 1st step | Episodic, delayed | Absent | | | −2 |
| Lumbalgia | Permanent | Serious crisis | Moderate | Absent | | −3 |
| Neurodeficit | Major | | Moderate | | Absent | −4 |
| Necessary treatment | Major drugs | Moderate | Absent | | | −2 |
| Normal life | Impossible | Very limited | Slightly limited | Normal | | −3 |

### Radiologic Results

A total of 64 (95.5%) of the arthrodeses were fused, this being verified each time on frontal, profile, and three-quarter view x-ray plates and in 16 cases by scanner (Fig. 6A,B). Repeat surgery was carried out on two pseudoarthroses. One graft fractured after a serious traffic accident.

Eight rods unfortunately broke, with widely varying consequences. Two breaks before the sixth month after the operation were the consequence of a pseudoarthrosis. Six breaks after the twelfth month did not produce any clinical signs and did not cause any modification of reduction (Fig. 7A–C). Two broken screws had no consequence.

Analysis of the x-ray plates did not reveal any loosening of the anchoring points (even in the sacrum). There have thus far been no reactions around the implants (Fig.

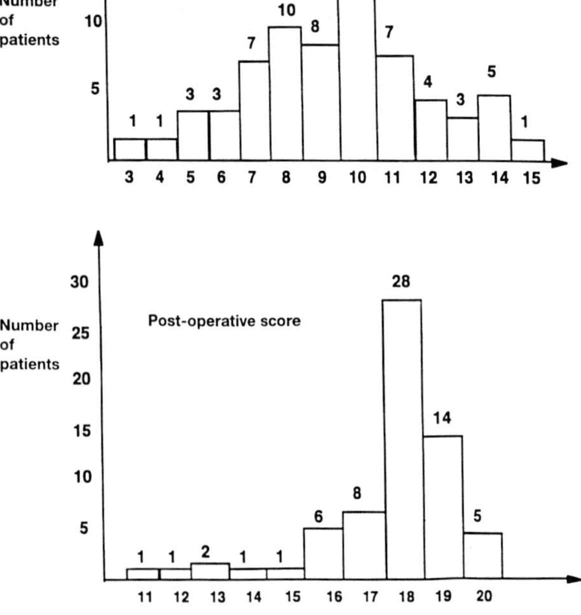


**FIG. 5.** Pre- and postoperative scores.

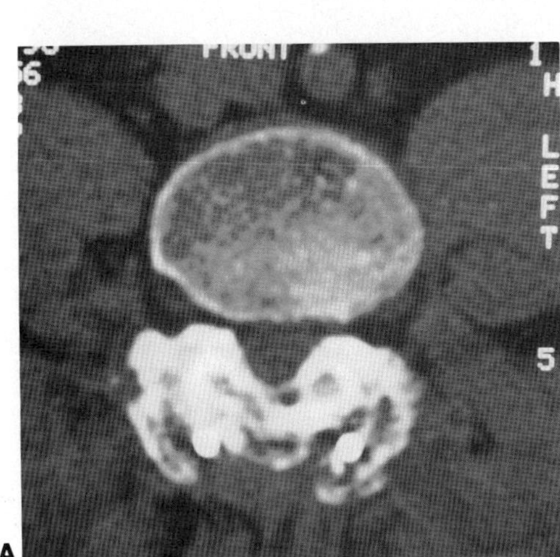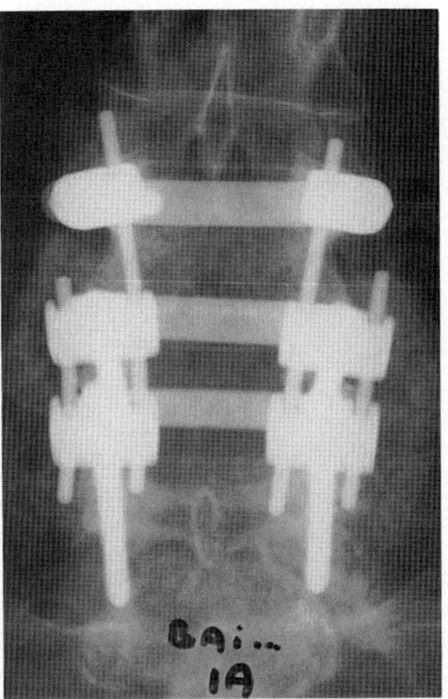

**FIG. 6. A:** Fused articular arthrodesis. **B:** Fused posterolateral arthrodesis.

8), nor any articular discopathies nor, it appears, any decalcification of the instrumented segment of the spine (Fig. 9A–D).

## ANALYSIS

The analysis of this first patient group is encouraging, despite the fact that the time that has elapsed since the operations is still too short for a proper assessment to be made. There is nothing out of the ordinary about the composition of the group as regards the mean age and the distribution of the sexes.

The etiologies deserve more particular attention. There is a substantial incidence of deformations, which indicates the need for a certain extension of spinal surgery to patients who have never yet undergone any such surgery. As Dubousset (3) and Guillaumat (6) have emphasized, development of this type of surgery demands the creation of reduction techniques different from those used in young people. The purpose of this surgery is to bring about re-equilibration of the spine, which guarantees a satisfactory and durable result. It must not be forgotten that the patient's age demands an operation which is as short as possible and causes the least possible trauma.

The technique of insertion of the New Orleans system fulfills these diverse conditions. The instrumentation is simple, the ancillary material permits a step-by-step (or vertebra-by-vertebra) reduction technique, and the results appear to confirm the relatively nontraumatic character of the effect of this type of material on the skeleton. The reductions obtained were of good quality, both for the frontal and sagittal deformations and for the spondylolistheses. No measurable angular loss or any lesions at the anchoring points have thus far been found. The absence hitherto of any bone reaction validates the concept of semi-rigidity.

The low incidence of morbidity is a serious argument in favor of the use of this

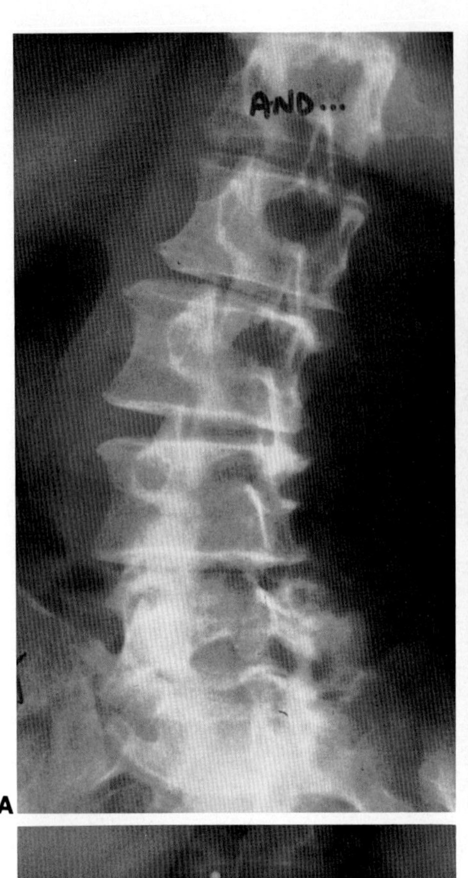


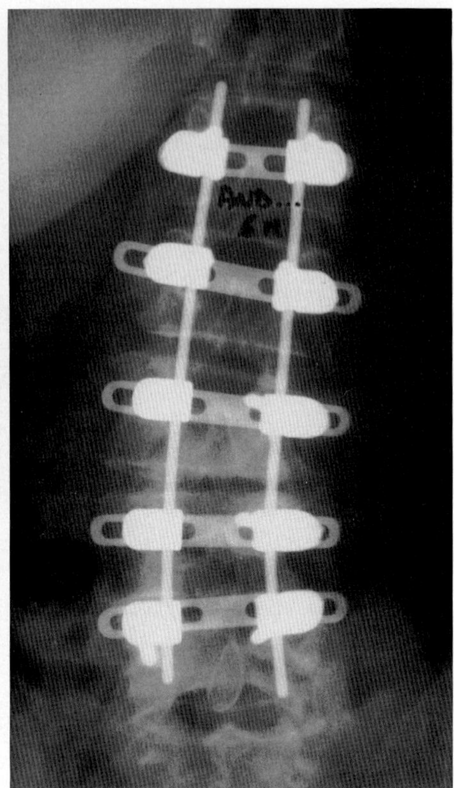


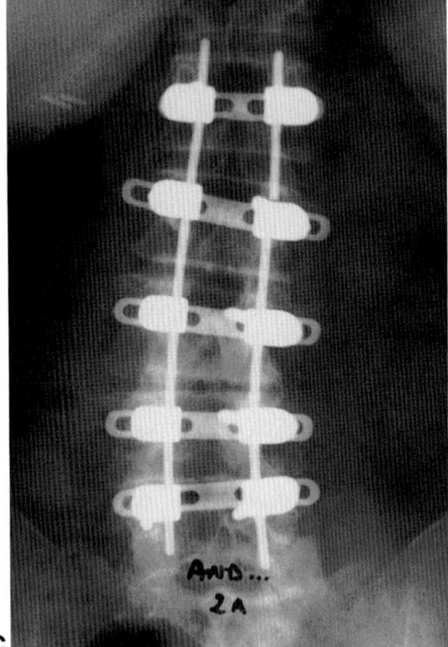


**FIG. 7. A:** A 61-year-old woman, preoperative x-ray plate. **B:** Check after 6 months. **C:** Check after 2 years. Broken rod produced no symptoms. Reduction was not modified.

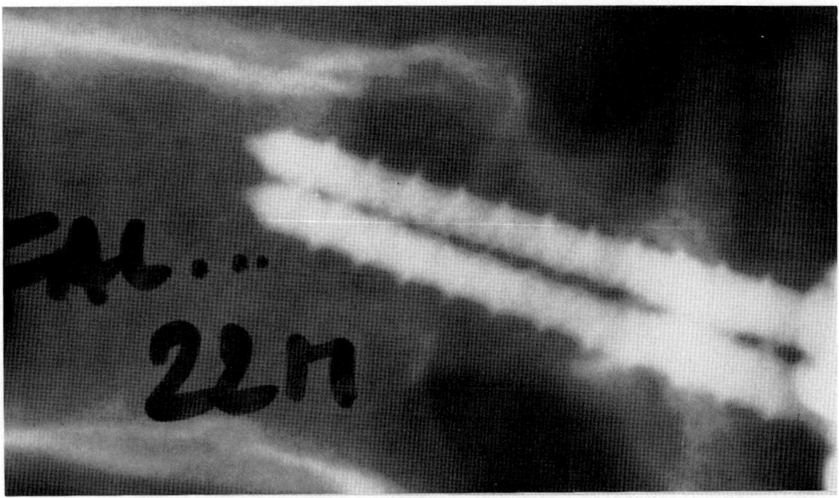

**FIG. 8.** A 80-year-old man, check after 2 years. No sign of intolerance of the material, no alteration of the adjacent disc above.

surgery in relatively elderly patients, as long, of course, as the general contraindications and a reliable surgical technique are respected. The clinical results obtained in this small group of surgical patients emphasize the quality of life after surgery. The Beaujon classification takes into account the neurologic signs, the lumbar pain, and the taking of analgesic medications. The postoperative gain clearly reveals a definite improvement in the comfort of these patients. Moreover, the degree of fusion of the grafts is identical to that reported by most authors who instrument their arthrodeses.

The technique of performance of a graft undoubtedly assumes considerable importance in the final result. The surfaces that are to be grafted must be carefully cleaned (although it has been possible to devote little discussion to this). In this group, whenever possible, the graft was articular and was performed by the Louis technique. The type of graft inserted was more debatable. The absence of taking of iliac graft material was motivated by the desire to reduce the operative time and also the bleeding.

The technique has recently been refined. The bone fragments collected during laminectomy or spinal resection are carefully cleaned, cut into small 4–5-mm cubes, mixed with a bone substitute, and granulated (Triosite), and then mixed with 20 ml of bone marrow taken from the posterior iliac crest. The entire mixture constitutes a conglomerate easily applicable to the previously cleaned surfaces.

The three failed arthrodeses were carefully analyzed. The first two were performed in active young patients (42 and 45 years old) who had already undergone surgery (laminoarthrectomy in both cases for disc pathology). One of them did not heed the advice given to take care after the operation. Both pseudoarthroses were revealed by breaking of the rods, with immediate reappearance of the lumbalgias. The operation was repeated in both patients, with an excellent final clinical result in one case and a poor result in the other (fusion of the arthrodesis was achieved in both cases). The third failure was more unusual because the arthrodesis had perfectly fused, but the patient was the victim of a serious road accident which fractured the graft and broke a rod.

The breakages of the materials were rigorously studied. Apart from the two

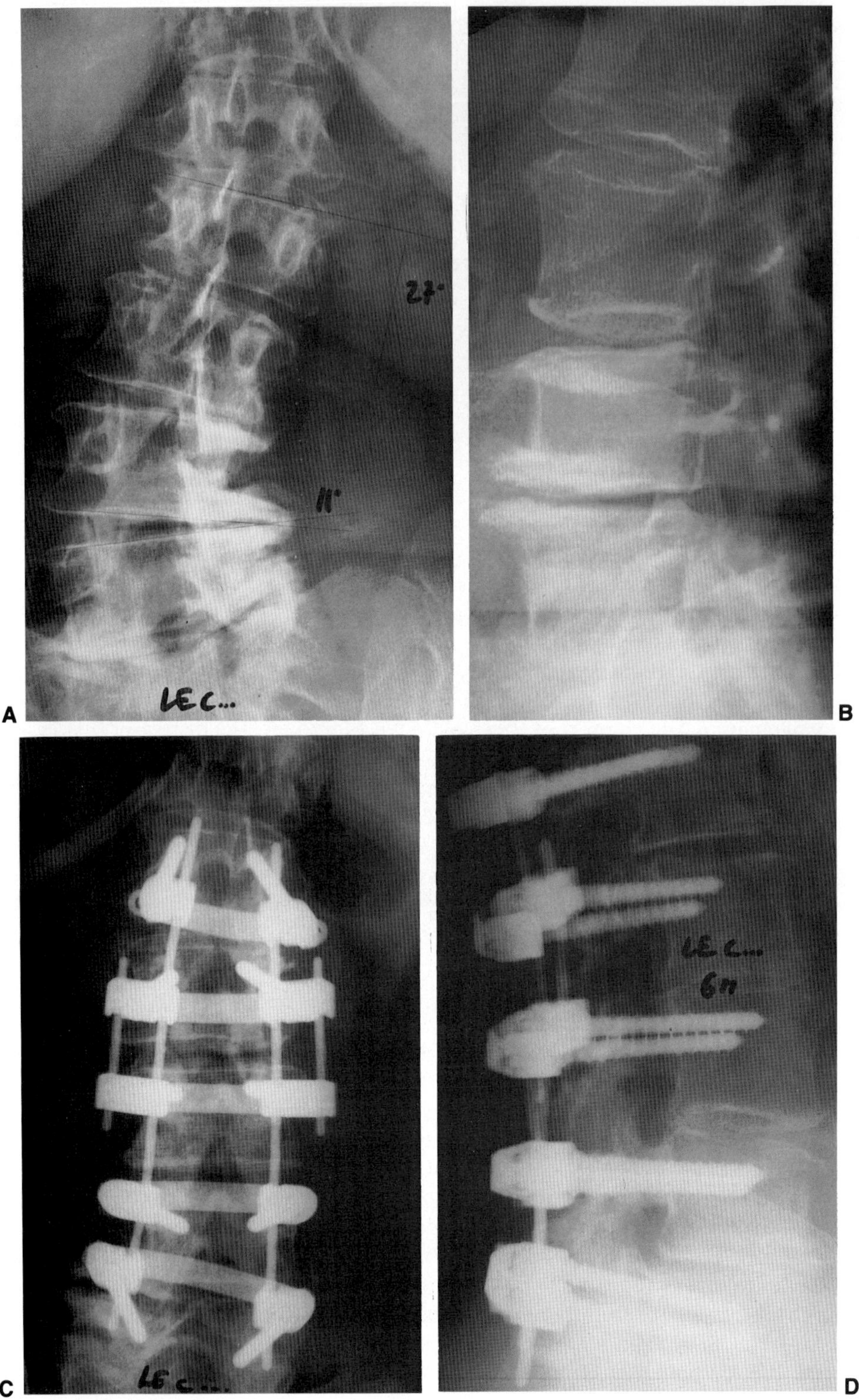

**FIG. 9. A, B:** Degenerative spine in a 67-year-old woman. **C, D:** Lumbar instrumentation by New Orleans material.

pseudoarthroses, breakage of the rod occurred in six other patients. These breakages were always discovered by x-ray more than 12 months after the operation and without reappearance of any clinical signs. In six cases the arthrodesis was fused, the clinical result good or excellent, and no patient underwent repeat surgery to remove the material.

Two screws broke, but this had no clinical effect. Both were on fused arthrodeses. These late material breakages without clinical signs and with fused arthrodeses in all probability indicate the difference in the elasticity module between the bone and the material, despite the fact that the latter is semi-rigid. This mechanical aspect of an instrumented arthrodesis is probably the cause of certain unexplained postoperative pain experienced as a result of the mechanical constraints to which the anchoring points are subject and which increase with increasing rigidity of the material.

## CONCLUSION

Once it has been decided, without going over the indications again, to perform a lumbar arthrodesis, this should be supplemented with instrumentation to increase its level of success. The performance of an arthrodesis is not without consequence, either for the instrumented spinal segment or for the adjacent segments. Development of a semi-rigid instrumentation had the objective of successful fusion of the arthrodesis yet at the same time of permitting reduction manipulations and limiting the harmful effects of any instrumentation. The satisfactory quality of the results obtained shows the validity of the concept of semi-rigidity in instrumentation of the degenerative spine.

## REFERENCES


1. Craven TG, Carson WL, Asher MA, Robinson RG. The effects of implant stiffness on the bypassed bone mineral density and facet fusion stiffness of the canine spine. *Spine* 1994;19:1664–73.
2. Dalenberg DD, Asher MA, Robinson RG, Jayatanan G. The effects of a stiff spinal implant and its loosening on bone mineral content in canines. *Spine* 1993;18:1862–66.
3. Dubousset J. Rachis scoliose. Aspects cliniques et abord bioméchanique. *Rachis* 1995;7:121–2.
4. Feighan JE, Stevenson S, Emery SE. Biologic and biomechanical evaluation of posterior lumbar fusion in the rabbit. The effect of fixation rigidity. *Spine* 1995;20:1561–7.
5. Gosi VK, Hong Lin T, Gogwow J, et al. Effects of rigidity of an internal fixation device. A comprehensive biomechanical investigation. *Spine* 1991;16S:155–61S.
6. Guillaumat M, Kreichati G, Tassin JL. La scoliose lombaire de l'adulte: traitement chirgical avec l'instrumentation Cotrel Dubousset. *Rachis* 1990;2:463–84.
7. Halvorson TS, Kelly LA, Thomas KA, Whitecloud TS III, Cook SD. Effects of bone mineral density on pedicle screw fixation. *Spine* 1994;19:2415–20.
8. Johnston CE II, Ashman RB, Baird AM, Allard RN. Effect of spinal construct stiffness on early fusion mass incorporation. *Spine* 1990;15:908–12.
9. Katz JN, Lipson SJ, Brick GW, et al. Clinical correlates of patients' satisfaction after laminectomies for degenerative lumbar spinal stenosis. *Spine* 1995;20:1155–60.
10. Kleiner JB, Odom JA, Moore MR, Wilson NA, Huffer WA. The effect of spinal instrumentation on human spinal mass. *Spine* 1995;1:90–7.
11. Lee CK. Accelerated degeneration of the segment adjacent to a lumbar fusion. *Spine* 1988;13:375–7.
12. Lin TH, Goel VK, Winterbottom JM, et al. A comparison of stress induced porosity due to a conventional and a modified spinal fixation device. *J Spinal Dis* 1994;1:1–11.
13. McAfee P, Farey ID, Sutterlin CE, et al. Device related osteoporosis with spinal instrumentation. *Spine* 1989;14:919–26.
14. McCullen M, Bernini PM, Bernstein SH, Tosteson TD. Clinical and roentgenographic results of decompression for lumbar spinal fusion. *J Spinal Dis* 1994;7:380–7.
15. Nazel DA, Edwards WT, Schneider E. Biomechanics of spinal fixation and fusion. *Spine* 1991;16S:151–4S.

16. Schwab FJ, Nazarian DG, Mahmud E, Michelson CB. Effects of spinal instrumentation on fusion of the lumbosacral spine. *Spine* 1995;20:2023–8.
17. Weinhoffen SL, Guyer RD, Hebert M, Griffith SL. Intradiscal pressure measurements above an instrumental fusion: a cadaveric study. *Spine* 1995;20:526–31.
18. Whiffen JR, Neuwirth MG. Spinal stenosis. In: Bridwell KH, Dewald RL, eds. *The textbook of spinal surgery*. Vol. 2. Philadelphia: JB Lippincott, 1991:637–56.
19. White AA, Panjabi MM. *Clinical biomechanics of the spine*. 2nd ed. Philadelphia: JB Lippincott, 1990:586–7.
20. Wood GG, Boyd RJ, Carothen TA, et al. The effects of pedicle/screw plates fixation on lumbar/lumbosacral autogenous bone graft fusions in patients with degenerative disc diseases. *Spine* 1995;20:819–30.
21. Zdeblieck TA. A prospective randomised study of lumbar fusion. *Spine* 1993;18:983–91.

*Instrumented Fusion of the Degenerative
Lumbar Spine: State of the Art, Questions,
and Controversies,* edited by M. Szpalski,
R. Gunzburg, D. M. Spengler, and
A. Nachemson. Lippincott–Raven
Publishers, Philadelphia © 1996.

# 10

# Instrumented Lumbosacral Fusion in Degenerative Spine Using the Universal Spine System

R. Khazim, M. Grevitt, C. Reckling, M. Harris, and J. Webb

*Centre for Spinal Studies and Surgery, Queen's Medical Centre,
Nottingham NG7 2UH, England*

Hibbs and Swift (28) first described spinal arthrodesis for painful lumbosacral "developmental abnormalities." Additional posterior and posterolateral fusion techniques have subsequently been developed. More recently, these operations have been used in the treatment of degenerative spinal disorders. Spinal instrumentation has been devised in an attempt to increase fusion rates. Several investigators have noted that rigid fixation increases the fusion rate as well as the rigidity of the fusion mass (22,34,39,54,61). Roy-Camille et al. (47,48) and Louis (37) described pedicle screw-and-plate fixation systems. Steffee (57) in 1986 reported his preliminary experience using a rigidly locked plate–screw system. Many pedicle fixation systems are now commercially available, but the risks and complications associated with this technique are now well recognized. Historically, decompression of the neural elements involved a total laminectomy. In such instances, the early techniques of spinal fusion (spinous process wiring/plating or sublaminar hooks and wires) were not applicable. The advent of pedicle screw fixation allowed stable fixation of the vertebra despite posterior element deficiencies.

The ASIF Universal Spinal System (USS) was launched in 1993. This new system was designed to simplify the surgical treatment of a wide range of thoracolumbar spinal disorders. A single range of instruments allows tumors, trauma, deformities, and degenerative conditions to be dealt with from either the anterior or the posterior approach. This chapter describes the use of the USS in instrumented lumbosacral fusion for degenerative spine conditions, including the indications, preliminary results, and complications. Its use in nondegenerative scoliosis and kyphosis, tumors, infections, fractures, and revision fusion/instrumentation is beyond the scope of this report.

## BIOMECHANICS OF THE USS

The USS was developed to meet the needs of both the patient and the surgeon. The system allows segmental or global three-dimensional correction of the spine.

The implants provide stable and rigid internal fixation. The system is made up of three modules (fracture, deformity, and low back). It is designed for use in a wide variety of clinical conditions and contains implants appropriate for use from the high thoracic spine to the sacrum. The instrumentation is also user-friendly. The USS is manufactured of unalloyed titanium (commercially pure) and titanium alloy. This material offers several advantages over spinal systems manufactured from stainless steel. The advantages of a titanium system are a more "physiologic" modulus of elasticity, lower density, improved biocompatibility, corrosion resistance, and magnetic resonance imaging (MRI) compatibility.

Modulus of elasticity is an important physical property of materials and can serve as a basis for comparison to other materials. It is an indication of the flexibility or rigidity of a component before permanent deformation occurs. The moduli of elasticity of pure titanium and titanium alloy implants are similar, and both are significantly lower than that of 316 stainless steel. The advantage of a material with a low modulus of elasticity is that stress shielding is reduced and increased stress will therefore be transferred to the bone (1). The modulus of elasticity of titanium (105 GPa) is more "physiologic" because it is closer to the modulus of elasticity of cortical bone (16.5 GPa) than is the modulus of elasticity of stainless steel (187 GPa) (3).

Titanium has a significantly lower density than does 316L stainless steel. Titanium implants weigh approximately 45% of stainless steel implants. This offers a theoretical advantage of titanium over stainless steel implants in older individuals and in children.

Titanium and titanium alloy implants contain no iron. These implants produce superior MRI resolution and significantly less "starburst" or signal interference during MRI scanning. Cadaver studies have shown that MRI resolution was greatly improved by the use of titanium spinal implants compared to stainless steel implants (10). MRI scanning is often the imaging modality of choice for investigating pathology of the spine.

The biocompatibility of titanium implants over stainless steel implants has been well documented in the total joint and in the dental literature. The bone–titanium interface undergoes a process called "osseointegration." The bonding of molecules (bone) to the titanium surface has been analyzed by sophisticated analytical techniques. Adell et al. (1) have documented the direct apposition of bone to unalloyed titanium. One advantage of this tissue integration at the surface is the potential for less bacterial colonization and subsequently reduced infection. Other advantages are the increased strength of the bone–implant interface and the limited formation of the fibrous tissue layer often seen at the interface with stainless steel implants.

The titanium alloy employed in the USS is Ti-6AI-7Nb rather than the more common Ti-6AI-4V used in many other orthopedic implants. The former is composed of nontoxic elements. In cell culture studies, vanadium salts exhibited toxicity of an order of magnitude greater than nickel, cobalt, or copper salts. No toxic reactions occurred with aluminum or niobium. Histologic analysis has shown that the Ti-6AI-7Nb alloy implants did not create adverse tissue tolerance reactions.

The USS contains both "hard" and "soft" rods for use as implants. The soft rods are annealed or heat-treated and the hard rods are cold-worked. Annealing produces a soft rod with maximal ductility, defined as the material's ability to permanently deform before fracturing. The advantage of the soft rods is that they are easier to contour. This is particularly useful in degenerative low back conditions, for which the rods must be contoured to the sagittal profile. The hard rod is more highly cold-worked and will withstand a much greater load before permanent deformation occurs. It is recommended to use the hard rods for cases of spinal fracture and deformity correction. The hard rods demonstrate a bending strength of 30 Nm compared to 26 Nm for the soft rods.

The minimal biomechanical strengths of spine instrumentation are not known, e.g., the required pull-out strength of a pedicle screw. The pull-out force of the USS 5-mm (405 Nm), 6-mm (598 Nm), and 7-mm (965 Nm) screws compare favorably to other pedicle screw systems in common use, such as the TSRH 6.5-mm (740 Nm) and ISOLA 6.25-mm (710 Nm) screws.

The USS has been tested against other popular spinal implant systems such as the TSRH, ISOLA, and CD in four-point bending tests and fatigue testing. The strength of the USS is comparable to the other systems mentioned as determined in ASTM (American Society for Testing and Materials) tests. The fatigue properties of the USS implants also compare favorably to these other systems in ASTM fatigue tests.

The USS-manufactured titanium offers unique advantages to the spinal surgeon. The material properties of titanium and titanium alloy allow a more "physiologic" modulus of elasticity, superior MRI compatibility, biocompatibility, and corrosion resistance. The mechanical properties of the USS titanium system for rigid stabilization of the spine are comparable in terms of mechanical performance to other available systems.

## INDICATIONS FOR INSTRUMENTED FUSION

The general clinical indications for surgery are disabling back and/or leg pain and diminished physical and social functioning with resultant reduced quality of life. These subjective indications can be supplemented with objective measurements that quantify disability and pain. We have used a visual analogue scale (VAS) to measure pain and the Oswestry Back Disability questionnaire (15) and Short Form 36 (SF-36) (17) as general health outcome measures.

In analyzing the results of spinal fusion, uncontrolled patient-related factors may act as confounding variables. Workers' compensation and preoperative psychological disturbance have a positive correlation with poor prognosis and surgical outcome (8,19,20,44,56). Smoking and previous spinal surgery are two additional variables associated with poor results after spinal fusion and should be considered before surgery.

Specific indications for USS instrumentation may include the following categories:

1. Isthmic spondylolysis or spondylolisthesis.
2. Degenerative spondylolisthesis.
3. Degenerative scoliosis.
4. Degenerative disc disease.
5. Fusion combined with decompression.

### Isthmic Spondylolysis or Spondylolisthesis

Indications for surgery in this group are: (a) persistent disabling pain despite adequate nonoperative treatment; (b) significant gait disturbance or postural deformity; (c) progressive neurologic deficit; and (d) progressive slip or slips more than 50%, particularly in a child or adolescent.

The following factors must be considered in assessing the risk of progressive deformity:

Type of slip (59). The Dysplastic (type 1) slip (25) is associated with much higher risk.

Degree of slip (24,49). Slips greater than 50% have increased potential for progression.

Sagittal rotation of L5 on S1 (5).

Instability on flexion–extension radiographs.

Slips at levels above L5–S1.

In patients older than 25 years with a spondylolysis, instrumented fusion is recommended because the results of direct lysis repair are unsatisfactory in this age group (32,45).

In patients less than 25 years of age, we consider an instrumented fusion rather than lysis repair if the MRI shows associated degenerative disc disease at the affected or adjacent motion segment or if there is a normal MRI but failure of a lysis block with local anesthetic to significantly relieve the patient's pain. In selected instances, provocative discography (with a strongly concordant pain response) is used to determine the levels to be fused. Instrumented fusion is also considered when there is a normal MRI but a wide lysis gap (greater than 7 mm).

When surgery is indicated for isthmic spondylolisthesis, the procedure and number of levels are dependent on the grade or degree of slip (40). In grades 1 and 2, the number of fusion levels is determined by the MRI findings and the results of discography. However, for higher grade slips a minimum two-level fusion is performed regardless of the MRI findings. USS instrumentation is used in these cases, usually augmented with an anterior fusion.

The surgical treatment of spondyloptosis is more complicated and is beyond the scope of this chapter. However, instrumented fusion is used regardless of whether or not reduction is performed. If the deformity is not reduced, this is done either in conjunction with anterior partial vertebrectomy and fusion or posterior surgery using fibular grafting between L5 and S1 (14,55). If reduction is planned, our present regimen is a three-stage procedure. The first stage is posterior decompression and external fixator application. The latter is used for gradual slow reduction over a 1–2-week period. This is followed by anterior discectomy and tricortical grafting, combined with removal of the external fixator. Posterior instrumented fusion is then performed as part of the third stage. The indications, advantages and disadvantages of reduction have been recently reviewed (11).

### Degenerative Spondylolisthesis

Displacement of the lumbar spine occurs with an intact pars. The instability is secondary to degenerative changes in the intervertebral disc and facet joints. The resultant disability may need surgical treatment in about 10% of patients (46). In these cases, the main goal of surgery is nerve root decompression. There is controversy about the role of fusion after decompression (21). Decompression without additional fusion may result in slip progression and severe mechanical back pain (30).

Decompression and fusion may yield less back and leg pain, reduced postoperative slippage, and significantly better results than decompression alone (16,26,33,36). Instrumented fusion should supplement decompression when there is:

Minimal anterior column spondylosis.
A steep lumbosacral angle.
Sacralization of L5 with L4–L5 spondylolisthesis.
Disruption of greater than 50% of each facet or a total facetectomy at the decompressed level.
Previous decompression at the same level.
Decompression with penetration of the disc space.

Satisfactory results can be obtained without fusion where there is no significant preexisting back pain; the slip is mild and the preoperative functional radiographs show no hypermobility (9,27). Adequate decompression of the neural elements should preferably be performed by bilateral laminotomies, preserving at least half of the facet joints.

### Degenerative Scoliosis

The main indication for surgery is disabling pain despite adequate nonoperative treatment. Most surgeons anticipate high complication rates and only fair clinical results in these patients. However, several reports describe good clinical results with minimal complications using posterior instrumented fusion (2,35,38,53). Most complications were device-related and secondary to osteoporosis; they did not significantly affect the general outcome. The posterior approach is preferred because it enables decompression and facilitates fusion to the sacrum compared with anterior surgery.

### Fusion Combined with Decompression

Decompression is usually achieved with single or multiple laminotomies, excising the ligamentum flavum and undercutting the facets but preserving the posterior osteoligamentous complex (7,18,51). Total laminectomy is reserved for several central/foraminal stenosis or revision surgery necessitating either complete facetectomies, pars excision, or instrumented distraction of the foramina. We combine decompression with instrumented fusion when the stenotic segments are unstable or rendered unstable after decompression in:

Patients in whom preoperative functional x-rays show hypermobility of the stenotic segment.
Patients with structural scoliosis (>10°) in the stenotic area or with marked retro- or lateral listhesis (>3 mm) at the stenotic segment.
Patients in whom total laminectomy is performed without preservation of at least one whole facet at the decompressed level.
Extensive multilevel decompressions.
Previous decompression at the same level with progressive spondylolisthesis.
Coexistent severe, disabling back pain.

### Degenerative Disc Disease

Degenerative disc disease, with or without neurologic abnormalities or deformities, constitutes the main pathologic group in which instrumented fusion is performed (50,56,60–62). The indications for surgery and the use of instrumentation in this group remain controversial. For successful surgical treatment, the segment(s) causing the symptoms must be identified.

The following investigations are helpful in deciding on the fusion levels, although each has limitations:

1. Plain x-rays: loss of disc height, traction spurs, osteophytes, and malalignment. However, there is poor correlation between these findings and the pain level on provocative discography.
2. Functional radiographs.
3. MRI scans: a very sensitive but much less specific study when used to determine fusion levels. The main disadvantage is the high incidence of abnormalities in asymptomatic individuals (4,43).
4. Provocative discography. Despite being invasive, this investigation plays an important role in demonstrating disc pathology and is one of the few methods presently available for identifying a pain source (23). It can also be used as a predictor of outcome after surgery. Controversy exists regarding discography's high false-positive rate (29,52). A recent well-controlled study has reported a false-positive rate of 0% (58). The precise pain source in those patients exhibiting a concordant pain response is a subject of investigation. The variability of reported results of surgery performed on the basis of an abnormal discography casts doubt on the role of discography (6,42,52).

   The indications for discography include:

   Multilevel degenerative disc disease.
   Intra-annular clefts/tears.
   Intermediate degenerative pattern on MRI.
   "Discogenic" back or nonradicular leg pain with normal or equivocal investigations.
   Assessment of the segment adjacent to the proposed fusion levels.
   Assessment after "failed" posterior spinal fusion.

5. Facet joint injections have not been found to be good predictors of spinal fusion outcome (13).
6. The response to external fixator application (12) is still infrequently used to determine fusion levels or as a predictor of outcome. The invasiveness and risks of the procedure limit its use to that of a last resort if all previous investigations give no clear indication of fusion levels.

### PATIENTS AND METHODS

The first 100 consecutive cases of posterior instrumented fusions of the degenerate lumbosacral spine using the USS system were reviewed. All operations were performed at the same center and the minimal follow-up was 1 year. All patients with degenerative lumbar spine disease were included (Table 1). We excluded cases of

**TABLE 1.** *Diagnoses of patients studied*

| Diagnosis | No. of patients |
| --- | --- |
| Spondylolysis/spondylolisthesis | 13 |
| Degenerative spondylolisthesis | 12 |
| Degenerative disc disease | 64 |
| Degenerative scoliosis | 2 |
| Spinal stenosis | 7 |
| Others | 2 |
| Total | 100 |

nondegenerative scoliosis and kyphosis, tumors, infections, fractures, and revision fusion with instrumentation.

Most data were collected prospectively; patients were seen at 6 weeks and at 3, 6, 12, 18, and 24 months postoperatively. A preoperative Oswestry Back Disability Questionnaire was completed by 60 patients. For this latest review, all patients were sent postal questionnaires, including the Oswestry disability and SF-36.

One patient had died from a complication of the back operation, six were not traced, and 80 of the remaining 93 responded. All living patients (99) were clinically assessed at a minimum of 1 year postoperatively. The patients' subjective assessments after surgery were documented as either better, worse, or same as preoperatively.

The SF-36 questionnaire was not available at the start of the study, but the results from the latest review were analyzed. This questionnaire has 36 items that measure eight variables:

1. Physical functioning (10 items)
2. Social functioning (2)
3. Role limitations due to physical problems (4)
4. Role limitations due to emotional problems (3)

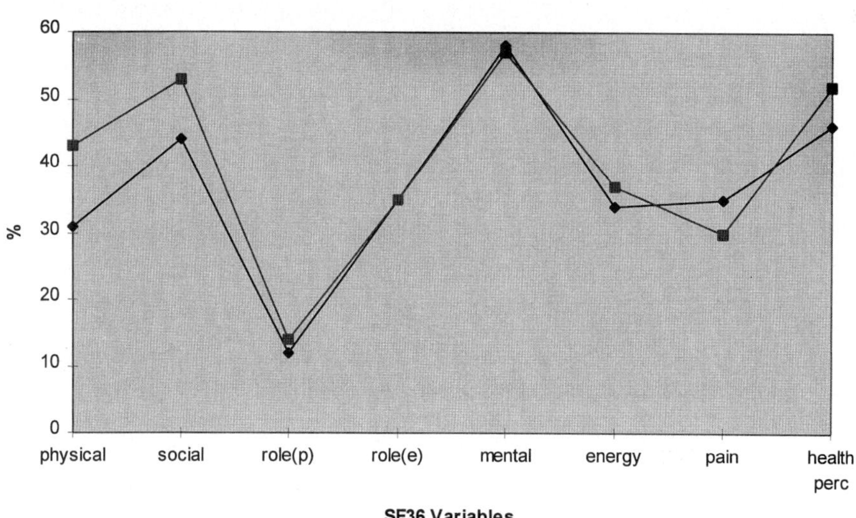


**FIG. 1.** SF-36 health profile of the study population at follow-up compared to normative data of British patients presenting to a back pain clinic (—♦—, fusion; —■—, low back). (From ref. 31, with permission.)

5. Mental health (5)
6. Energy and vitality (4)
7. Pain (2)
8. Perception of general health (5)

For each variable, items are coded, summated and transformed to a score from 0 (worst possible health) to 100 (best possible health). Each transformed score may be linked to form a "health profile." Profiles vary among chronic medical disorders (17). The SF-36 has been validated on large patient populations (31).

The fusion status was assessed with plain radiographs (anteroposterior, lateral, oblique, and functional x-rays), tomograms, and computed tomography (CT) scans as necessary. Fusion determination by radiologic means is very difficult and is far from being accurate. The gold standard is re-operation with inspection and testing of the fusion mass. This was done, for different reasons, in 18 patients. Fusion status at this review was judged as either consolidated, pseudarthrotic or indeterminate.

### Statistical Evaluation

Where appropriate, comparisons were made using two-tailed $t$ tests and $\chi^2$ tests. The level of significance was 0.05. All were performed with a commercial statistical package (Minitab for Windows, v9.0).

### RESULTS

There were 50 men and 50 women, ranging in age from 21 to 73 years (average 46 years). Twenty-one patients had undergone previous spinal surgery; 15 had a previous decompression, five had more than one previous decompression, and another a lysis repair. Forty-six percent were smokers.

Symptom duration before surgery averaged 5.7 years. Forty-two patients had radicular symptoms; 29 had mono- and 13 multiradicular symptoms.

The approaches used were posterior midline in 67, Wiltse in 28 and combined in five. The numbers of levels fused were one level in 48 cases, two in 47, and three or more in five. Of the patients with one-level fusion, 13 had L4–L5 and 35 had L5–S1 fusion. Blood loss averaged 836 ml/case (range 0–4,500 ml). Average hospital stay was 9 days. Sixteen patients were braced for 12 weeks postoperatively.

Intra-operative complications occurred in 10 patients. These were eight dural tears and two pedicle screw misplacements (one of which was recognized and removed in the same procedure).

Postoperative complications occurred in nine patients. Two patients had a proven deep venous thrombosis. There were two deep and two superficial infections, and one wound hematoma that required evacuation. There was one wound dehiscence that required secondary closure, and one patient died of pulmonary complications. Fourteen had removal of implants. Implant failures appeared in eight cases. These included one rod fracture, two screws pulled out, and five screws were loose radiologically. There was no screw breakage in the 518 screws inserted.

A total of 99 patients were reviewed at an average of 15 months after surgery (range 12–36 months). At latest follow-up, 63 patients were subjectively better, 26 were the same, and 10 were worse than preoperatively. The preoperative Oswestry

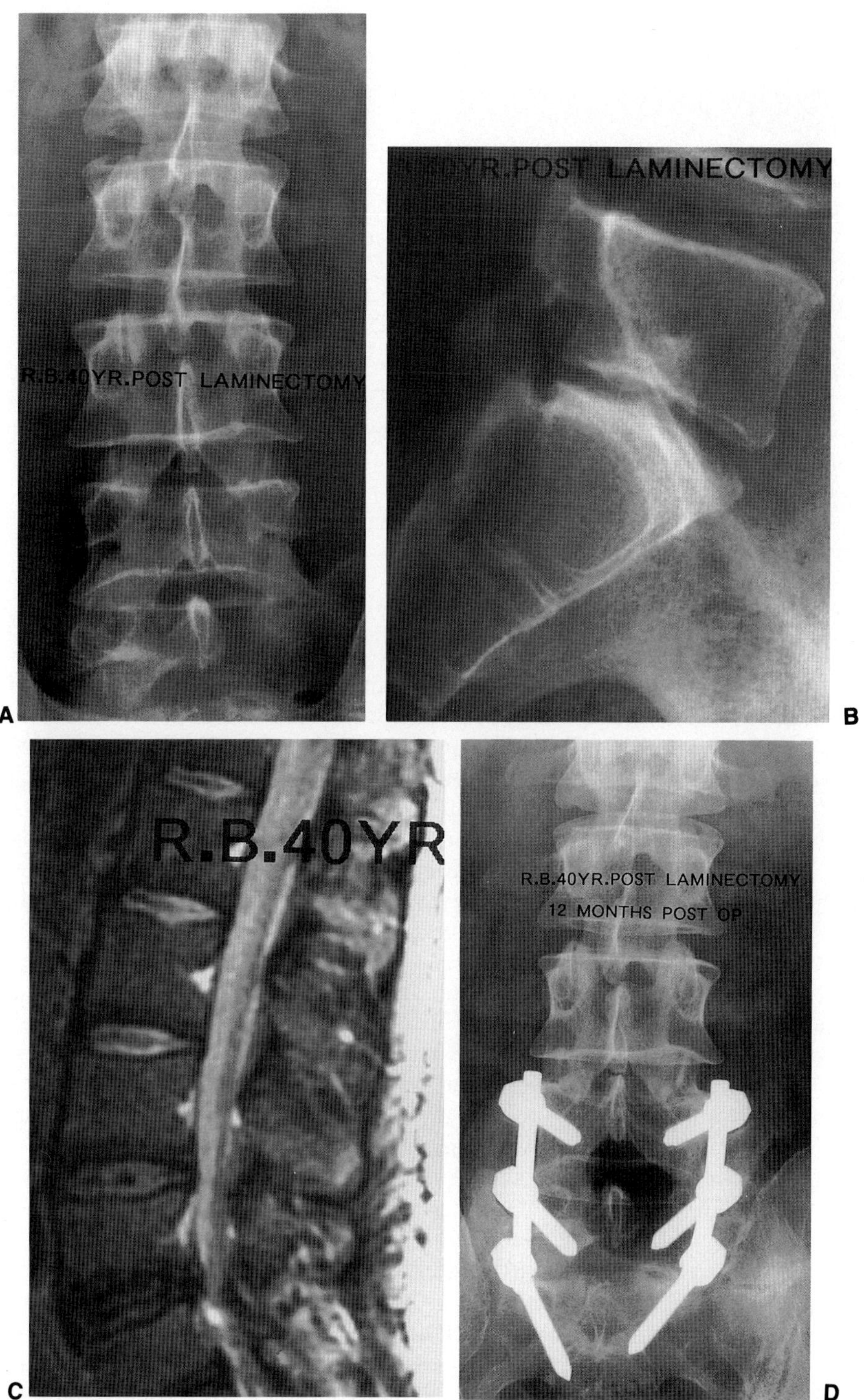



**FIG. 2.** A 40-year-old man with severe back pain after a hemilaminectomy. **A:** Anteroposterior radiograph. **B:** Lateral radiograph. **C:** MRI scan. **D:** Twelve-month postoperative AP x-ray shows a solid fusion. **E:** Postoperative lateral radiograph.

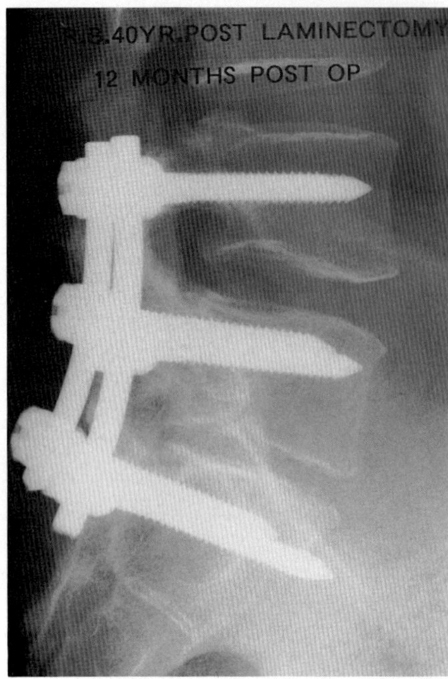


**E**  **FIG. 2.** *Continued.*

score averaged 56% (100% being worst health and 0% normal health). At this review, the average Oswestry score was 52% but the difference was not statistically significant. The SF-36 health profile for our patients is plotted in Fig. 1. For illustration, this is compared with normative data on British patients presenting to a back pain clinic (31). The two profiles are not statistically different.

There was statistically significant association between a good outcome and solid fusion. There was a significant association between smoking and poor outcome and pseudarthrosis. There was no significant association between clinical outcome or fusion status with diagnosis, previous surgery, duration of symptoms, or number of levels fused. The surgical approach, associated decompression, and fusion level had no influence on outcome. There was no significant difference in the fusion rates between single-level L4–L5 and L5–S1 fusions. At latest follow-up, 15 had obvious or suspected pseudarthrosis. Of the 18 patients who underwent revision surgery, only eight were found to have pseudarthrosis. A few examples are presented in different indications: severe pain after previous hemilaminectomy in a 40-year-old male (Fig. 2), spondylolisthesis with back and leg pain in a 53-year-old female (Fig. 3), and degenerative disc disease and disc herniation presented in a 33-year-old male (Fig. 4).

## DISCUSSION AND CONCLUSION

This preliminary study of the use of USS instrumentation in degenerative spine fusion shows that the instrumentation is safe, with few implant-related complications. It achieved an acceptable rate of fusion and allowed early mobilization without bracing in most cases. The clinical results are similar to those of other series. The very high rate of smoking in our patients (46%) should be stressed, as this could have seriously affected the results.

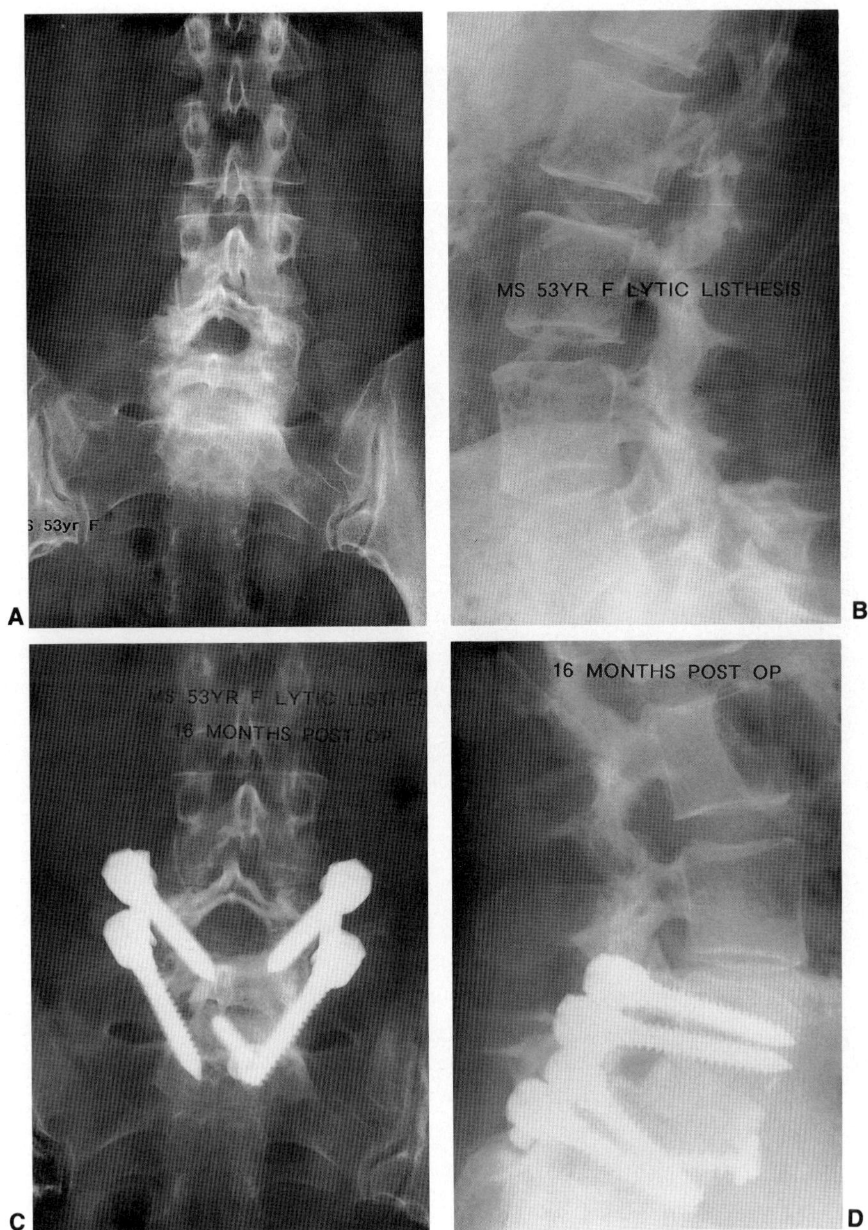


**FIG. 3.** A 53-year-old woman with back and leg pain. AP view **(A)** and lateral view **(B)** radiographs show a grade 2 spondylolisthesis. The patient underwent anterior and posterior fusion and instrumentation. Sixteen-month postoperative AP view **(C)** and lateral view **(D)** radiographs.

There is increasing interest in developing valid outcome measures in spinal surgery. The SF-36 is being increasingly used in other orthopedic subspecialities. We are now prospectively collecting SF-36 data on patients before surgical fusion. This subgroup may have significantly worse disability and health profiles than other spinal groups (e.g., surgical decompression or disc herniation) so that the above results

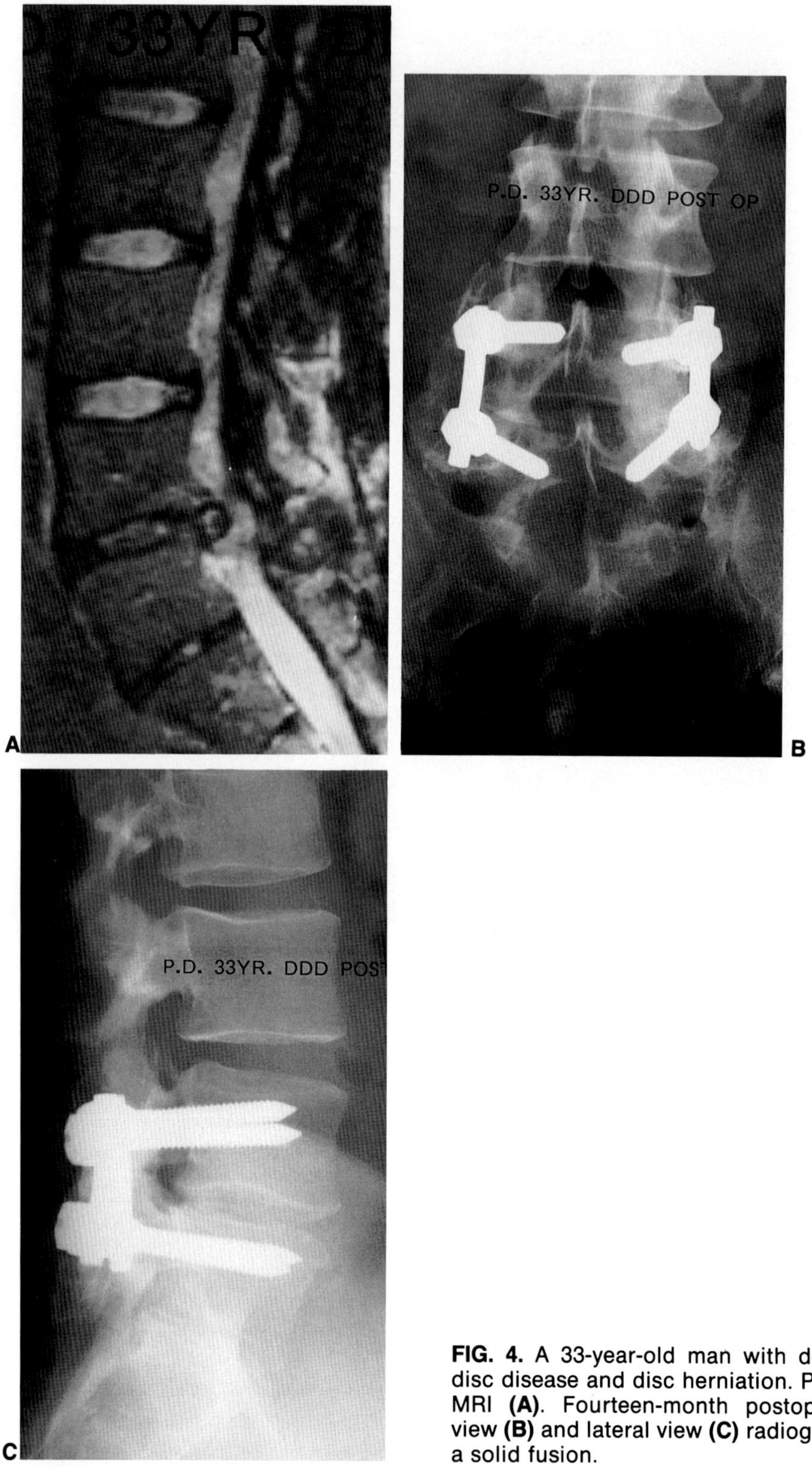

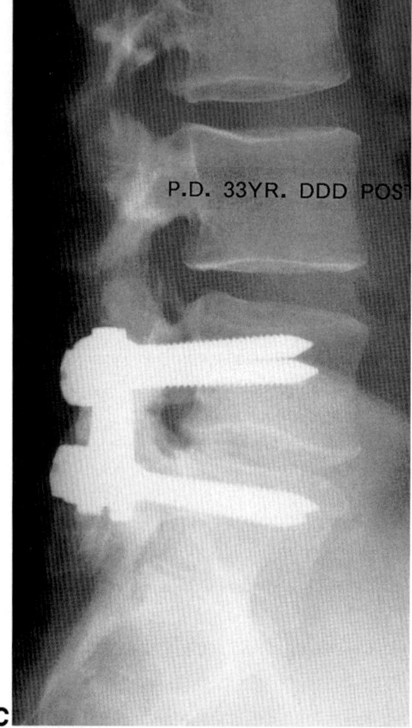


**FIG. 4.** A 33-year-old man with degenerative disc disease and disc herniation. Preoperative MRI **(A)**. Fourteen-month postoperative AP view **(B)** and lateral view **(C)** radiographs show a solid fusion.

may represent *improved* health after surgery. Unfortunately, the SF-36 was not available at the start of this study and we are unable to compare pre- and postoperative profiles.

This chapter does not seek to answer the wider questions of the correct indications for instrumented lumbar spine fusion and the selection of levels. The long-term effect of this procedure on general health parameters and the level of disability are yet to be determined.

## REFERENCES

1. Adell R, Lekholm U, Rockler B, Branemark P. A 15 year study of osseointegrated implants in the treatment of the edentulous jaw. *Int J Oral Surg* 1981;10:387–416.
2. Aebi M. Correction of degenerative scoliosis of the lumbar spine. A preliminary report. *Clin Orthop* 1988;232:80–6.
3. Bannon BP, Mild EE. Titanium alloys for biomaterial application: overview. In: Luckey HA, Kubli F Jr, eds. *Titanium alloys in surgical implants, ASTM STP 796*. American Society for Testing and Materials, 1983:206–19.
4. Boden SD, Davis DO, Dina TS, Patronas NJ, Wiesel SW. Abnormal magnetic resonance scans of the lumbar spine in asymptomatic patients. A prospective investigation. *J Bone Joint Surg [Am]* 1990; 72:403–8.
5. Boxall D, Bradford DS, Winter RB, Moe JG. Management of severe spondylolisthesis in children and adolescents. *J Bone Joint Surg [Am]* 1979;61:479–95.
6. Colhoun E, McCall IW, Williams L, Pullicino VNC. Provocation discography as a guide to planning operations on the spine. *J Bone Joint Surg [Br]* 1988;70:267–71.
7. Crock H, Crock M. A technique for decompression of the lumbar spinal canal. *Neuro-orthopaedics* 1988;5:96–9.
8. Currey HLF, Greenwood RN, Lloyd CG, Murray RS. A prospective study of low back pain. *Rheumatol Rehab* 1979;18:94–104.
9. Dall BE, Rowe DE. Degenerative spondylolisthesis. Its surgical management. *Spine* 1985;10:688–72.
10. Disegi J. Magnetic resonance imaging of AO/ASIF stainless steel and titanium implants. *Injury* 1992;23(suppl 2).
11. Edwards CC, Bradford DS. Controversies in instrumented reduction of spondylolisthesis. *Spine* 1994;94:1535–7.
12. Essess SI, Botsford DJ, Kostuik JP. The role of external spinal fixation in the assessment of low back disorders. *Spine* 1989;14:594–600.
13. Essess SI, Moro JK. The value of facet joint blocks in patient selection for lumbar fusion. *Spine* 1993;18:185–90.
14. Essess SI, Natout N, Phelps K. Posterior interbody arthrodesis with a fibular strut graft in spondylolisthesis. *J Bone Joint Surg [Am]* 1995;77:172–6.
15. Fairbank JC, Couper J, Davis JB, O'Brien JP. The Oswestry low back pain disability questionnaire. *Physiotherapy* 1980;66:271–3.
16. Feffer HR, Wiesel SW, Cuckler JM, Rothman RH. Degenerative spondylolisthesis. To fuse or not to fuse. *Spine* 1985;10:287–9.
17. Garrat AM, Ruta DA, Abdalla MI, Buckingham JK, Russell IT. The SF 36 health survey questionnaire. An outcome measure suitable for routine use within the NHS. *BMJ* 1993;306:1440–4.
18. Getty CJ, Johnson JR, Kirwan EO'G, Sullivan MF. Partial undercutting facetectomy for bony entrapment of the lumbar nerve root. *J Bone Joint Surg [Br]* 1981;63:330–5.
19. Greenough CG. Recovery from low back pain. 1–5 year follow up of 287 injury-related cases. *Acta Orthop Scand* 1993;251:126–9.
20. Greenough CG, Taylor LJ, Fraser RD. Anterior lumbar fusion. Results, assessment techniques and prognostic factors. *Eur Spine J* 1994;3:225–30.
21. Grob D, Humker T, Dvorak J. Degenerative lumbar spinal stenosis. Decompression with and without arthrodesis. *J Bone Joint Surg [Am]* 1995;77:1036–42.
22. Gurr KG, Mcafee PC, Warden KE, Shih CM. Roentgenographic and biomechanical analysis of lumbar fusions. A canine model. *J Orthop Res* 1989;7:838–48.
23. Guyer RD, Ohnmeiss DD. Lumbar discography. Position statement from the North American Spine Society Diagnostic and Therapeutic Committee. *Spine* 1995;20:2048–57.
24. Harris IE, Weinstein SL. Long term follow up of patients with grade III and IV spondylolisthesis. Treatment with and without posterior fusion. *J Bone Joint Surg [Am]* 1987;69:60–9.
25. Hensinger RN, Lang JR, MacEwen GD. Surgical management of spondylolisthesis in children and adolescents. *Spine* 1976;1:207–16.

26. Herkowitz HN, Kurz LT. Degenerative lumbar spondylolisthesis with spinal stenosis. A prospective study comparing decompression with decompression and intertransverse process arthrodesis. *J Bone Joint Surg [Am]* 1991;73A:802–8.
27. Herron LD, Trippi AC. L4–L5 degenerative spondylolisthesis. The results of treatment by decompressive laminectomy without fusion. *Spine* 1989;14:534–8.
28. Hibbs RA, Swift WE. Developmental abnormalities at lumbosacral juncture causing pain and disability. Report of 147 patients treated by spine fusion operation. *Surg Gynecol Obstet* 1929;48:604–12.
29. Holt EP Jr. The question of lumbar discography. *J Bone Joint Surg [Am]* 1968;50:720–6.
30. Hopp E, Tsou PM. Postdecompression lumbar instability. *Clin Orthop* 1988;227:143–51.
31. Jenkinson C, Coulter A, Wright L. Short form 36 (SF36) health survey questionnaire. Normative data for adults of working age. *BMJ* 1993;306:1437–40.
32. Johnson GV, Thompson AG. The Scott wiring technique for direct repair of lumbar spondylolysis. *J Bone Joint Surg [Br]* 1992;74:426–30.
33. Johnsson K, Willner S, Johnsonsson K. Postoperative instability after decompression for lumbar spinal stenosis. *Spine* 1986;11:107–10.
34. Johnston CE, Welch RD, Baker KJ, Ashman RD. Effect of spinal construct stiffness on short segmental fusion mass incorporation. Presented at the Scoliosis Research Society annual meeting, Kansas City, MO, 1992.
35. Krismer M. Multisegmental fusions for degenerative scoliosis of the lumbar spine. In: Wittenberg RH, Steffen R, eds. *Instrumented spinal fusion*. Stuttgart: Georg Thieme Verlag, 1994:107–12.
36. Lombardi JS, Wiltse LL, Reynolds J, Widdel EH, Spencer C. Treatment of degenerative spondylolisthesis. *Spine* 1985;10:821–7.
37. Louis R. Fusions of the lumbar and sacral spines by internal fixation with screw plates. *Clin Orthop* 1986;203:18–33.
38. Marchesi DG, Aebi M. Pedicle fixation devices in the treatment of adult lumbar scoliosis. *Spine* 1992;17:S304–9.
39. McAfee PC, Farey ID, Sutterlin CE, Gurr KR, Warden KE, Cunningham BW. Device-related osteoporosis with spinal instrumentation. *Spine* 1989;14:919–26.
40. Meyerding HW. Spondylolisthesis. *Surg Gynecol Obstet* 1932;54:371–7.
41. Mulholland RC. Lumbar spondylolisthesis. In: Findlay G, Owen R, eds. *Surgery of the spine*. London: Blackwell, 1992:737–53.
42. Nachemson A. Lumbar discography—where are we today. *Spine* 1989;14:555–7.
43. Paajanen H, Erkintalo M, Kuusela T. Magnetic resonance study of disc degeneration in young low-back pain patients. *Spine* 1989;14:982–5.
44. Pheasent HC, Gilbert D, Goldfarb J, Herron L. The MMPI as a predictor of outcome in low-back surgery. *Spine* 1979;4:78–84.
45. Ricciardi JE, Pflueger PC, Isaza JE, Whitecloud TS III. Transpedicular fixation for the treatment of isthmic spondylolisthesis in adults. *Spine* 1995;17:1917–22.
46. Rosenberg NJ. Degenerative spondylolisthesis. *J Bone Joint Surg [Am]* 1975;57:467–74.
47. Roy-Camille R, Roy-Camille M, Demeulenaere C. Osteosynthese du rachis dorso-lombaire et lombo-sacre par plaques metalliques visseas dans les pedicules vertebraux et les apophyses articulaires. *Presse Med* 1970;78:1447–8.
48. Roy-Camille R, Saillant G, Mazel G. Internal fixation of the lumbar spine with pedicle screw plating. *Clin Orthop* 1986;203:7–17.
49. Saraste H. Long-term clinical and radiological follow-up of spondylolysis and spondylolisthesis. *J Pediatr Orthop* 1987;7:631–8.
50. Schwab FJ, Nazarian DG, Mahmud F, Michelsen CB. Effect of spinal instrumentation on fusion of the lumbosacral spine. *Spine* 1995;20:2023–8.
51. Senegois J, Etchevers JP, Vital JM, Boulny D, Grenier F. Widening of the lumbar vertebral canal as an alternative to laminectomy in the treatment of lumbar stenosis. *French J Orthop Surg* 1988;2:93–9.
52. Simmons JW, Aprill CN, Dwyer AP, Brodsky AE. A reassessment of Holt's data on "the question of lumbar discography." *Clin Orthop* 1988;237:120–4.
53. Simmons ED, Simmons EH. Spinal stenosis with scoliosis. *Spine* 1992;17:S117–20.
54. Smith KR, Hunt TR, Asher MA, Morris DC. The effects of stress bypass on canine vertebral cancellous bone resorption. Presented at the Scoliosis Research Society Annual Meeting, Amsterdam, The Netherlands, September, 1989.
55. Smith MD, Bohlman HH. Spondylolisthesis treated by a single-stage operation combining decompression with in situ posterolateral and anterior fusion. An analysis of eleven patients who had long-term results. *J Bone Joint Surg [Am]* 1990;72:415–21.
56. Stauffer RN, Coventry MB. Posterolateral lumbar spine fusion. Analysis of Mayo clinic series. *J Bone Joint Surg [Am]* 1972;54:1195–1204.
57. Steffee A. Segmental spine plates with pedicle screw fixation. *Clin Orthop* 1986;203:45–53.
58. Walsh TR, Weinstein JN, Spratt KF, Lehmann TR, Aprill C, Sayre H. Lumbar discography in normal subjects. A controlled prospective study. *J Bone Joint Surg [Am]* 1990;72:1081–8.

59. Wiltse LL, Newman PH, McNab I. Classification of spondylolysis and spondylolisthesis. *Clin Orthop* 1976;117:23–9.
60. Wood GW, Boyd RJ, Carothers TA, et al. The effect of pedicle screw/plate fixation on lumbar/lumbosacral autogenous bone graft fusions in patients with degenerative disc disease. *Spine* 1995;20:819–30.
61. Zdeblick TA. A prospective, randomized study of lumbar fusion. Preliminary results. *Spine* 1993;18:983–91.
62. Zucherman J, Hsu K, Picetti G, White A, Wayne G, Taylor L. Clinical efficacy of spinal instrumentation in lumbar degenerative disc disease. *Spine* 1992;17:834–7.

*Instrumented Fusion of the Degenerative Lumbar Spine: State of the Art, Questions, and Controversies,* edited by M. Szpalski, R. Gunzburg, D. M. Spengler, and A. Nachemson. Lippincott–Raven Publishers, Philadelphia © 1996.

# 11

# The GDLH System in Degenerate Lumbar Disorders

## Eduardo R. Luque

*Hospital Dr. Germán Díaz Lombardo, Mexico City, 01000 Mexico*

In degenerative lumbar disorders, there are three main reasons for provoking an arthrodesis:

1. Instability: lateral, as in spondylolisthesis, rotational, as in degenerative scoliosis, or longitudinal, as in loss of intervertebral space.
2. Deformity, such as loss of lumbar lordosis or asymmetry of the pelvis.
3. Lack of support, as in severe osteoporosis.

Not all degenerate lumbar spines are candidates for arthrodesis. Most patients can obtain excellent results from physiotherapy and gentle mobilization. In our experience, approximately two-thirds can improve over 50% with this type of treatment. The other one-third are candidates for surgery and can be divided into two categories: (a) those who need support and whose symptoms are mainly due to soft-tissue invasion of the neural canal, with or without laxity of the perispinal ligaments; and (b) those who need decompression of the lumbar canal and in addition have instability deformity or lack of support due to a previous extensive surgical procedure. Instrumentation should be used not as a corrective device but to immobilize the spine in the desired physiologic position while an adequate arthrodesis matures.

### RATIONALE FOR THE GDLH SYSTEM DESIGN

The GDLH System permits incremental millimetric segmental translation. Its open, top-tightening connectors allow easy assembly, as do its adjustable component attachments. Finally, it is a universally applicable system with fewer components than other such systems.

The GDLH System has a 5-mm rod with offset engagement connectors that are equal in strength to a quarter-inch Cotrel or SRH soft rod. On testing all components of the GDLH System are equal to other existing systems on the market in parameters of rotation, tension, load, sheer, and slip. Parameters of stiffness and fatigue life are shown in Figs. 1–3 and Table 1.

**TABLE 1.** *GDLH hook fatigue testing*

| No. | Type of hook | Loading condition | No. of cycles |
| --- | --- | --- | --- |
| 1 | GDLH single | 10–150 lbf. | 500,000 no failure |
| 2 | GDLH single | 10–150 lbf. | 500,000 no failure |
| 3 | GDLH single | 10–150 lbf. | 500,000 no failure |
| 4 | GDLH single | 10–150 lbf. | 500,000 no failure |
| 5 | GDLH single | 10–150 lbf. | 1,000,000 no failure |
| 6 | C–D closed | 10–150 lbf. | 100,000 no failure |
| 7 | C–D closed | 10–150 lbf. | 200,000 no failure |
| 8 | C–D open | 10–150 lbf. | 1, hook slipped |
| 9 | C–D open | 10–150 lbf. | 1, hook slipped |

The main differences between the GDLH System and other existing systems are, first, that the GDLH System brings the spine to the bar. The claws and hooks (Figs. 4 and 5) are designed for translation rather than for distraction of compression as in all other systems (although distraction–compression hooks are available). The interpeduncular bolts (Fig. 6) are conical and self-locking, and permit some degree of orientation (with wedge wafers for easy assembly). The cross-links are designed for either a distraction or a compression modality. A multiangle screw can aid in cases that require awkward positioning. Finally, implants can be removed or added at any time throughout the procedure.

## PROCEDURE

After subperiosteal dissection and neurological procedures, a decision must be made about the use of hooks or interpeduncular screws. Screws should be used, when absolutely rigid fixation is required. Claw hooks can protect against screw loosening or breakage and can control transverse correction, rotational forces, and flexion–extension instability.

Screws and/or hooks (claw or, in distraction, compression) are put in place to maintain the position of the spine, corrected for the particular pathology. Rods are cut to size and bent to a physiologic curves. Connectors are preloaded and the rod

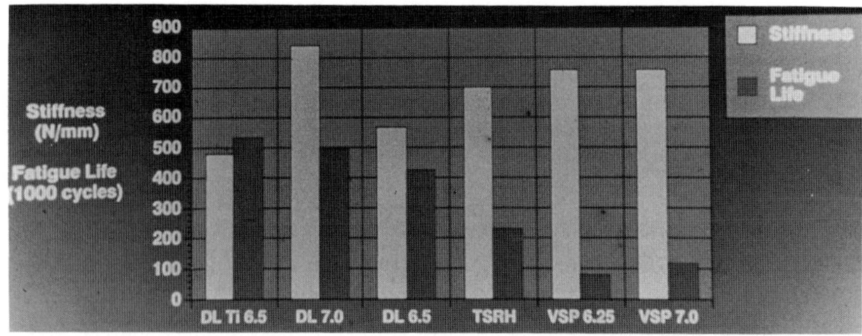


**FIG. 1.** Parameters of stiffness and fatigue life for the GDLH System (□, stiffness; ■, fatigue life).

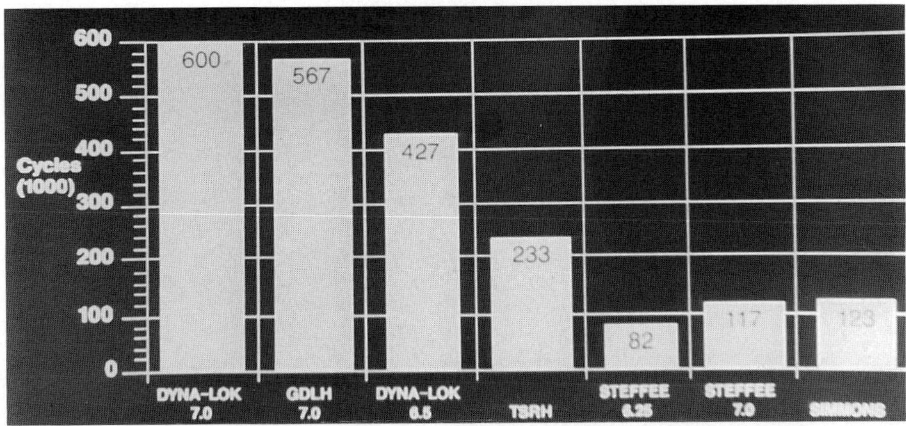

**FIG. 2.** GDLH bolt connector. Life under cyclic load compared to similar systems (loading, ±300 N axial).

shaped for size and form. Rod and connectors are then dropped over the top of the implants and tightened to maintain position (Fig. 7; see also Fig. 6). Next, incremental millimetric adjustment (or correction) is made, and finally the system is locked into place (Figs. 8 and 9). Any hook, screw, or crosslink can be added or removed at this time, as necessary (Fig. 10). Once the implants are in place, introducing the rods and connectors and locking them should not take more than 10 min (Fig. 11).

Despite the rigidity of the GDLH System and the ease of insertion, it is not a substitute for a careful, well-executed arthrodesis technique. Sacral fixation in degenerate pathology is usually obtained by large Dyna-lock bolts, inserted into the sacrum running in the sacral intervertebral plane.

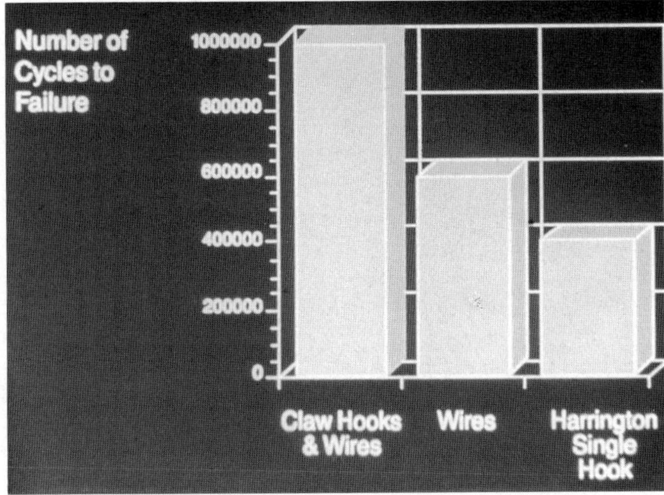

**FIG. 3.** Fatigue analysis, various configurations.

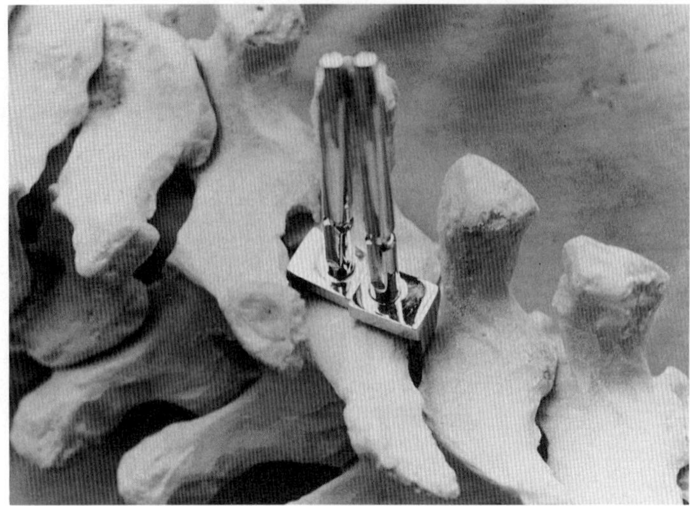

**FIG. 4.** Sublaminar insertion of double claw hook.

## CLINICAL EXPERIENCE

Between 1990 and 1994, 122 consecutive cases received the GDLH System, 72 women and 50 men. The diagnoses were stenosis of the neural canal with instability (81 patients) deformity (31), and pseudoarthrosis (10). The patients were followed for at least 16 months.

The GDLH System can be tailored to the individual patient. For the most part it is used for alignment and compression, and normal lordosis is always created. Dynalock bolts were used in the sacrum in 74 patients, as interpeduncular fixation in 76, and double claw hooks were used in 61 patients. There were 82 lumbosacral fusions, and the average number of spaces arthrodesed was three (range one to five).

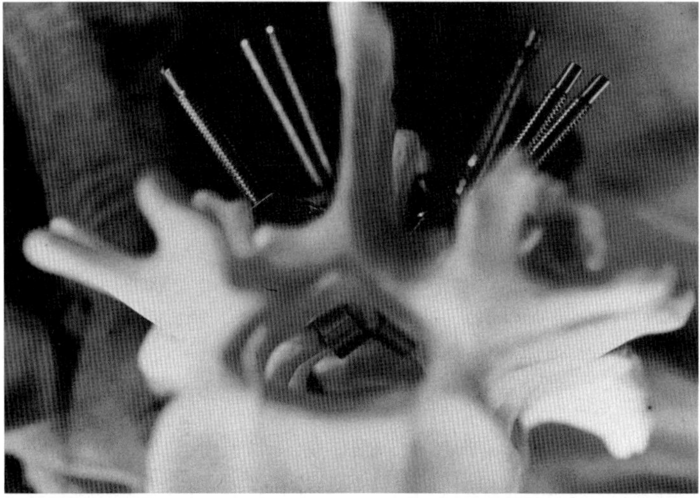

**FIG. 5.** Sagittal view of sublaminar double claw hooks.

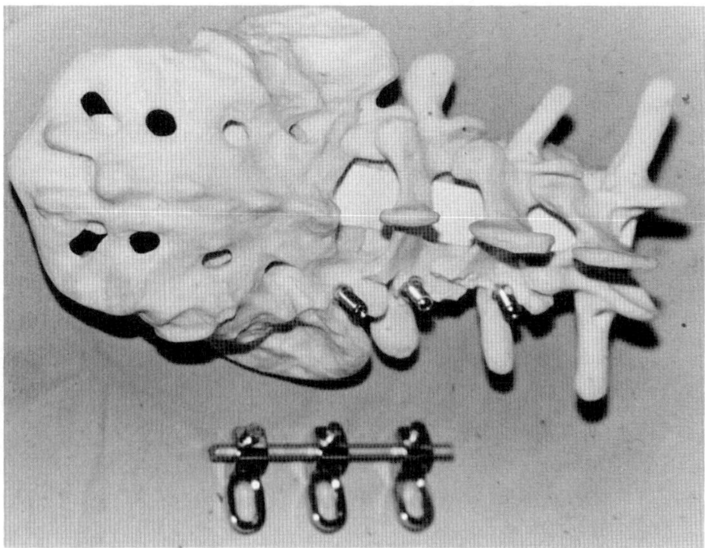

**FIG. 6.** One sacral screw and two interpeduncular screws in place, with rod and bolt connectors premounted on bar.

All cases were decorticated in the entire area of the instrumentation. Facetectomy was performed only when necessary. Autogenous graft was always used in the posterolateral suture. Anterior arthrodesis was not performed in any of these cases.

## Complications

A total of 32 patients experienced excessive bleeding (over 2,000 ml); the average blood loss was 1,200 ml. The surgical time ranged from 1 h and 30 min to 6 h. There were no intraoperative complications.

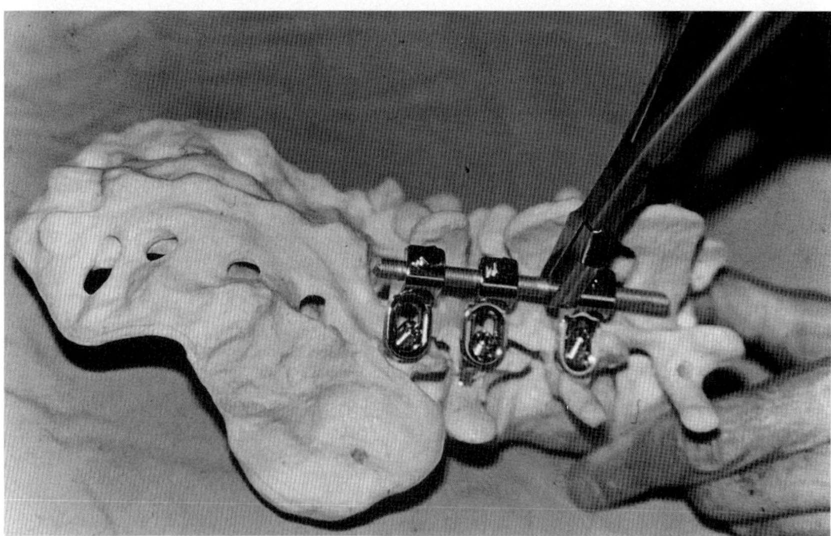

**FIG. 7.** Bar and rod connectors are placed overhead on Dyna-lock bolts.

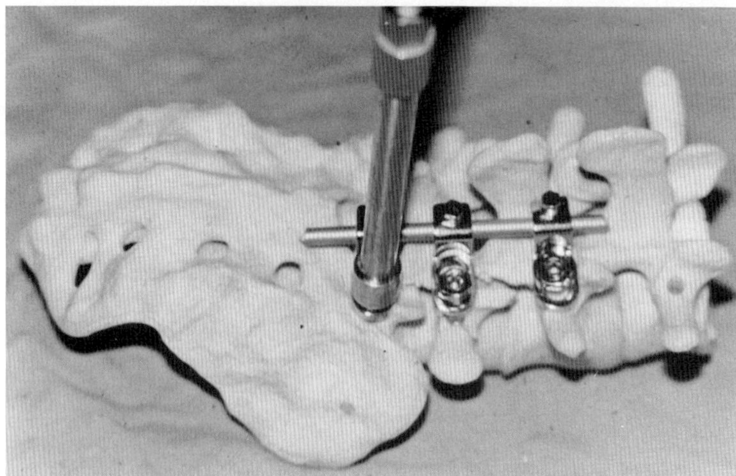

**FIG. 8.** Insertion of locknut over Dyna-lock bolts. The nut is tightened to 150 pounds.

A total of 24 patients experienced postoperative paresthesias that lasted from 2 weeks to 3 months. These patients were treated with mild mobilization and corticosteroids. Tomograms were taken of all the patients, and no visible evidence of encroachment was found. There was one proven pseudoarthrosis that was subsequently corrected in compression.

Eleven patients experienced minor infections that were corrected by debridement and antibiotics; none was severe enough to require removal of the implant. Medical complications in these patients included depressive symptoms, paralytic ileus, pneumonia, and thrombophlebitis, none of which had any lasting consequences. Ten patients had their instrumentation removed after a year, mostly because of minor pain.

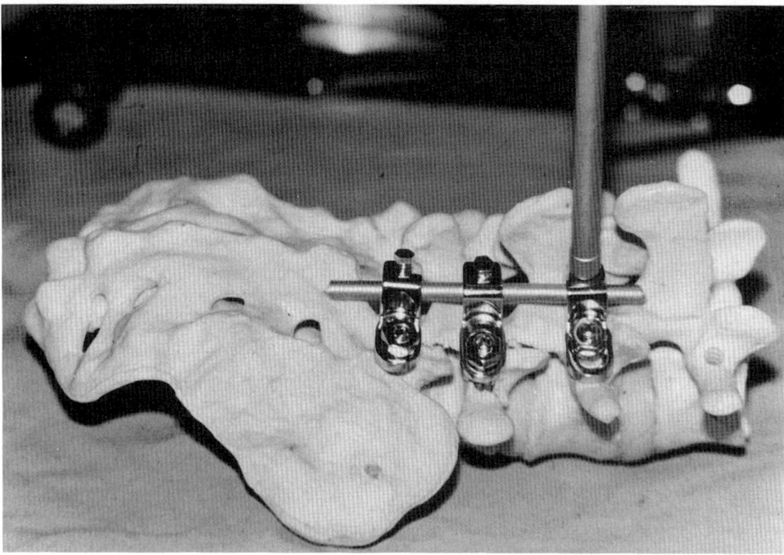

**FIG. 9.** Bolt connector, head screw tightened to 80 pounds, and engaging rod.

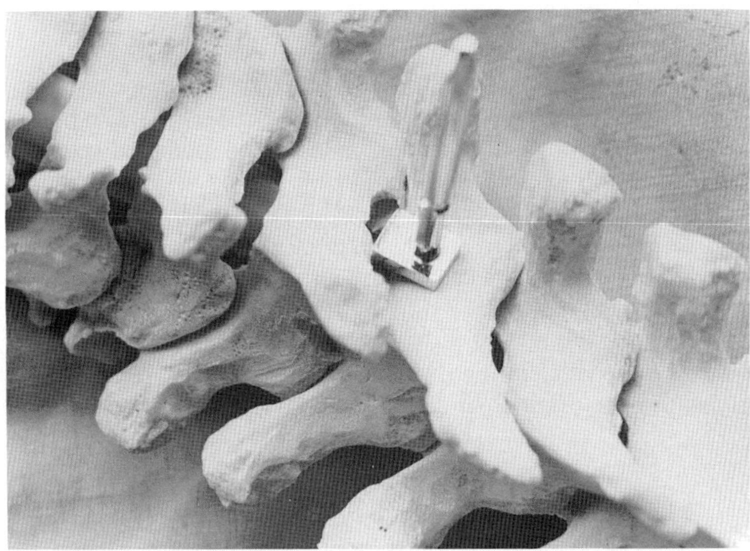

**FIG. 10.** A single sublaminar hook can be inserted at any time during the procedure.

Preoperatively, patients graded their pain and discomfort on a scale from 0 to 10 at an average of 8.3. On final postoperative follow-up the range was 0 to 7, with an average of 3.2. Neurologic signs had coverted to normal in 79 patients at final follow-up.

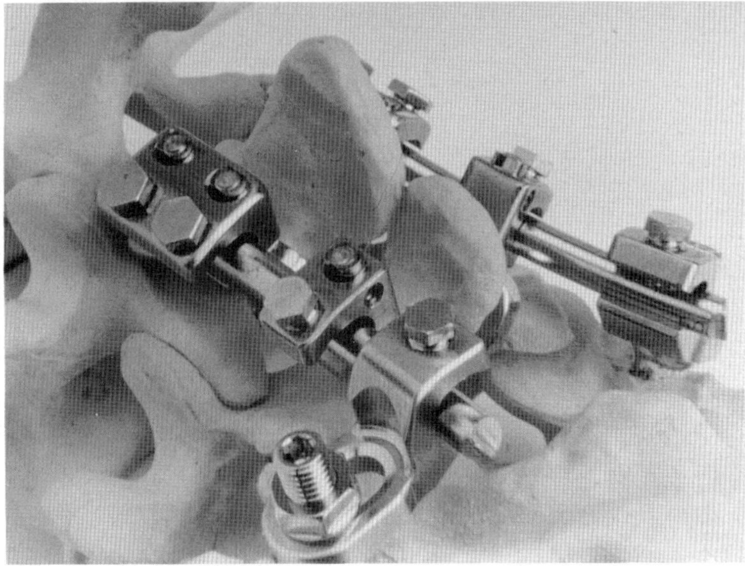

**FIG. 11.** System in place. Dyna-lock bolts are in S1, a single sublaminar compression hook at L5, and a sublaminar double hook on L4. Note that the L3–L4 facet joint has not been disturbed.

## DISCUSSION

In short instrumentation of the lumbar spine, no crosslink is necessary unless more than three spaces are covered. A single sacral screw appears adequate in these short fusions. Longer fusions may need to be extended to the ilium and stabilized at L5 or L4 with instrumentation in compression. Double claw hooks are slightly less rigid than interpeduncular screws but are excellent for applying forces such as translation and flexion–extension movements (for control of lordosis).

The GDLH System not only is easy to use but is the only system approved on the market that brings the spine to the rod in millimetric increments, making final placement mechanical and simple. The capability for addition or removal of implants at any time during the instrumentation adds an advantage for correction, stabilization, or reinforcement of the original strategy at any given moment.

## CONCLUSION

The GDLH System performs equally well in degenerate lumbar pathology as any other recognized method. The fact that it is easier to insert is translated into less operative time and, consequently, fewer complications.

The fact that not all patients were totally cured can be attributed to other factors, such as age, generalized arthritis, diabetes, or chronic smoking. Certainly, our low rate of pseudoarthrosis shows that the GDLH System is an efficient adjunct for producing an arthrodesis.

*Instrumented Fusion of the Degenerative Lumbar Spine: State of the Art, Questions, and Controversies*, edited by M. Szpalski, R. Gunzburg, D. M. Spengler, and A. Nachemson. Lippincott–Raven Publishers, Philadelphia © 1996.

# 12

# Diapason Posterior Spinal Osteosynthesis in Degenerative Pathology

P. Lapresle and G. Missenard

*Clinique Arago, 75014 Paris, France*

The Diapason Posterior Spinal Osteosynthesis was designed in 1987 and the first patients were operated on in October of 1988. The purpose of this device was to associate the advantages of transpedicular fixation with a rod linkage. Transpedicular fixation, promoted for 25 years and popularized worldwide by Roy-Camille (5,12,13) may be segmental, is always possible even after a large laminectomy, and is mechanically interesting because the pedicle is located in the middle of the vertebrae. Its efficiency has been demonstrated by routine use in traumatic and tumor pathologies. Nevertheless, it appeared that the plates were not the most convenient system in cases of degenerative disease. They were difficult to fit in view of the very different interpedicular spaces and lumbosacral shapes among the patient population. Moreover, the plates provided good fixation but had a poor reduction effect. Rods, on the other hand, offer the greatest possibility for individual adjustment. Dubousset (2,7,10) described the results that could be obtained by distraction, contraction, and sagittalization to reduce extremely severe deformities. However, rods were used exclusively with hooks because this method derived from scoliosis surgery. Surgery in degenerative pathologies, with its need for frequent decompressions and corrections of slight or more severe deformities, appeared to require both screws and rods.

Increasing interest in new imaging, such as computed tomography (CT) scanning and magnetic resonance imaging (MRI), has led to a preference for titanium over stainless steel. Titanium is particularly appreciated for the semi-rigidity of 6–mm-diameter rods, which appear to provide a good compromise between the stiffness necessary to correct deformities and the elasticity required because bones are often porous. Titanium is also preferred for its special compatibility with bone, as already demonstrated by long-term applications in other fields, such as stomatology. Nevertheless, titanium has been criticized for its lack of resistance to friction, resulting in the release of metallic dust. This metallosis might cause some side effects that are not yet clearly identified.

Examinations have demonstrated that titanium spinal implants are very well tolerated when the graft has fused, as long as there is no movement among the various parts of the device. We did, however, observe some metallosis in a small area around locations of mechanical problems, such as blocker loosenings or rare rod breakages. This metallosis was in all cases much more restricted than that observed during revision of some titanium total hip or knee prostheses, and we have not noted any clinical consequences. Nevertheless, in view of the doubts concerning the long-term effects of this complication, we suggest removing titanium implants when x-rays show any mobility between two pieces. Moreover, to meet the very specific requirements of different spinal pathologies, the Diapason, like other devices, should be available in stainless steel (for young patients, scoliosis, or lytic spondylolisthesis) when the device is intended to stay in place for many decades and in titanium (for tumors, trauma, and degenerative diseases) when MRI postoperative control is essential.

## IMPLANTS

Difficulties encountered in training with other systems, which involved too many implants and highly specific ancillary items, convinced us that the Diapason had to be very simple. Screws are usually of only one length (40 mm in lumbar), as it was considered that only transpedicular crossing provided significant strength. The five screws used are different only in their transpedicular part: the diameters increase from 4 mm in thoracic to 6.7 and 7.7 mm in lumbar and 8 and 9 mm in sacrum. This diameter is measured below the screw head, as the screws are conical. This shape was initially criticized for the risk of immediate loosening if screwing back is required. However, it was chosen because of the very specific situation of the transpedicular screw, which is quite exceptional in orthopedic surgery: Stresses on pedicular screws are different from those on cortical screws, which cross two cortices in all cases, and cancellous bone screws, which are always quite low in strength. Although pedicular screws penetrate some cancellous bone, they are surrounded by cortical bone. A slightly conical shape was chosen to increase the press–fit effect of the screw's core throughout its length. Of course, an adequate diameter is required and the screw must be set at the correct depth without any possibility of unscrewing. All the screw heads are similar, and their shape led to the name ''Diapason'' which means ''tuning fork.'' The U-shaped head receives inside a hexagonal-holed blocker and outside a cap to prevent the two arms from spreading apart. This cap makes it possible to apply very high torque to the blockers. At the same time, the cap is self-secured. Rods are smooth surfaced to facilitate reduction maneuvers. They end in a hexagonal hole that provides the rod handles with great derotation efficiency.

Ancillary devices were initially reduced to a screwdriver, a blocker driver, and a rod bender. All the other necessary instruments were presumed to be available in a general orthopedic operating room. Year after year, a more complete range of instruments was added to the ancillary box, including distraction forceps, contraction forceps, derotation keys and, more recently, a screw blocker that makes it possible to apply a very high torque while the blocker is tightened.

In February of 1990, the Diapason was significantly improved by the design of the ball-ring. This is a small sphere around the rod, one for each screw, which gives the possibility of a 30° angle between rod and screws (Fig. 1). During the first 2 years,

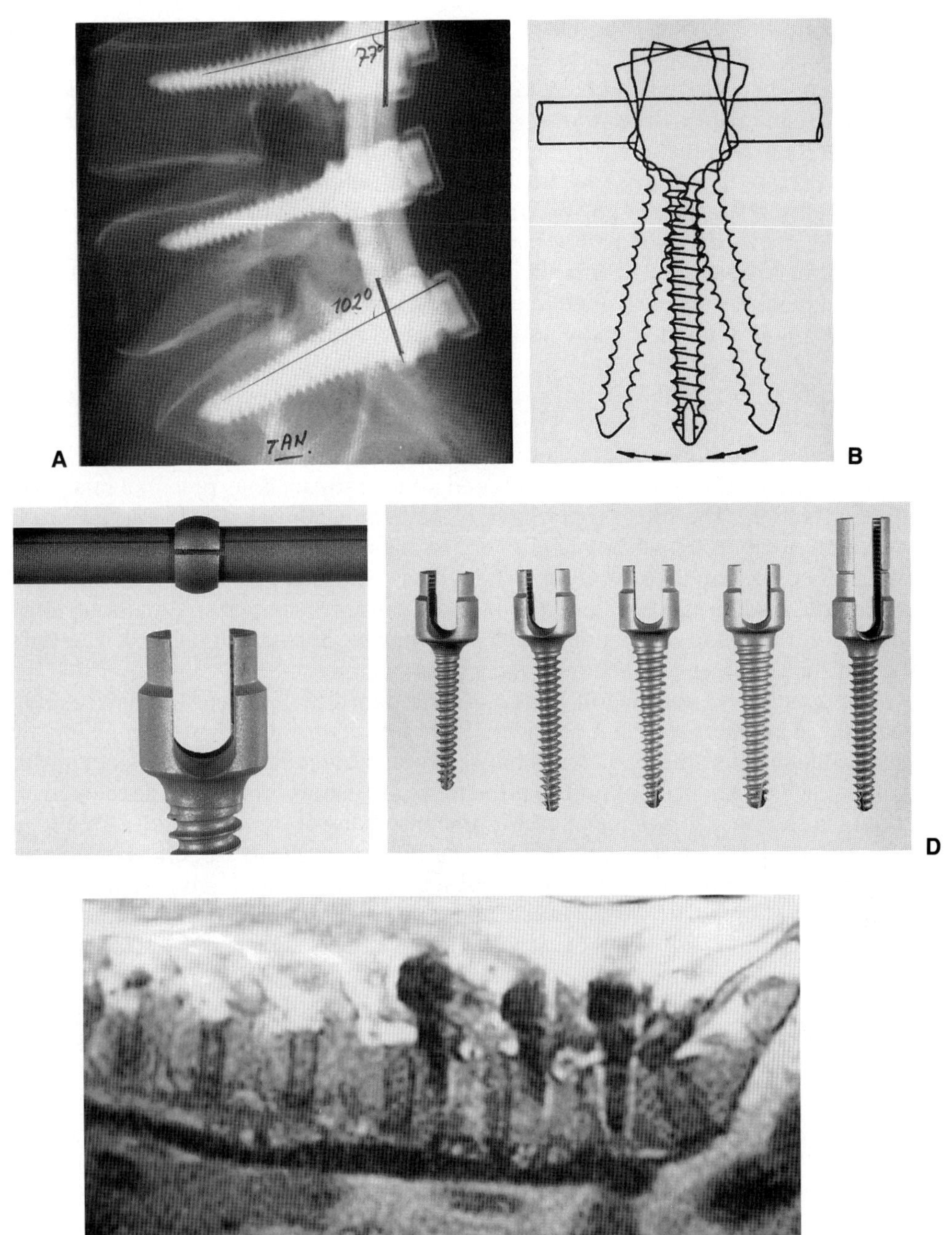

**FIG. 1.** **A:** In the lumbosacral area, rod–screw angulation is rarely strictly 90°. **B:** Diapason allows a 30° rod–screw angulation. **C:** A ball-ring around the rod provides angulation. **D:** Thoracic, lumbar, and two sacral screws are commonly used. Long-armed screws are employed to reduce SPL and in any case of long fusion. In scoliosis concavities, they provide an efficient pull-back effect. **E:** Foraminal RMI lecture always remains possible, even with implanted transpedicular titanium screws.

like many other devices, the Diapason blocker could be locked only in a strictly perpendicular position. Because this configuration is very rare in the lumbosacral area, even when the rod had been meticulously bent either the blocker could not be properly tightened or there was stress bending of the screws, with a high risk for fatigue fractures in the implant. The mechanical results demonstrated that this concept was valid. From a screw fracture rate of approximately 8% when the first orthogonal screws were used, we observed only one screw breakage in over 1,100 angulated screws implanted for straightforward degenerative pathologies. Moreover, the ball-ring appeared to absorb micromobility between screws and rods, so that the loosened blockers that had sometimes been observed in 1989–1990 also disappeared. The ball-ring is actually the key point of the device and constitutes its main advantage.

All screws, except the sacral screws, are available either with normal heads or with easy-to-break long arms. These were initially designed to reduce displaced spondylolisthesis, following the long-threaded-head corkscrew of Dr. Roy-Camille. These long-armed screws were soon found to have tremendous potential in all types of long fixation. The rods do not have to be bent accurately for the screws to fit. Moreover, long-armed screws have a very strong reduction power in scoliosis, as the rod is less bent than the curvature. When the system is implanted in the deformity's concavity, gradual tightening of the blocker causes an impressive pull-out effect, which contributes to derotation of apical vertebrae. Sagittalization or derotation of the rod then achieves reduction in the normal manner.

More recently (2 years ago), hooks were designed to complete the device. For 5 years these implants were not considered as a priority for many reasons, mainly that of maintaining the transpedicular philosophy and avoiding any nonsegmental long fixation, which might be unsafe with semi-rigid titanium rods. We developed this project in response to comments from surgeons, many of whom are still afraid to use thoracic pedicular fixations above T10, especially in scoliosis surgery. However, as described below, this fixation may well be as safe as in the lumbar spine. From a mechanical standpoint, we observed that screws and hooks can be employed not only as competitors but together, according to their specific qualities. To summarize, a screw may avoid the medial or lateral slippage of an adjacent subpedicular or laminar hook. Conversely, a hook will be more efficient than a screw for dealing with distraction or contraction stresses, because in this situation a transpedicular screw may loosen. Simultaneous use of screws and hooks had already been developed by J. Dubousset in thoracolumbar fractures after he observed some early screw breakages (2,3). Only nine hooks were designed so that the device would remain reliable even if used by less highly trained surgical teams. Most of the hooks are offset, following the idea of a combined use with pedicular screws. Because hooks offer natural mobility, the ball-ring is not employed. Its omission reduced bulk by 3 mm and consequently made it possible to design very "low-profile" implants. The hooks are all made with long arms. An efficient push-down effect on the rods can be obtained without any need for many sophisticated, unstable forceps.

Initial clinical reports in 1991 clearly determined that the device's earlier problems had been completely eliminated. The only problem noted with any significant frequency was loosening around some screws. Some of these were obviously related to a pseudoarthrosis but, in many cases, loosening appeared within the first months after the operation and did not prevent later fusion. Loosening was most commonly seen in the sacrum, specifically in connection with certain critical mechanical situations: old age with its bone porosity, long fixations with excessive loading on S1 screws, and lytic spondylolisthesis, with its specific instability and well-known difficulty in fusing. Nevertheless, the principle of only two screws in the sacrum should be discussed. Many prototypes were designed to provide a multipoint sacral fixation. This implant had to be efficient and safe but not too bulky, to avoid local pain and to leave enough room for grafting. Unfortunately, biomechanical tests did not show an increasing resistance to fatigue tests. We now apply C. Argenson's findings on S1 screws. He demonstrated after many pull-out tests that optimal location was just below the S1 plateau, parallel to the disc, with a 15° convergency. The goal is to reach a stronger bone than that inside the sacral wing. Nevertheless, there is still a critical 3-month gap between the implantation of the device and the fusion of the graft. For this reason, on the basis of successful results of hydroxyapatite (HA)-coated acetabular components, some Diapason screws were coated with HA. A first series was reported in 1994 after a 2-year experiment (8). The selected 29 patients each had one factor against fusion. The conclusions were that HA appeared to represent a real improvement for normally loaded screws (porousness and lytic spondylolisthesis) but not for overstressed screws (e.g., distal screws with very long fixations, lumbosacral arthrodesis below former fusions). Sacral fixation in these extreme situations remains a pending issue.

Fixation of HA screws on dog vertebrae was recently studied by Matsuzaki and colleagues (12). HA screws were compared to normal Diapason screws, stainless steel screws, and titanium porous-coating screws. A total of 120 screws were implanted. Dogs were sacrificed immediately or at 2, 4, 6, or 8 weeks after operation. The torque necessary to extract screws was measured and a histologic examination was performed on the bone–screw interface. The results confirmed what we hoped: HA coating improved the quality of screw fixation. Histologically, the fibrous gap observed between implant and bone was narrower with titanium screws than with stainless steel. This is evidence of titanium's excellent bone compatibility. Moreover, no fibrous gap could be seen at 6 weeks with HA-coated screws, in which newly formed bone tissue was first observed only 2 weeks after implantation.

Logically, the force required to remove HA Diapason screws was greater than for normal screws (and much greater than for stainless steel screws). The difference was 1.5-fold 2 weeks after implantation and increased to 2.4-fold after 8 weeks.

These experimental data suggest that, to be efficient, HA-coated screws must maintain excellent and complete primary stability for at least the first 3 to 4 weeks.

## BIOMECHANICS

The Diapason was biomechanically tested in different countries (12). This revealed a particular type of behavior which may limit its indications. After the blocker was tightened, the average force necessary to achieve a displacement along the rod was very high. Conversely, it was easier to observe a flexion–extension or rotation displacement. This suggests that the ball-ring–rod union is very strong but that the ball–ring–screw union is somewhat weaker. Consequently, the Diapason probably has some degree of adaptability after tightening, which is a positive factor in degenerative pathologies because it protects the device from excessive stresses. Conversely, a too-short fixation could lead to some loss of correction in lordosis in cases of severe anterior instability (tumor or traumatic). In these situations, additional anterior stabilization must be provided or a posterior long fixation must be performed (1–3).

## PROCEDURE

Because transpedicular fixation is now in worldwide use, it is unnecessary to describe it. We will merely point out some details that make screw implants as safe as total hip prosthesis replacements (14,15).

In lumbar cases, the point of entry is chosen more medially than the beginning of the transverse process but at the same level. The small cortical crest below the facet joint is removed with the rongeur to reveal the cancellous bone of the pedicle. The hole is initiated with a big brad-awl to avoid drilling in the wrong direction. The hole itself is made with long curved hemostatic forceps (Bengolea) by turning on itself and crushing cancellous bone rather than pushing down. The concavity of the Bengolea is turned to the canal to fit with the convergence of the pedicles. A small elastic, ball-ended pin tests the path; bone must be felt everywhere. A thoracic screw is driven in to transform the curved path into a straight one and to determine the porousness of the bone. Then the definitive lumbar screw (6.7 and 7.7 mm) is positioned at the correct depth (all thread must be hidden in the bone) with the proper orientation.

In thoracic cases, the pedicle's point of entry is located below the joint, at the upper third of the transverse process. Cortical bone must be removed with a rongeur from a 1-cm$^2$ surface. Then subjacent cancellous bone is carefully removed with a small neurosurgical curette, following the medial wall of the pedicle. One centimeter deeper, the vertebral body is reached. The hole may be enlarged using Bengolea forceps (until T6–T7) or with the thoracic screw itself. The hole is checked with the elastic tester once more before fixation of the implant. In the sacrum, the point of entry is just below the facet joint. The direction of the screw must be 15° convergent.

Positioning the rod does not normally present any difficulty. The blocker must be engaged in exactly the right direction. After reduction maneuvers, the screw must be locked in position with the special instrument to avoid pedicle breakage or a rightward sliding of the upper vertebra. X-rays are not usually performed before the incision is closed.

According to specific different spinal situations and pathologies, some details may be helpful. In lumbosacral arthrodesis, we usually use a distraction of about 2 mm before ultimate locking in order to open the foramina of the root. In very short fixations, a windshield wiper effect may be observed, resulting from a rightward translation of the upper vertebra while the blocker is firmly tightened. An oblique transverse union system may provide greater rigidity to the construct.

In grades I, II, or III lytic spondylolisthesis, we always begin with a typical Gill procedure and a full bilateral root release. Then we fix with or without reduction. Fixation is proposed essentially to improve the fusion rate (grade I or II) or to restore a better lumbosacral shape (grade III). The disc must have a significant thickness and the bone must be sufficiently firm. Complete disc collapse or severe osteoporosis is a contraindication to reduction. If fixation is proposed without reduction, the length of the arthrodesis must be as short as possible (L4–L5 or L5–S1) (Figs. 2 and 3) after an MRI determines the quality of adjacent discs. If arthrodesis is proposed with reduction (Fig. 4), we think that, in the great majority of cases, a three-point fixation is more efficient than the two-point system. Long-armed screws are implanted in the olisthetic vertebra. The diameter must be very carefully chosen, as it will have to bear a very high pull-out stress. Usually, 7.7-mm lumbar screws are more often employed than 6.7 mm. Normal-headed screws are implanted in other vertebrae. HA

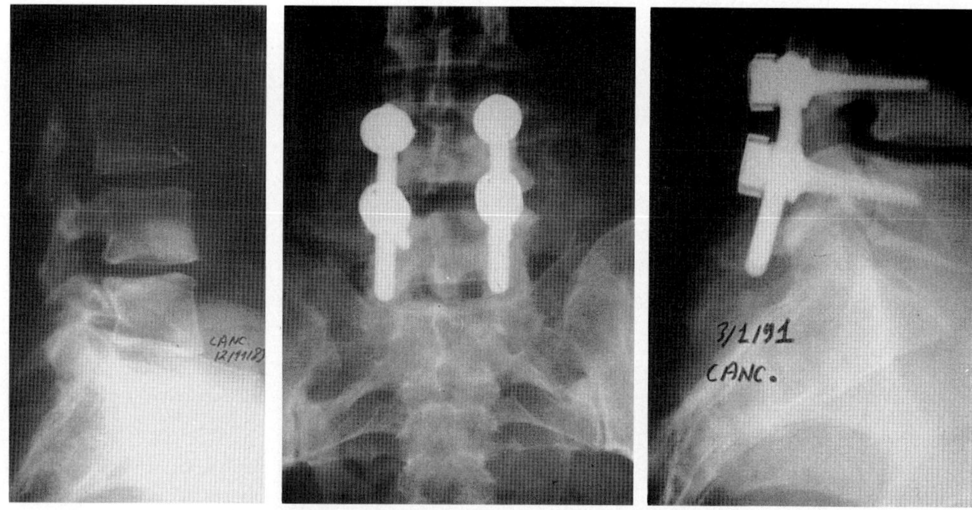

**FIG. 2. A–C:** L4–L5 fusion for low back pain on postdiscectomy discopathy.

screws are currently employed exclusively in the sacrum. Rods are bent so as to allow a maximal 1.5-cm pull-back. Simultaneously and mainly for an L5–S1 SPL (Fig. 5), both progressive distraction and blocker tightening will achieve the reduction. Root control must be constant during this stage. Once the blockers are locked, the long-armed screws are broken.

In every case, we must insist on the mandatory quality of the graft. It requires good decortication of the transverse process and sacral wings and a plentiful amount of cancellous bone fragments. In cases of extensive reduction, we believe that an associated PLIF may increase stability and fusion rate.

Lumbar degenerative scoliosis is one of the best indications for Diapason fixation. According to the Cobb angle, balance or imbalance of the trunk, and age of the patient, it is advisable to perform short or long fixations. Short fixations (L3–sacrum or L2–L5, for example) may be proposed when stenosis is in the clinical foreground, the patient is older than 70–75 years, and the main curvature's Cobb angle is less than 30°. Associated with a highly focused laminectomy or fenestration led by the myelogram, the main goal of fixation is to avoid destabilization induced by laminectomy. Nevertheless, in many cases a partial reduction can be obtained by derotation of rods and distraction of the lumbosacral concavity. This distraction must be carried out using a very "lordotic bent" rod to avoid creating a flat back.

Long fixations are more logical and widely used in scoliosis surgery. This involves younger patients (50–75 years) whose increasing deformity is in the foreground (while signs of stenosis are in the background) and in whom the main curvature's Cobb angle is greater than 30–35° (Fig. 6). Although the border between former idiopathic and degenerative de novo scoliosis is not clear, long fixations are indicated for the first type. Reduction efficiency is improved by segmental fixation (which reduces the risk for implant loosening), the pull-back effect of long-armed screws in the concavity and the sagittalization of the rods.

If a fenestration is necessary, this operation may be performed in two stages, 1 week apart (decompression and fixation on the first day, full spine x-rays at the sixth day, and improvement of balance correction and graft at the seventh day). A per-

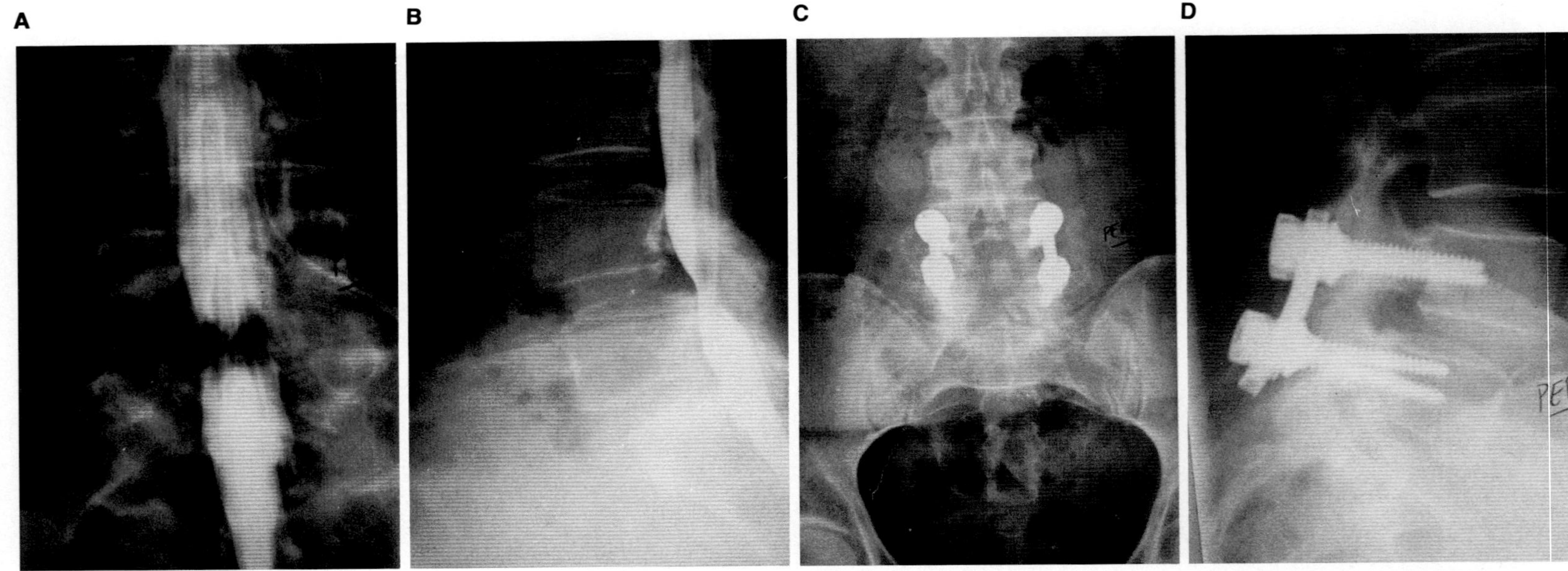


**FIG. 3. A–D:** L4–L5 fusion and laminectomy on stenosis determined by a degenerative spondylolisthesis.

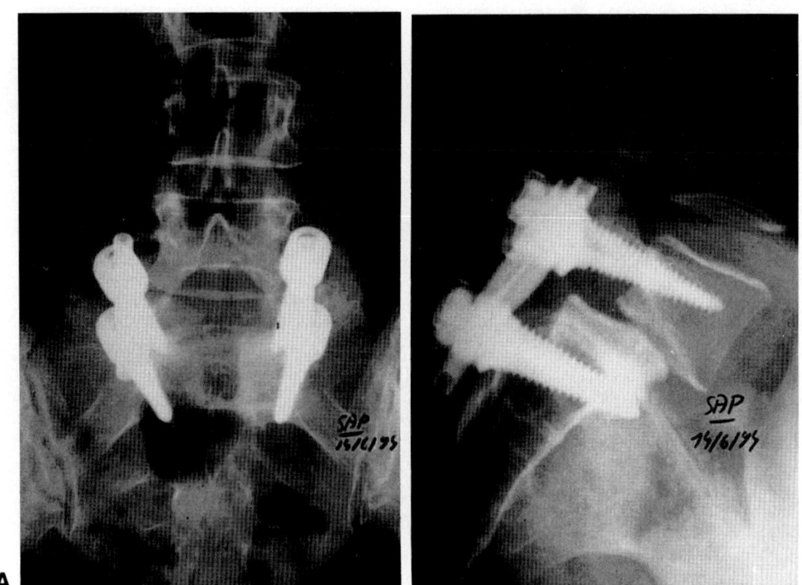

**FIG. 4. A,B:** In situ L5–S1 fusion for arthrotic lytic spondylolisthesis.

sonal report of 45 cases reviewed in 1993 (9) showed that this type of long fixation, even in old age, could provide over 70% reductions. Conversely, short fixations appeared to have mainly a stabilization effect but did not correct any imbalance. In addition, correction and main concavity did not exceed 40%.

## INDICATIONS

Indications for fixation in degenerative pathology are highly controversial (4,10, 13,14). Arguments against surgical fusion include: useless (arthrosis will restabilize

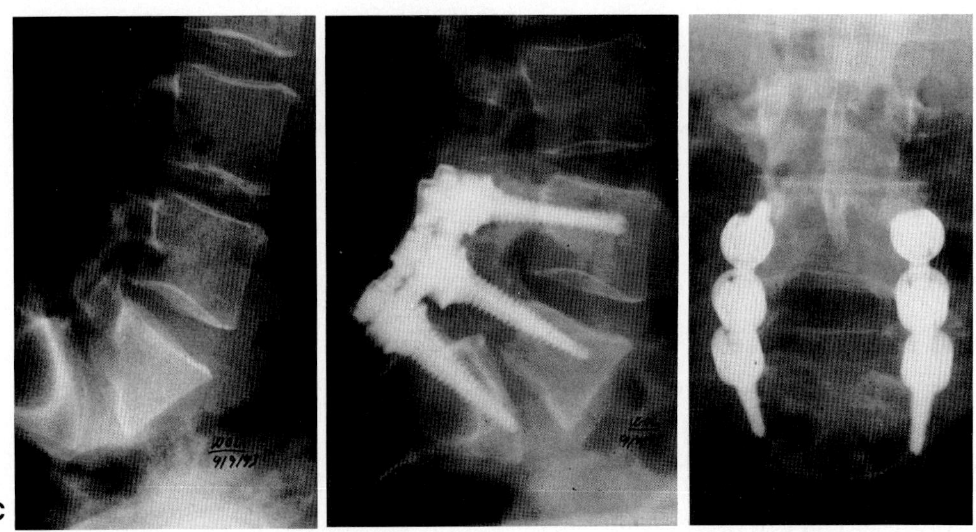

**FIG. 5. A–C:** L4–S1 fusion with reduction for a grade II lytic SPL.

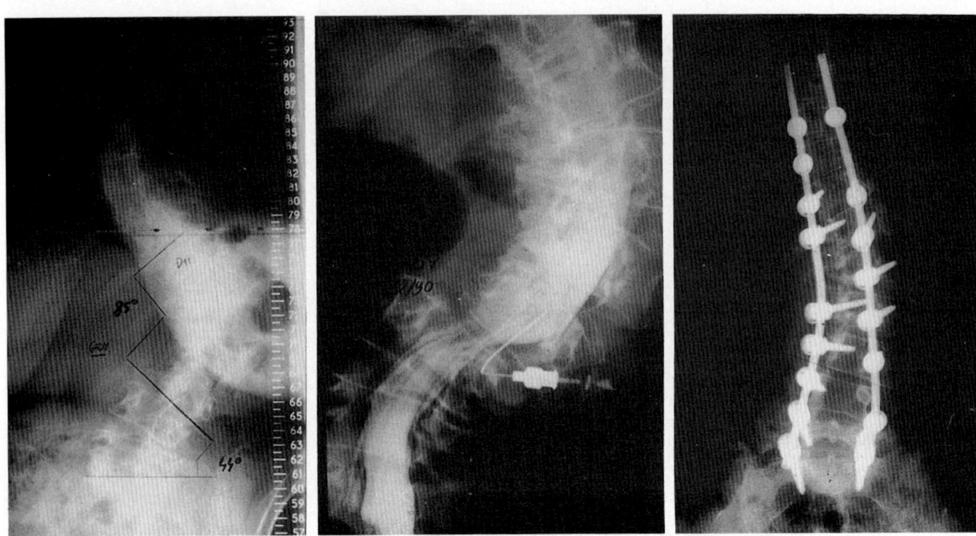

**FIG. 6. A–C:** Former idiopathic thoracolumbar scoliosis with stenosis at dislocation level in a 66-year-old patient, with treatment by L3–L4 laminectomy and T8-sacrum arthrodesis. Curvature was reduced from 85° to 31°.

sooner or later), dangerous (perioperative complications), frequently disappointing (bad functional results after long arthrodesis), or potentially iatrogenic (early degeneration of new junctional levels). After 12 years of experience, we believe that the majority of these criticisms are valid. However, perioperative morbidity can be reduced by better training. We now consider that there are only four indisputable indications for fusion with fixation in degenerative pathology. Three of them must be very short fixations (two or three vertebrae): lytic spondylolisthesis with root pain, degenerative spondylolisthesis with signs of stenosis (Fig. 7) and a thick disc (if collapsed, there is almost no risk of increased slippage), and at least some very rare primary or postinvasive-treatment one-level discopathies with disabling low back pain and good adjacent discs. A similar indication in cases of degenerative spondylolisthesis is fusion for synovial facet joint cyst. One indication for long fixation is also indisputable, in our opinion: lumbar stenosis on scoliosis with a Cobb angle greater than 30°, in cases where the patient's age and good general condition permit this type of surgery (Fig. 8).

We believe that there are hardly any indications for the four- or five-vertebra fixations in uncomplicated degenerative pathology and that these fixations were performed too frequently in the 1990s.

## RESULTS

The first 278 Diapason Posterior Spinal Osteosynthesis on straightforward degenerative spinal pathology (October of 1988 to July of 1994) were recently reviewed. A total of 252 patients were correctly followed. They had a total of 257 fixations, as five had undergone two operations. Primary indications were lumbalgia in 63, fixation on stenosis in 152, and lytic spondylolisthesis in 37. The average preoperative Beaujon functional score (10) was 10.5/20. A total of 64 were a single arthrodesis; 193 were

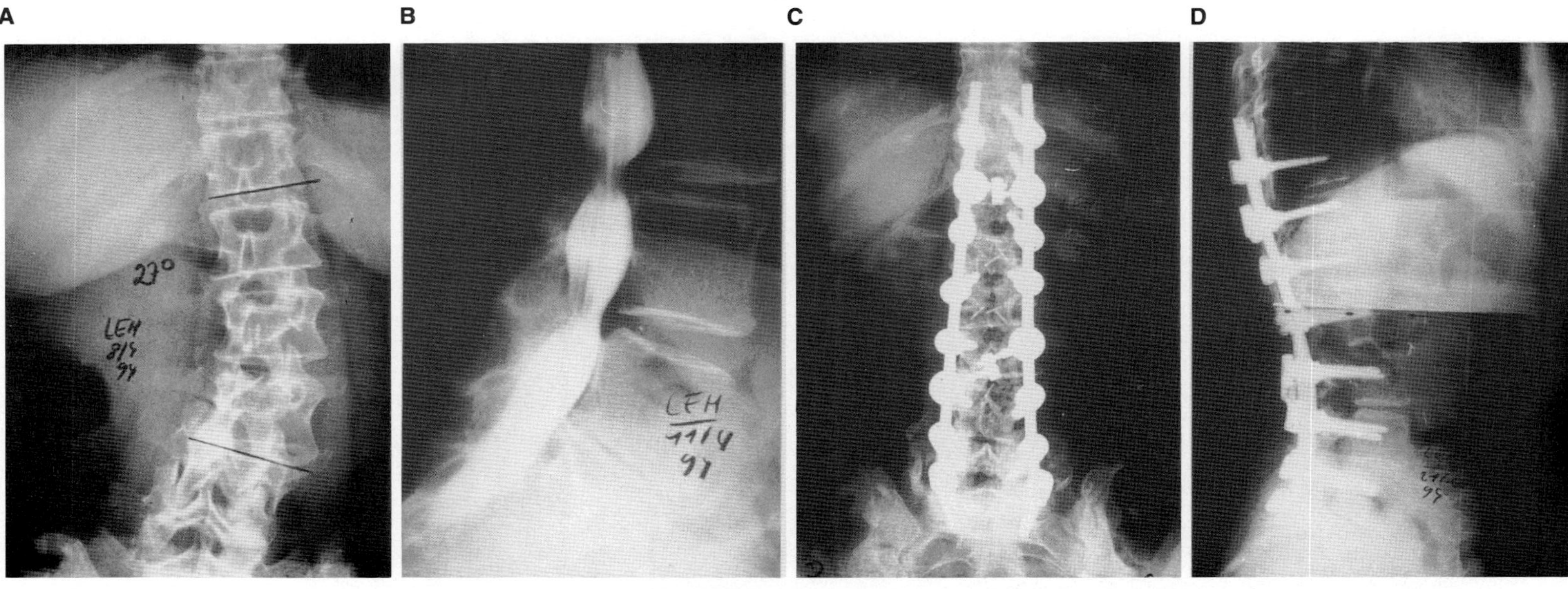

**FIG. 7. A–D:** Degenerative lumbar scoliosis with stenosis on myelogram. T10–sacrum arthrodesis, Cobb angle reduced from 27° to 5° with good lateral and sagittal balances.

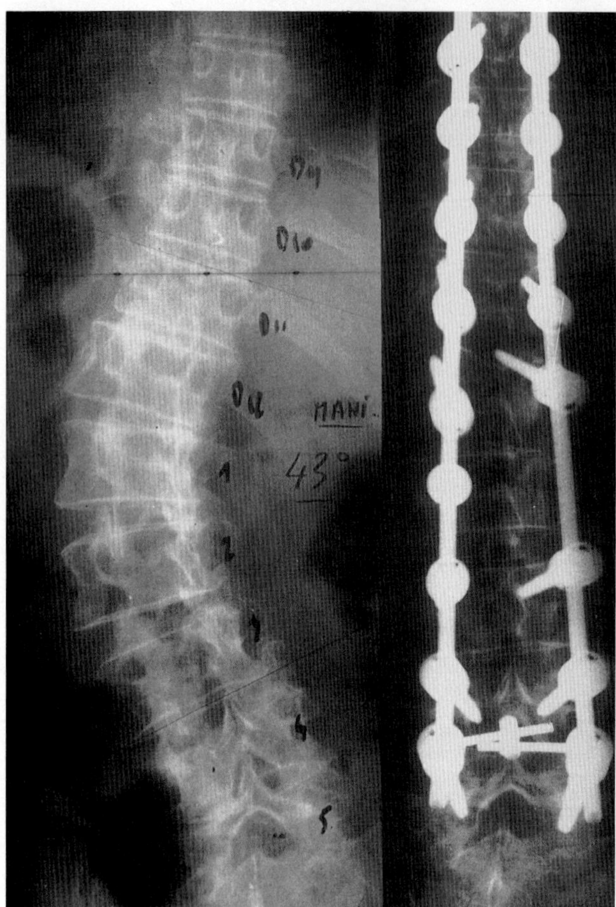

**Fig. 8.** A 43° degenerative lumbar scoliosis in a 59-year-old patient. Complete reduction with a segmental Diapason fixation.

associated with decompression. Length of arthrodesis was two vertebrae in 114 cases, three in 112, four in 22, five in five, and six in four cases. A total of 93 were float arthrodesis; 164 were lumbosacral arthrodesis. Grafts were exclusively autologous (iliac crest or product of laminectomy) and were posteriorly or posterolateraly located. Finally, 37 fixations were made using the Diapason system without angulation (Mark I) and 220 using the Diapason with angulation, after March of 1990 (Mark II). The mean follow-up was 32.6 months (range 12–72 months). Average postoperative functional score was 17.6/20. An interesting aspect is the percentage of functional improvement (Functional Benefit, FB) that patients could expect from surgery

$$(FB = Postop\ score\ -\ Preop\ score)/20\ -\ Preop\ score$$

Over 70% is an excellent result (E); between 40 and 70% is good (G); between 10 and 40% is insufficient (I); and below 10% is a failure (F). Our results were as follows: E = 165 (64%), G = 70 (27%), I = 18 (7%), and F = 4 (2%). The various pathologies gave quite similar functional results. The average functional scores were 17–17.6/20. FB ranged from 51% for revisions to 68% for lumbalgia and 75% for lytic SPL and fixations for stenosis (Table 1).

**TABLE 1.** *Functional benefit*

| Pathology | Results | | | |
|---|---|---|---|---|
| | Failure | Insufficient | Good | Excellent |
| General | 4 | 18 | 70 | 165 |
| ($n$ = 257) | (2%) | (7%) | (27%) | (64%) |
| Lumbalgia | 2 | 7 | 19 | 35 |
| ($n$ = 63) | (3%) | (11%) | (30%) | (56%) |
| Lytic SPL | 1 | 2 | 8 | 26 |
| ($n$ = 37) | (3%) | (5%) | (22%) | (70%) |
| Fixation on stenosis | 1 | 8 | 41 | 102 |
| ($n$ = 152) | (0.6%) | (5%) | (27%) | (67%) |
| Reoperation ($n$ = 5) | — | 1 | 2 | 2 |

Fusion was probably obtained in 240 cases (93.4%). There was some doubt in three cases, and 14 cases certainly had pseudoarthrosis. Early complications were observed in 17 cases and none in 240 (93.4%). Eight were perioperative (five dural tears, two asymptomatic extrapedicular screws, and one S1 symptomatic too laterally placed screw). Nine were immediately postoperative: six transient pains or paresis related to monoradicular root decompression and three infections (two leading to removal of the device).

No mechanical complications were noted in 228 cases (89%). One or more were reported in 29 instances. In 11 they were related to the device (three blocker loosenings, four screw breakages, three rod breakages, and two transverse rod breakages, of which two were on the same construct). In 18 they were related to many factors (two L4 screws loosened and 16 S1 screws loosened). All of the loosened screws, some of which were observed only several weeks after fixation, did not signify pseudoarthrosis, as was demonstrated in some cases by a thick posterolateral graft and by late spontaneous interbody fusion. A total of 21 patients underwent revision surgery (six of them for pseudoarthrosis).

## DISCUSSION

Our results demonstrated a significant relationship between mechanical failures and the possibility of angulation: 8 cases/37 D Mark 1 (21.6%) versus 3/220 D Mark 2 (1.4%) ($p$ = 0.001). We noted only one breakage among 1,147 implanted screws in the Diapason with a ball-ring (D Mark 2). Only loosenings in porotic bone continued to be observed (15 of 220 = 6.8%). The fusion rate is related to obviously known factors. These are mainly pathology, arthrodesis level, and possibly laminectomy and, consequently, the location of the graft.

The most interesting factor appears to be the nature of the pathology. We observed only 29 sure fusions among 37 lytic spondylolisthesis (78.4%). This should be compared with 95 and 96% for lumbalgia (60 of 63) and fixations on stenosis (146 of 152), respectively ($p$ = 0.01) (4). The second is the location of the arthrodesis. No pseudoarthrosis was noted among 93 lumbar float arthrodeses. Conversely, 17 lumbosacral arthrodeses (17 of 164 = 10%) presented a possible (3) or certain (14) pseudoarthrosis. All concerned the L5–S1 level ($p$ = 0.006). L5 laminectomy that requires a single posterolateral graft, without a posterior graft, still lowers the rate of lumbosacral fusion. Among 164 L–S arthrodeses, in 36 the L5 posterior arch was

**TABLE 2.** *Fusion rate in arthrodesis*

| Arthrodesis length | Number of cases | Fusions | % |
| --- | --- | --- | --- |
| 2 vertebrae | 114 | 114 | 100 |
| 3 vertebrae | 112 | 99 | 88 |
| 4 vertebrae | 22 | 20 | 91 |
| 5 vertebrae | 5 | 4 | 80 |
| 6 vertebrae | 4 | 3 | 75 |

saved. A total of 34 cases fused (94.4%). In 128, it was removed and only 113 certainly fused (88.3%) ($p = 0.459$), but this is not significant.

We believe that the nature of the graft has an influence on fusion: 97% with Hibbs graft (30/31), 94% with iliac cancellous bone graft (163/172), and only 89% with a product of laminectomy (48/54) fused, although this is not statistically significant ($p = 0.241$). The reason is that the nature of the graft is not an isolated factor in the prognosis of fusion. Hibbs decortications have been proposed for single-level arthrodesis without laminectomy and a high probability of fusion. Cancellous iliac crest bone grafts, conversely, have been proposed in more risky patients (e.g., long fixations, laminectomy). Graft with fragments of laminectomy were indicated for old patients needing rapid surgery after a long and sometimes large laminectomy. Finally the length of arthrodesis influenced the fusion rate, but without true statistical significance (Table 2).

## CONCLUSION

Rod–screw angulation introduced in 1990 with the ball-ring has dramatically eliminated mechanical complications related to the device. Instead of six screw fractures or blocker loosenings among 226 orthogonally implanted screws (2.6%), only one screw breakage was observed among 1,147 angulated screws (<1‰) ($p = 0.001$).

Although there is some risk of sacral screws loosening. HA coating and bigger screw diameters may reduce this complication, but a multipoint sacral fixation is necessary for some critical situations.

Lytic spondylolisthesis and, more generally, single posterolateral graft in L5–S1 present the highest rate of pseudoarthrosis. Posterior or posterolateral autologous iliac crest graft usually gives a high fusion rate. This does not indicate that it is advisable to extend indications for interbody fusion farther than lytic SPL and L5–S1 level in long fusions.

## REFERENCES


1. Alibenali M, Franck B., Moreau JJ, et al. Thoraco-lumbar spine osteosynthesis using the tuning fork system. A preliminary report. *Rachis* 1992;4:169–76.
2. Argenson C, Cambas PM, Loset J, Nasr ZG, de Peretti F, Puch JM. The use of the C.D. modular construct −(2 HS − 1 SH) for fixation of comminuted fractures of the thoraco-lumbar junction. A comparison with other constructs. *Rev Chir Orthop* 1994;80:205–16.
3. Asgler MA, Ebelcke DC, Kraker DP, Neff JR. Survivorship analysis of VSP spine instrumentation in the treatment of thoraco-lumbar and lumbar burst fractures. *Spine* 1991;16(suppl 8):428–32.
4. Boos N, Marchesi D, Heitz R, Aebi M. Surgical treatment of low grade spondylolisthesis in adults with pedicular fixation and postero-lateral fusion. *Rev Chir Orthop* 1992;78:228–35.
5. Demeulenaere C, Roy-Camille R, Roy-Camille M. Ostéosynthèse du rachis dorsal, lombaire et lom-

bosacré par plaques métalliques vissées dans les pédicules vertébraux et les apophyses articulaires. *Presse Med* 1970;78:1447–8.

6. Dhi N, Emoto K, Iwasaky Y, Kalsakabe T, Yamagushi Y. M.R. Imaging evaluation of the spine with titanium alloy pedicular screw fixation. *J Spinal Dis* 1995;8(suppl 1):S15–S22.

7. Dubousset J, Cotrel Y, Guillaumat M. New universal instrumentation in spinal surgery. *Clin Orthop* 1988;227:10–23.

8. Lapresle P, Missenard G. Hydroxyapatite coated Diapason. First clinical report. *J Spinal Dis* 1995; 8(suppl 1):S31–9.

9. Lapresle P, Missenard G, Pupin P. Management of adult and old age lumbar scoliosis with stenosis: 6 years of experience with the spinal osteosynthetic Diapason device. *Orthopaedics Intl Ed* 1995;3.

10. Lassale B, Bitan F, Bex M, Deburge A. Resultats fonctionnels du traitement chirurgical des sténoses lombaires dégénératives. *Rev Chir Orthop* 1988;74(suppl 2):85–8.

11. McAfee PC, Gurr KR. Cotrel Dubousset instrumentation in adult: a preliminary report. *Spine* 1988; 13:510–20.

12. Matcuzaki et al. H.A. screws biomechanical study: an experimental work on dogs. First International Stryker Symposium, Paris, 1995.

13. Motegi M, Musha Y, Okojima Y. Lumbar fusion using the Diapason system. *J Spinal Dis* 1995;8 (suppl 1):S7–S14.

14. Roy-Camille R, Saillant G, Mazel C. Internal fixation of the lumbar spine with pedicle screw plating. *Clin Orthop* 1986;203:7–17.

15. Saillant G. Etude anatomique des pédicules vertébraux. Applications chirurgicales. *Rev Chir Orthop Traumatol* 1976;2:151.

16. Van Heeswijk WHJC, Stengs C, Slot GH, Van Tiel W. Spinal fusion for low back pain using H.-frame instrumentation. *Orthop Int Ed* 1993;5:471–8.

*Instrumented Fusion of the Degenerative
Lumbar Spine: State of the Art, Questions,
and Controversies,* edited by M. Szpalski,
R. Gunzburg, D. M. Spengler, and
A. Nachemson. Lippincott–Raven
Publishers, Philadelphia © 1996.

# 13

# Our Indications, Methods, and Results of Treatment in Degenerative Disorders of the Lumbar Spine with Kluger's Spine Fixator

Patrick Kluger, Friedrich Weidt, and Andreas Korge

*Orthopädische Klinik, Universität Ulm, D-89081 Ulm, Germany*

In 1982 and 1983, Dick (1) and Kluger (3), independently of each other, developed an internal fixator for the spine. They had the goal of respecting the anatomic and mechanical characteristics of the vertebral column. Implants should fulfill the following requirements: the shortest possible range of fusion; stable transpedicular anchorage; three-dimensional stability for rotation and translation; and the possibility of using the device for reduction.

As early as 1977, Schläpfer and Magerl (8) had already developed an external spinal fixator. Initially, they described transpedicular instrumentation with Schanz screws. These screws can be used as leverage for the reduction as well as part of a bridging device. Reduction in the form of distraction, compression, lordosis, or kyphosis was possible by three threaded rods seated in three ball-and-socket joints. Compared with other existing methods of stabilization, the fused distance was as short as possible. The transpedicular anchorage led to optimal stability, corrections of malpositions were easily performed, and percutaneous explantation was possible.

The advantages of the principles of external spine fixation have been obvious. The consequence was the development of an internal fixator based on the same principles. According to physical laws, the force affecting the stabilization device decreases with shortening of the transpedicular leverage. Therefore, the implant could be reduced in size.

In 1983, Dick (1) introduced the so-called AO-Spine Fixator. Two threaded bars were connected with a system of clamping jaws. The length was continuously adjustable. The rotation of the longitudinal bars was variable in 6° steps. The Schanz screws were fixed to the clamping jaws with bolts as an additional safety device. However, the AO-Fixator system exhibited some disadvantages:

Because of the fixed length of the threaded bars, they often irritated soft tissue and
the facet joints

The threaded bars had to be assembled before the reduction and interfered with the
surgical field. Moreover, approaches to the spine for laminectomy or PLIF were
blocked by the device

In the depth of the surgical field, a large amount of fine adjustment for fixation of the
bolts was necessary

The fixator required a lot of space; above the level of T8 it could be used only if there
was enough soft tissue to cover it

Shortening of the Schanz screws was complicated, and sharp edges caused irritation
of soft tissue.

Dick developed a mechanically powerful device that transferred the principles of
external spine fixation to internal use. With an internal fixator and with good reduction of malpositions, there is no need for further correction or dynamization.

## DEVELOPMENT OF THE KLUGER SPINE FIXATOR

Consideration of the procedure led to a comprehensive concept of basic principles
and procedures. First was the process of reduction and retention, and then the
process of final stabilization. These steps had to be kept in mind in the development
of an instrumentation system for the spine. The disadvantages of the classical AO-
Fixator had to be eliminated. The results of this development were the following:

Self-tapping transpedicular bone screws: these are available in diameters of 4, 5, and
6 mm; their length varies in 5-mm steps from 30 to 75 mm according to the
diameter. The bone screw top has a serrated connecting square for the longitudinal
bars. So-called grub screws in the head of the bone screw lock the bolts after the
union bars are assembled. Since 1993, the pedicle screws have had a slope of 30°
and therefore assembly of the longitudinal bar is facilitated (Fig. 1).

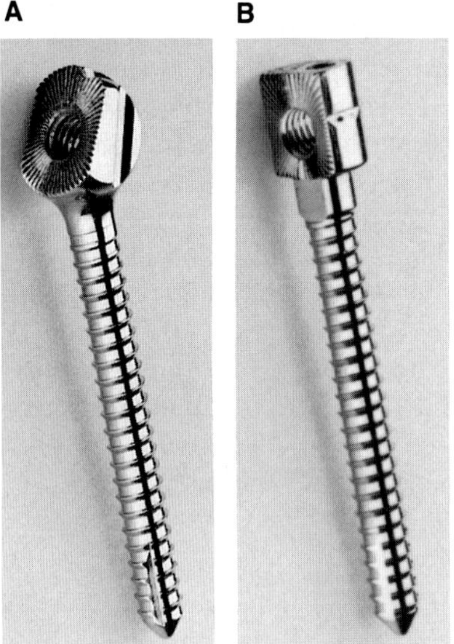


**FIG. 1. A:** Transpedicular bone screw with a
slope of 30° and a serrated surface. **B:** Conventional transpedicular bone screw.

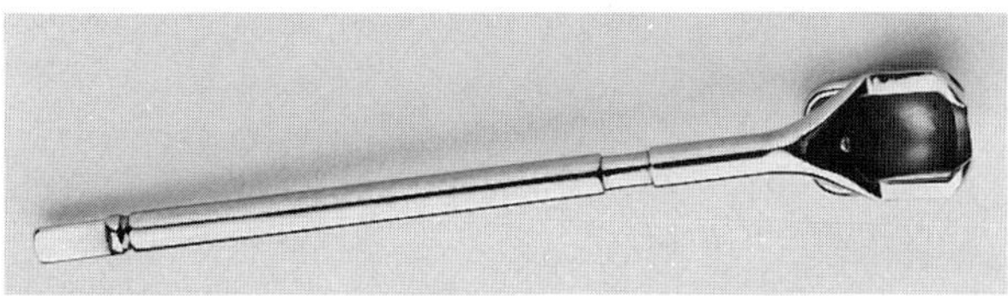

**FIG. 2.** Extension rod, which is clamped to the bone screws.

Extension rods which are clamped on the bone screws: these are used to manipulate the screws and to receive the distractor for reduction (Fig. 2).

The spine distractor for reduction and retention. This consists of a threaded rod, extended with two articulated arms, each ending in a universal connecting joint of the distractor. Reduction maneuvers in all planes are possible (distraction, compression, angulation, and lateral movements in sagittal and frontal planes). The spinal canal can be approached without interference of this instrument (Fig. 3).

Special union bars to connect the bone screws. Monobloc bars are available for very short assemblies, in 10 different lengths (20–38 mm) with an increment of 2 mm. Their rotation is set by contouring handles. The telescopic bars consist of a male and a female cylindric portion. They allow free adjustment of length and axial rotation. Then the female component is crimped onto the male component with special pliers and a template. The longitudinal bars are connected to the bone screws by union bolts. The connected areas of both sides are serrated to maintain a stable angle (Fig. 4).

Since July of 1995, a multisegmental spinal fixator has become available. It is based on the pedicle screws with its 30° slanting top square. Using special brackets at each pedicle screw, a threaded longitudinal rod can brace several screws. Indications for this system are long series of lumbar stenoses or multisegmental instabilities (Fig. 5).

## APPLICATION OF THE KLUGER FIXATOR

Initially, the internal spine fixator was used in patients with fractures of thoracic or lumbar vertebrae. Unlike the external fixator, the Kluger fixator could also be used in treatment of patients with spinal cord injuries and paraplegia (5). After surgical stabilization of a vertebral fracture nursing is easier and mobilization in a

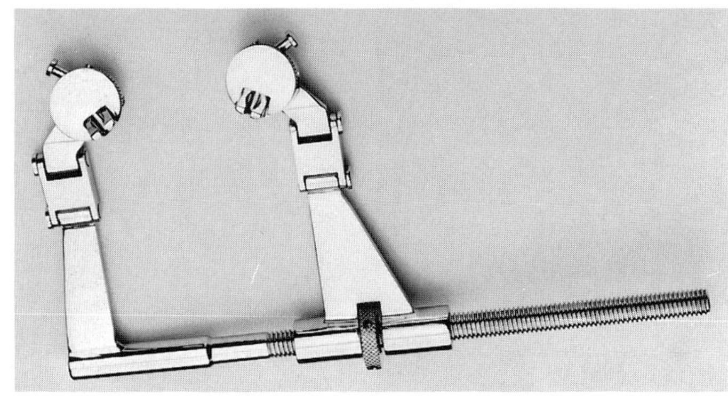

**FIG. 3.** The spine distractor.

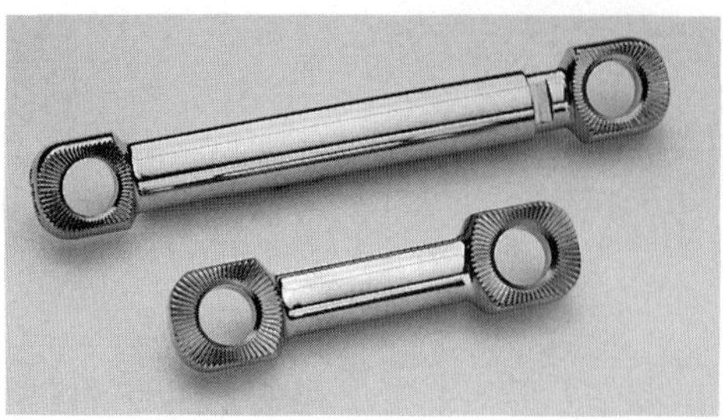

**FIG. 4.** Telescopic union bar and mono-bloc bar.

wheelchair is possible. After wound healing, training in swimming pools becomes possible, and the rehabilitation time is considerably shortened (Fig. 6).

Because the Kluger System allows distraction and reclination, we often corrected post-traumatic malpositions (4) with the patient lying on his flank. Autologous bone is taken from the pelvis, the vertebral column is prepared from the dorsal approach. Under an image intensifier, the vertebrae adjoining the fracture are instrumented. After installation of the spine distractor, a laminectomy, including the facet joints, is

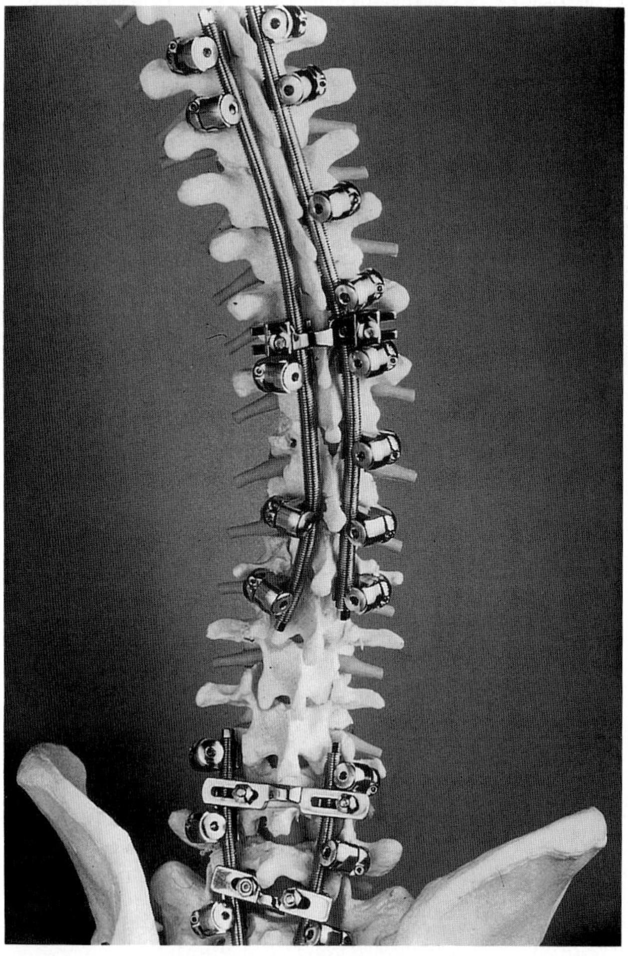

**FIG. 5.** Multisegmental spine fixator.

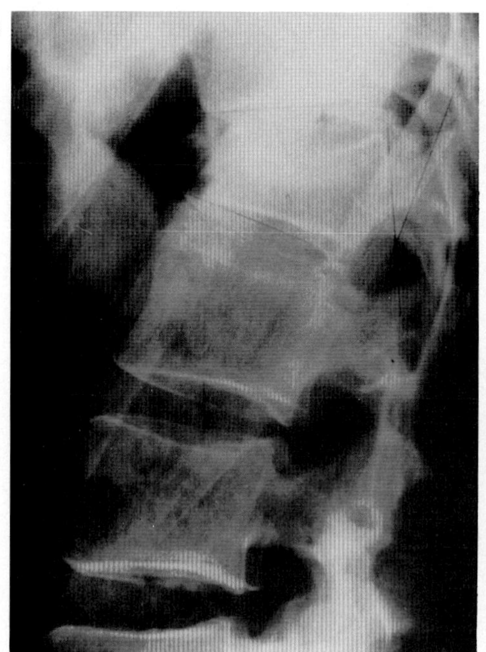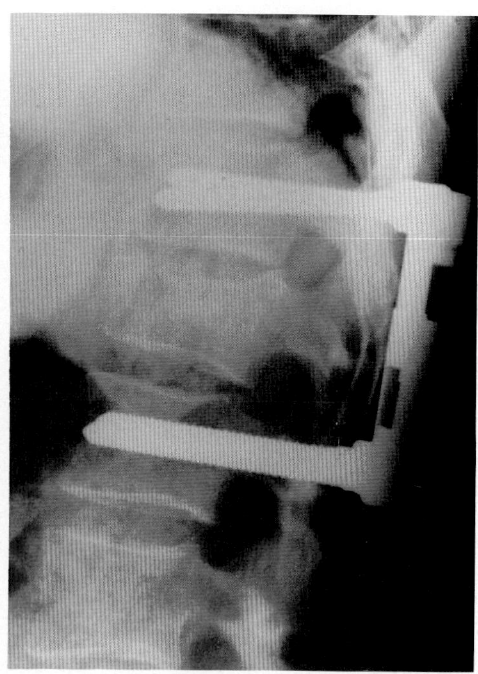

**FIG. 6. A:** A 45-year-old man with a fracture at T12. **B:** Same patient 1 year later, showing fusion without a kyphotic angle.

performed to avoid traction or compression on the spinal cord during reduction. A columnotomy can be performed by the ventrolateral approach. After exact reduction, the ventral defect of the vertebra is filled with spongiosa or bony chips. The union bars are assembled, and after disconnection of the extension rods and removal of the distractor the wound is sutured. In this procedure, the force for reduction is applied only from the dorsal side. Ventrally, the surgical field is not obscured by distraction rods. Ventrally sited instrumentation is not necessary because of the efficiency of the transpedicular system (7) (Fig. 7).

In cases of vertebral tumor or metastasis with the risk for instability caused by a pathologic fracture, we use the internal fixator as a bridging device. If only one vertebra is affected by a somewhat indolent tumor, a ventral approach with resection of this vertebra and replacement of the vertebral body is indicated (Fig. 8).

## THE PLIF INSTRUMENTATION SET

This set consists of the following parts:

1. Hollow drills with inside diameters of 8–18 mm in steps of 2 mm. They must be connected with a power drill. Centimeter scaling is on the outer side of the drills.
2. A chisel tube with an inside diameter up to 18 mm, cut tip up to 18 mm, conical outside thread, and reinforced hexagonal head.
3. A socket wrench fitting onto the chisel tube with a strong shaft and handle.
4. Spiral drills with diameters of 8–18 mm, coupling for the power drill.

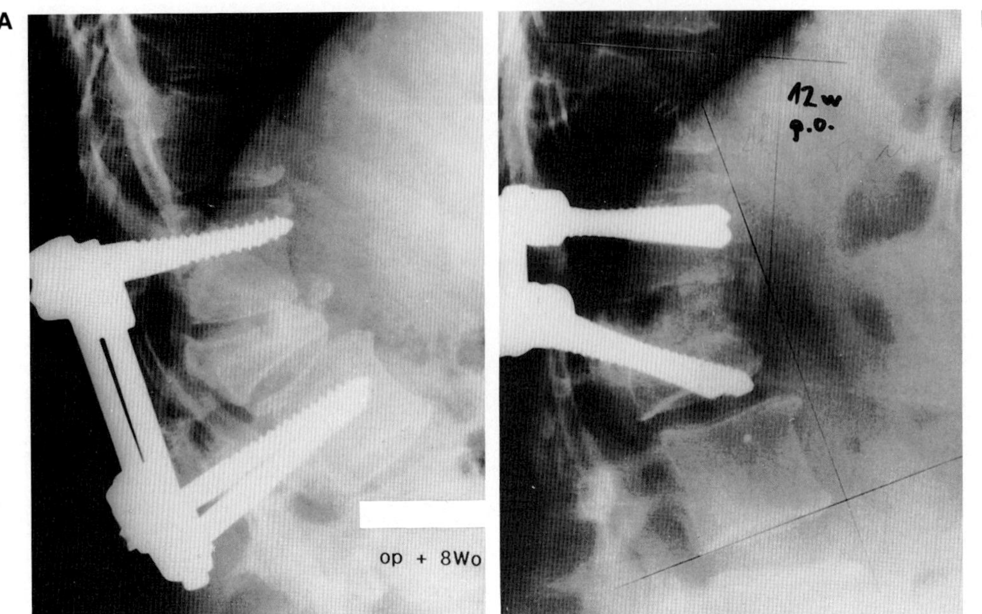



**FIG. 7. A:** A 40-year-old woman with serious kyphotic malposition 8 weeks after stabilization of a fracture of the first lumbar vertebra (fixator type Socon). **B:** Same patient 12 weeks after double approach and reduction; Kluger fixator from T12–L1.

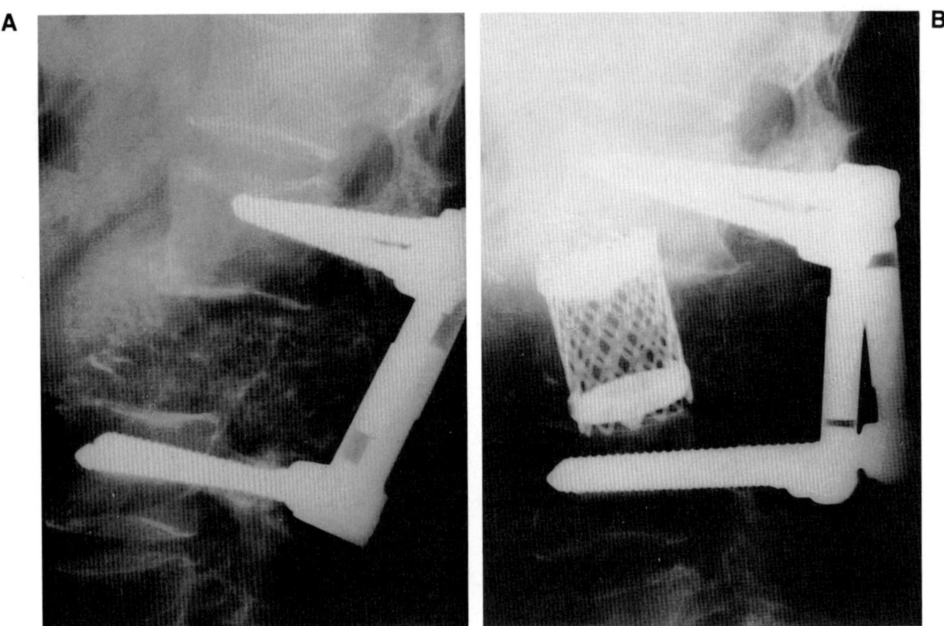

**FIG. 8. A:** A 54-year-old man with relapse of a hemangioma in the entire vertebral body 2 years after resecting surgery. **B:** Same patient 2 weeks after resection of the vertebral body with vertebral body replacement and spinal fixator.

5. A milling cutter with outside diameter of 10 mm, spiral shaft, coupling for power drill.
6. Push rods of 8–18 mm.

### Technique

After exposure of the posterior iliac crest, two bony cylinders are produced by using the hollow drill in a oblique direction tangentially to the iliac bone. Corresponding to the centimeter scale on the outside of the hollow drill, a corticotomy is performed perpendicular to the outside cortex of the os ileum to obtain bony blocks. The blocks are kept moist. Cancellous bone is harvested with a curved chisel and a milling cutter.

## MATERIALS AND METHODS

Since 1988 we have performed a total of 1,667 spinal operations in our hospital. In 361 cases we implanted Kluger's spinal fixator (SF); 279 of those were assembled in the lumbar spine and at the lumbosacral junction. We treated 79 traumatic lesions, 6 post-traumatic malpositions, 15 inflammatory lesions of vertebral bodies, and 128 degenerative disorders in 118 patients. The age range was 14 to 80 years. Most patients were between 31 and 60 years (41 men, 49 women).

The indications for spinal surgery in degenerative disorders of the spine were ($n$ = 118) spondylolisthesis (55 cases), spinal stenosis (10 cases), failed back surgery (35 cases), segmental instability (10 cases), or nonunion (18 cases). The following procedures were chosen: SF and AIF simultaneously (19 cases); SF and AIF not simultaneously (41 cases); posterior SF and bone chips (19 cases); SF and PLIF (32 cases); facet joint screws (in addition to SF in another segment) (10 cases); and second anterior intervention of patients treated in another hospital (7 cases).

## RESULTS

### Group 1: Simultaneous Combined Procedure with SF and AIF

A total of 19 patients underwent this combined procedure at L4–L5 or at L5–S1. After fusion they were additionally treated with a removable body brace for 12 weeks. All patients were mobilized in their braces for 2 days after intervention. At 12 weeks, routine postoperative x-rays were taken. When the bone graft showed a tendency toward interbody fusion, the plaster jacket was removed step by step. Further follow-up examinations were performed 6 and 12 months postoperatively. In all, 13 of 19 patients showed a bony fusion and three had a nonunion and underwent revision surgery. Three cases were followed in other hospitals and we do not have further information about them. The fusion rate in the combined SF/AIF group was 70%.

### Group 2: Spinal Fixator and AIF, Not Simultaneously

A total of 41 patients first underwent a posterior instrumentation with the spinal fixator and 6 to 12 weeks later an AIF was performed. Eighteen of these patients had a spondylolisthesis, 18 a failed back syndrome, and five a segmental instability. The segments to be fusioned were the following: one case L2–L3, another one L3–L4, 13 cases L4–L5, and 14 cases L5–S1. A total of 11 patients had to be fusioned in two segments, four cases L3–L5 and seven cases L4–S1. In one case the fusion range included L3–S1. On follow-up, the radiologic outcome showed 24 interbody fusions and one nonunion. In nine cases we have no follow-up, and seven patients underwent surgery less than 1 year ago. Excluding these latter cases, the fusion rate was at least 71% (Fig. 9).

### Group 3: Posterior Fusion with Spinal Fixator and Bone Chips

A total of 19 patients were fusioned with an SF only. Seven of them are scheduled for future AIF. In nine cases we have no postoperative follow-up for 1 year. In two cases a posterior fusion with bone chips was achieved. In another case, a revision after nonunion (posterior only) was performed. In cases of spinal stenosis in elderly patients after laminectomy, a merely posterior procedure is possible.

### Group 4: Spinal Fixator Combined with PLIF by a Single Posterior Approach

Since 1988, we have operated on 32 patients using the PLIF technique. The patients had the following diagnoses: two post-traumatic segmental instabilities, 19 cases of spondylolisthesis (L3–L4 one; L4–L5 eight; L5–S1 10), nine cases of failed back surgery of L4–L5 and L5–S1, and two cases of spinal stenosis. In the radiologic follow-up, 18 interbody fusions could be seen. In five cases revision for nonunion was necessary. Since 1993, the hollow drills of the PLIF set have had diameters of up to 18 mm. From 1993 to the first 6 months of 1995, 19 patients underwent SF and PLIF. At present there are 13 cases of radiologic fusion and two cases of nonunion. Three patients are in early follow-up and one patient is lost to follow-up. Without including the three cases of early follow-up, the fusion rate of these cases was approximately 81% (Fig. 10).

In one case, because of the dislocation of a bony cylinder due to the insertion of the second dowel, an early revision was necessary (Fig. 11).

### Groups 5 and 6

In seven cases, previous fusion procedures had been performed in other hospitals. These patients underwent anterior revisions. The radiologic outcome showed four fusions, and in three cases the SF is still in situ.

In addition to the implantation of an SF in 10 cases, we blocked the facet joints of another segment when there was a pain reduction in the preoperative evaluation. Using Kluger's spinal fixator and AIF or PLIF, we achieved interbody fusion in 68–71% of all cases. Considering only the results of the PLIF technique from 1993 to 1995, the fusion rate appears to be about 80%. In all cases the patients were mobilized 2 days after surgery.

In the cases of spondylolisthesis, good correction of malpositions was achieved. Normally, we performed an exploration of the spinal canal with decompression of nerve roots that were affected. Because of the stable-angled dorsal internal fixation, we did not have to use ventrally positioned instrumentation for osteosynthesis.

In 11 patients a revision in our hospital was necessary for nonunion. Five of these

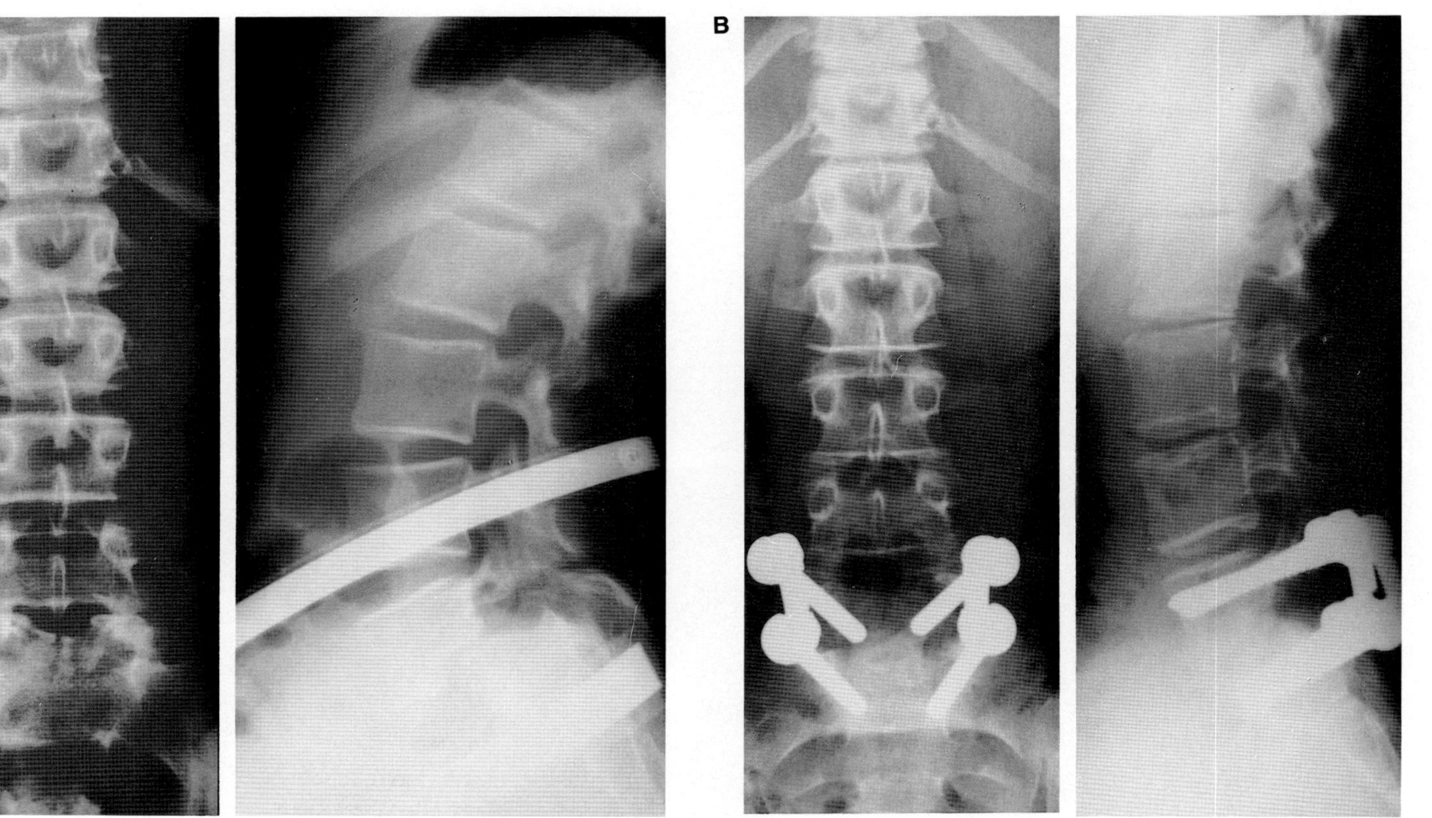

**FIG. 9. A:** A 14-year-old girl with spondylolisthesis. **B:** Same patient 3 months after SF and AIF.

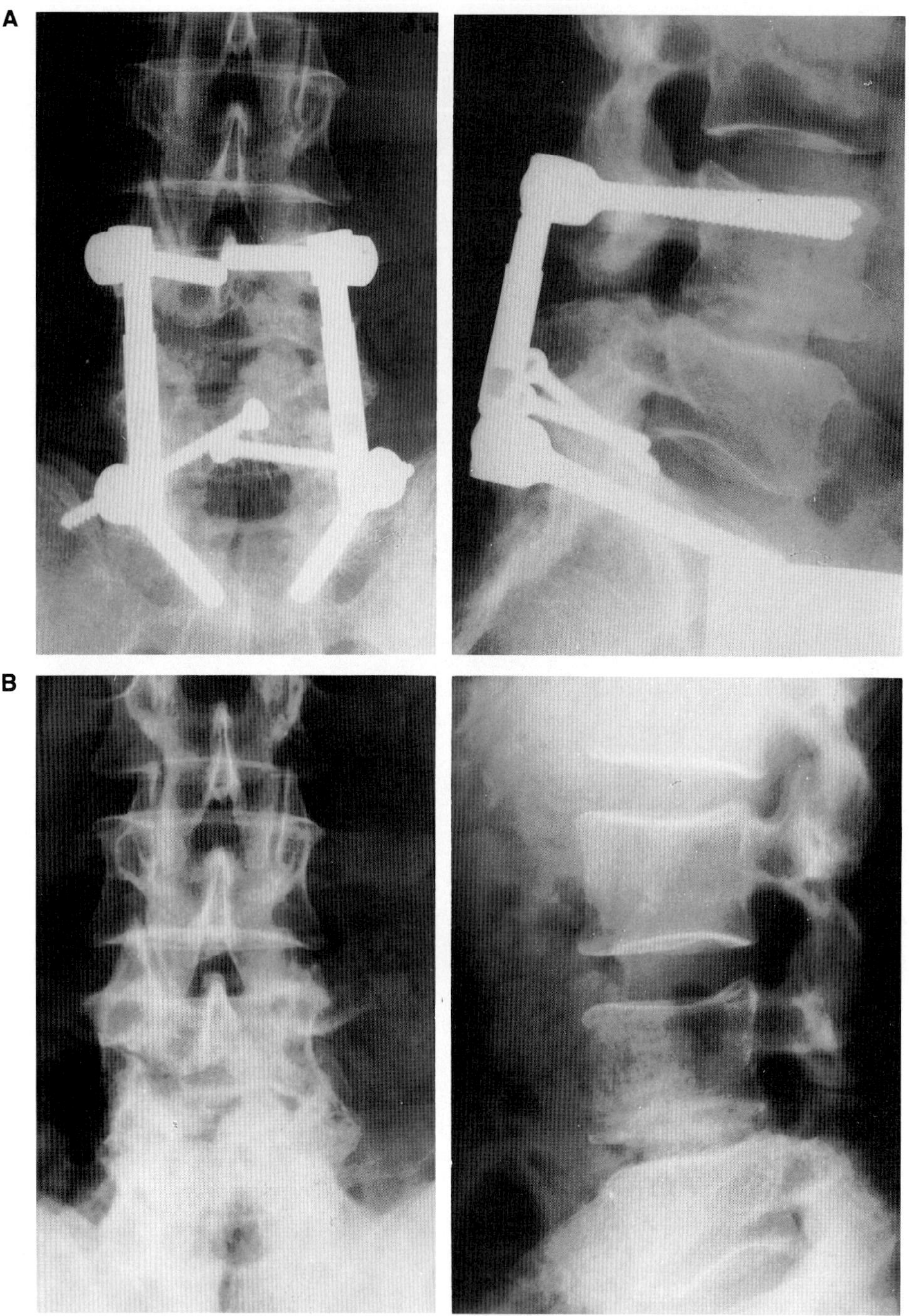

**FIG. 10. A:** A 52-year-old man at 8 weeks after PLIF L4–L5; the bone graft contacts L4 and L5 sufficiently. **B:** Same patient at 15 months postop. L4–L5 are fusioned and the patient has no pain.

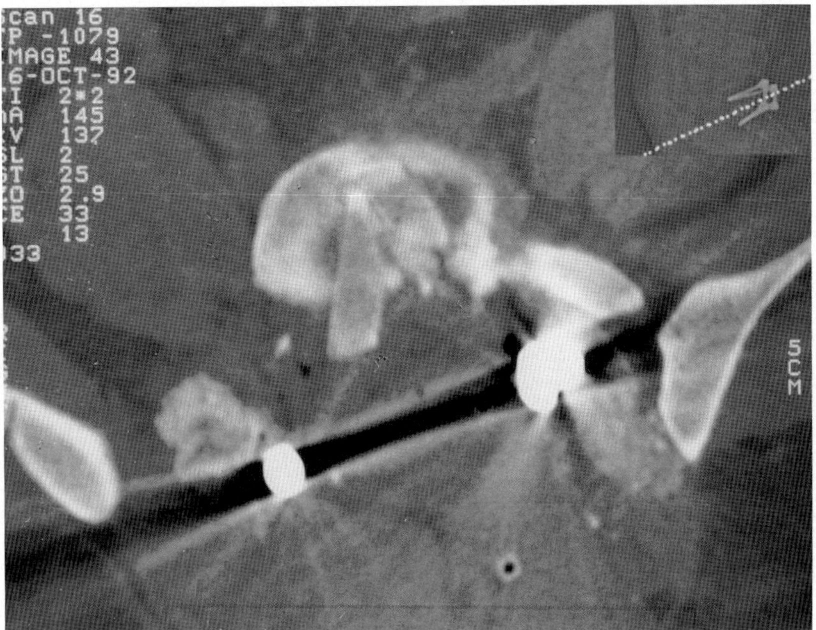

**FIG. 11.** A 28-year old man. Several days after PLIF a CT scan shows the bone graft compromising spinal structures; a revision was necessary.

cases had undergone PLIF before 1993, at which time only bone grafts with a maximal diameter of 12 mm were available.

We are convinced that the theory of stress protection by rigid dorsal fixation systems to explain nonunions is invalid. McAfee et al. (6) found a higher fusion rate when the rigidity of implants was increased. They compared the Harrington system, the Luque system, and the CD implant. Johnston et al. (2) observed that callus formation had a better quality and that the fusion had greater rigidity. In a prospective randomized study in patients with degenerative disorders of the lumbar spine and lumbosacral junction, Zdeblick (9) achieved a fusion rate of 95% with a rigid device, whereas a semi-rigid device had fusion rates of only 77%. In our opinion, the term "dynamic" used in context with transpedicular fixation systems has to be understood as making an excuse for the fact of "substability."

## REFERENCES

1. Dick W. Die operative Behandlung der thorakalen und lumbalen Wirbelfrakturen unter besonderer Berücksichtigung des Fixateur interne. Thesis, Universität Basel, 1983.
2. Johnston ChE, Ashman RB, Baid AM, Allard RN. Effect of spinal construct stiffness on early fusion mass incorporation. Experimental study. *Spine* 1990;15:908–12.
3. Kluger P. Vorrichtung zum Einrichten einer Wirbelsäule mit geschädigten Wirbelkörpern. German Patent No. P 3414374.2, 1984.
4. Kluger P. Das Fixateurprinzip an der Rumpfwirbelsäule–sein Einsatz beim kombinierten ventralen und dorsalen Eingriff. In: Stuhler TH, ed. *Fixateur externe—fixateur interne*. Berlin, Heidelberg: Springer-Verlag, 1989:36–58.
5. Kluger P, Gerner HJ. Das mechanische Prinzip des Fixateur externe zur dorsalen Stabilisierung der Brust und Lendenwirbelsäule. *Unfallchirurgie* 1986;12:68–79.

6. McAfee PC, Farey JD, Sutterlin CE, Gurr KR, Warden KE, Cunningham BW. Device-related osteoporosis with spinal instrumentation. *Spine* 1989;14:919–26.
7. Nolte LP, Steffen R, Krämer J, Jergas M. Der Fixateur interne: eine vergleichende biomechanische Studie verschiedener Systeme. *Aktuelle Traumatol* 1993;23:20–26.
8. Schläpfer F, Magerl F. Fixateur zum Fixieren von Knochen oder Knochenbruckstüken, inbesondere Wirbeln. Swiss Patent No. 7031–78, 1978.
9. Zdeblick TA. A prospective, randomized study of lumbar fusion. Preliminary results. *Spine* 1993;18: 983–91.

*Instrumented Fusion of the Degenerative Lumbar Spine: State of the Art, Questions, and Controversies,* edited by M. Szpalski, R. Gunzburg, D. M. Spengler, and A. Nachemson. Lippincott–Raven Publishers, Philadelphia © 1996.

# 14

# Instrumented Fusion of the Lumbar Spine with the Rogozinski Spinal Rod System

Abraham Rogozinski and Chaim Rogozinski

*Rogozinski Orthopedic Clinic, Jacksonville, Florida 32216*

Studies conducted during the past 10 years have demonstrated the value of rigid fixation over less rigid methods in support of arthrodesis of the lumbar spine (3, 12,14,15,18,21,24,25,27,30). Less rigid fixation has included the use of wires and hooks for capture of vertebral elements, sometimes incorporated into constructs employing flexible or inflexible rods. Rigid fixation includes multiple systems employing various combinations of pedicle screws or bolts attached to longitudinal plates or bars, sometimes with transverse cross-connections between longitudinal elements.

Rigid fixation has proved most valuable to enhance fusion in degenerative disease, instability, spinal trauma (fracture), isthmic and degenerative spondylolisthesis, and deformity (scoliosis, kyphosis). However, complications of excessively rigid fixation have been identified, including stress shielding, osteopenia, and possible premature degeneration of adjacent vertebral levels (7,17). Complications of the earliest systems (screw pullout, breakage, and bending) have largely been eliminated by biomechanical adjustments as our understanding of instrumented spinal fusion has advanced. The need to employ impeccable surgical technique when placing instrumentation with pedicle screws and to adhere to well-established surgical principles that promote arthrodesis remain prerequisites for surgical success.

The advantages of implants employing pedicle screws have been widely described and can be summarized as providing (a) appropriate stabilization of the fused segment, (b) improved bony fixation, (c) correction of deformity and maintenance of correction, and (d) support of the healing fusion in patients with the appropriate surgical indications.

This chapter documents outcome in terms of fusion rate and complication rate in patients undergoing spinal fusion with Rogozinski spinal rod instrumentation. Results with more and less rigid constructs employing the instrumentation are presented for comparison. Additional factors that affect the fusion result are identified.

## DESIGN RATIONALE

The degree of rigidity of spinal instrumentation systems varies by product. The Rogozinski system was designed to provide the surgeon with a range of constructs of various degrees of rigidity so that modulations of the system could be adapted to a variety of clinical presentations. To that end, posterior instrumentation can include an all-hook construct (less rigid), combined hook and pedicle screw construct (moderately rigid), or a pedicle screw construct (more rigid).

### Components

Components include hooks with variously shaped openings (C, up-angle, down-angle), pedicle screws (of both offset and in-line types), smooth rods, crossbars, couplers, and set screws (Fig. 1). System implants are composed of screws and/or hooks attached to bilateral rods linked by crossbars at each level, forming a quadrilateral or ladder-shaped configuration.

Pedicle screws are available with major diameters of 5.5, 6.4, and 7.0 mm and corresponding minor diameters of 4.8 and 5.5 mm. Screw lengths are from 35 mm to 55 mm. The in-line (direct) screws allow direct attachment of the rod to the screw. Offset screws are best used in longer fusions in which pedicles at multiple levels do not align evenly and various offset lengths are needed.

Instruments have been designed to facilitate pedicle screw insertion. Because this step is critical to success and influences the potential for complications, appropriate attention was directed at instrument design. The reamer probe is an example of design development of an instrument; it is a hybrid combination of gear shift probe, pedicle drill, and x-ray depth marker. A long-handled inserter allows the reamer probes to be left in the spine at multiple levels without impinging on themselves for subsequent use as x-ray markers. The reamer probe is designed with a blunt tip which expands into a drill portion designed with a very nonaggressive side-cutting profile, enabling the instrument to "bounce" off the endosteal surface of the pedicle and follow the path of least resistance down the medullary canal of the pedicle. This design minimizes the likelihood of accidental screw cut-out. When performed in

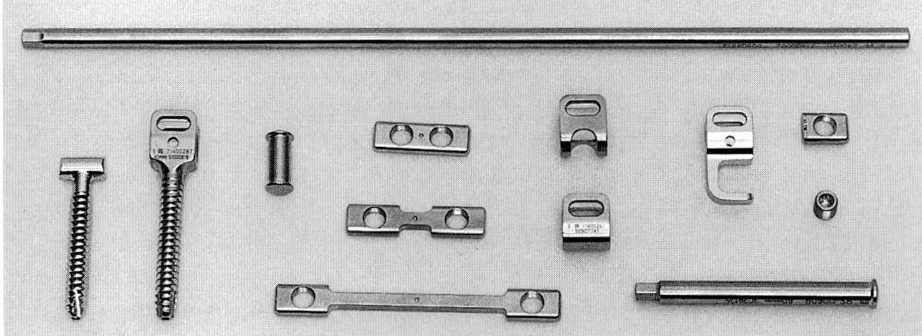

**FIG. 1.** Rogozinski spinal rod system components. Smooth hex-end rod (top) or short hex-end rod with flared end (bottom right). Left to right: Offset screw and direct screw; double-flared rod; crossbars, rigid crossbars (top) and modified crossbars for contouring (bottom); couplers, slotted and solid; neutral hook, hook bar, and set screw.

conjunction with available self-tapping pedicle screws, the task of pedicle preparation and screw insertion is greatly streamlined without increasing associated risks.

### Modularity of the System for Varying Rigidity

System rigidity is adjusted by taking advantage of design features, i.e., different means of bone implant attachments (hooks versus screws), thus affording a variety of constructs of various intrinsic rigidities (Figs. 2–4). Additional modulation is provided with transverse connectors between rods.

The modularity of the system enables surgeons to make choices on the basis of the pathology, including the number of affected surgical levels. For example, in treatment of a burst fracture the surgeon can choose a posterior procedure with pedicle screw instrumentation after reduction. The surgeon can incorporate additional motion segments in the posterior instrumentation and fusion, or, if a combined anteroposterior procedure is preferred, a short-segment posterior instrumentation and fusion can be used in conjunction with anterior fusion.

With these types of options, the surgeon can more specifically design the instrumentation to match the amount of instability present. Although preoperative planning can correctly anticipate the implant needed, the modularity of the Rogozinski system gives the surgeon the ability to revise implant design when an intraoperative change in strategy is required. In this way, the system helps to optimize rigidity and to produce an improved rate of fusion, while minimizing concerns of instrument-related stress shielding and adjacent level degeneration.

## PATIENT PROFILE

Between 1988 and 1992, 150 posterolateral spinal fusions with fixation were performed on 139 patients. The average age of all patients was 37 years (range 21–63

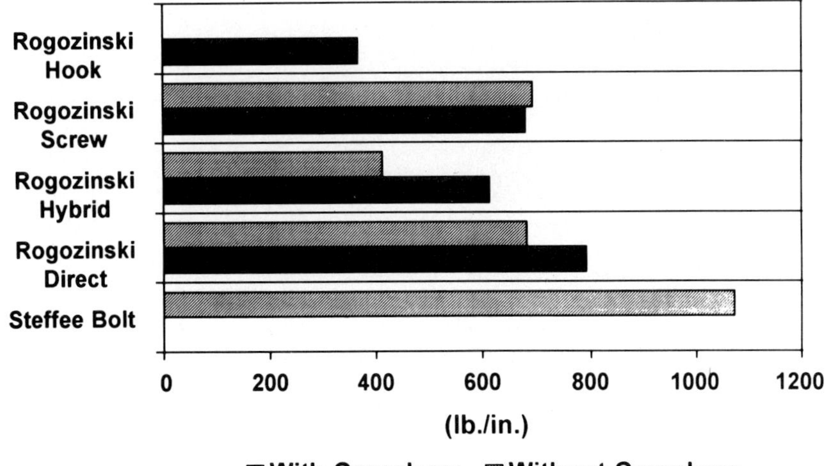


**FIG. 2.** Comparison of stiffness in tension of various Rogozinski system constructs (with and without crossbars) and the Steffee bolt/plate system.

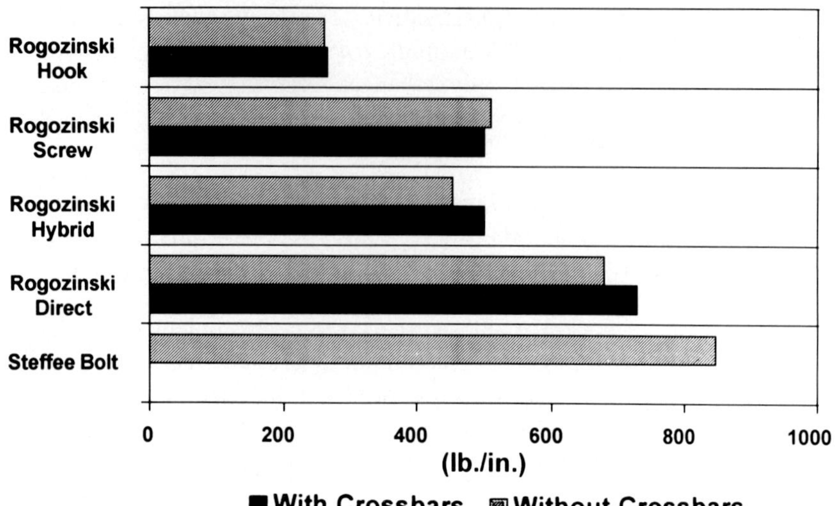



**FIG. 3.** Comparison of stiffness in compression of various Rogozinski system constructs (with and without crossbars) and the Steffee bolt/plate system.

years). Men constituted 72% (100 of 139) of the group and women 28% (39 of 139). Most patients (90%) were Worker's Compensation recipients; the remainder held private insurance.

Presenting diagnoses included degenerative disc disease (25%) with chronic hypermobility or instability of the spine. Degenerative disc disease in combination with herniated nucleus pulposus was the diagnosis in 29% of the study group; degenerative disc disease combined with spinal stenosis was present in 2%. An additional 29% were diagnosed as having failed back surgery syndrome (previous laminectomy,

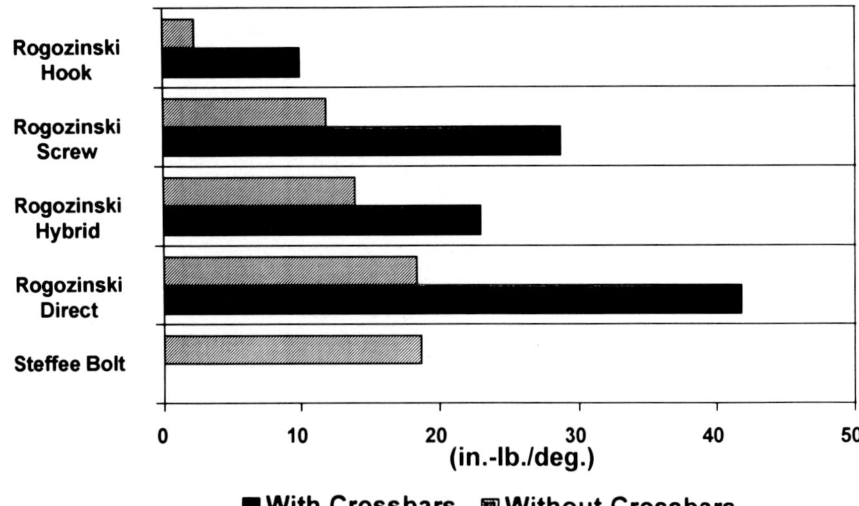



**FIG. 4.** Comparison of stiffness in torsion of various Rogozinski system constructs (with and without crossbars) and the Steffee bolt/plate system.

discectomy, or failed fusion) combined with degenerative disc disease. Other categories were spondylolisthesis in 7% of study patients and pseudarthrosis in 8%.

Fusion using bone graft was employed in all cases, using either banked bone (freeze-dried or cadaveric) and autologous graft or autologous graft alone. In 54 procedures involving 51 patients, the surgeons supplemented the fusion with all-hooks instrumentation posteriorly. In 19 procedures, a combination of hooks and screws (so-called hybrid constructs—pedicle screws in the sacrum and hooks elsewhere) instrumentation was employed posteriorly. In 60 procedures, all-screws instrumentation was used posteriorly. In 17 procedures, combined simultaneous anteroposterior (360°) spinal fusion was undertaken, in which a variety of instrumentations were employed posteriorly and banked bone dowels were grafted anteriorly.

Some cases (90) were simultaneously subjects of an investigational device exemption (IDE) study as required by the U.S. Food and Drug Administration (FDA) for the instrumentation system (Rogozinski Spinal Rod System, Smith & Nephew Spine, Memphis, TN). Use of pedicle screws above the sacrum was investigational at the time of surgery. [At the time of this writing (December, 1995) use of the system with pedicle screws above S1 has received FDA 510k approval limited to application in grades 3 and 4 spondylolisthesis using autograft only at L5–S1 and removal of instrumentation when bony fusion occurs. Expanded indications and usage are investigational.] After full disclosure of risks and FDA status of the device and pedicle screw usage, all patients signed consent forms and subsequently completed pre- and postoperative follow-up questionnaires in accordance with FDA guidelines.

## PREOPERATIVE PROTOCOL

Adult patients who had undergone rigorous attempts at conservative treatment for 6 months or longer were included in the group. In many cases, conservative treatment was pursued for 1 year or longer. Conservative treatment includes physical therapy and reconditioning, judicious use of selected analgesics, nonsteroidal anti-inflammatory drugs, and epidural steroid and trigger point injections. Trials of thoracolumbosacral orthoses were attempted when indicated.

Patients whose level of pain and physical limitation remains unacceptable to them after conservative treatment and who request consideration for surgery are referred for baseline isokinetic testing and extensive psychological evaluation. Patients who smoke are required to discontinue smoking before surgery, and cessation is confirmed by preoperative carboxyhemoglobin testing.

Clinical signs of limited range of motion, pain, and neurologic impairment are documented and quantified, where possible. Patients are queried as to the presence of bowel and bladder dysfunction, sexual impairment, or cauda equina syndrome. Questionnaires are completed by patients for the purpose of providing a baseline rating of their pain and functional levels (10-point analogue scale and expanded Oswestry scale).

Radiologic work-up includes plain radiographs and magnetic resonance imaging (MRI) of the lumbar spine. Gadolinium-enhanced studies are obtained in patients who have undergone previous spine surgery. Provocative discography and computed tomography (CT) scans are performed in most patients. Those whose pathology warrants further investigation have at least one additional study performed from among the following: myelography, bone scan, stress films, selected nerve root blocks, or electromyogram/nerve conduction studies.

## SURGICAL APPROACH

All surgery was conducted by the same two surgeons. Chronologically in their experience, all-hooks constructs were the earliest procedures undertaken (1988), followed by "hybrid" constructs (January, 1990) and all-screws constructs (May, 1990). The 360° techniques were initiated in April of 1990.

All-hooks instrumentation was composed of laminar hook/rod constructs (Fig. 5). Rods spanned the length of the construct, with hooks placed superiorly and inferiorly. Crossbars linked rods at various levels as deemed necessary. Constructs extended the length of the affected segment. All patients were immobilized postoperatively with TLSO, and if fusion included L5–S1 a hip spica was attached.

So-called hybrid instrumentation was composed of a combination of pedicle screws in the sacrum inferiorly in the construct and laminar claw hooks superiorly (Fig. 6). The screw and hook combinations were secured to rods with crossbars linking the rods at various levels.

All-screws instrumentation was composed of pedicle screw/rod constructs (Figs. 7 and 8). Pedicle screws were inserted at each affected vertebral level, and crossbars

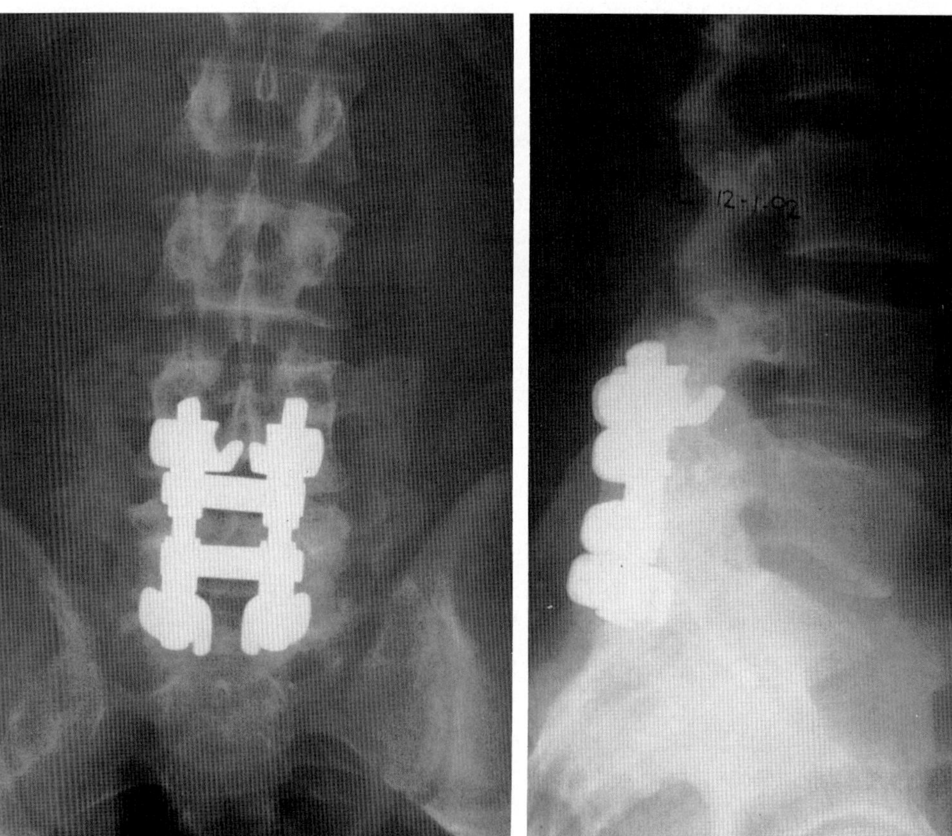

**A**                                                                                          **B**

**FIG. 5.** All-hook Rogozinski spinal rod system construct; AP view **(A)** and lateral view **(B)**.

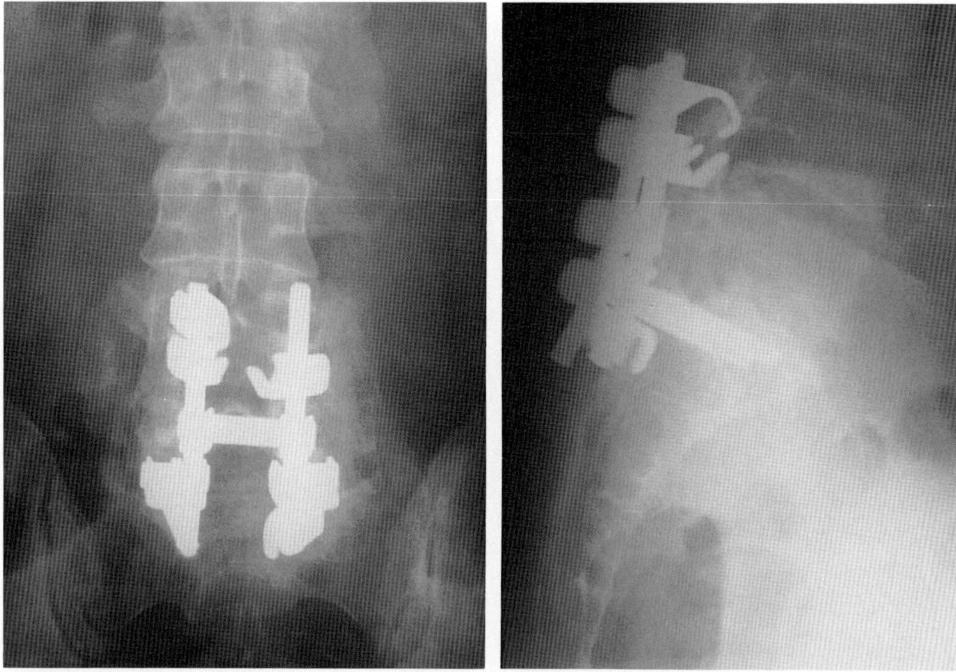

**FIG. 6.** Hybrid (both offset screws and laminar hooks) Rogozinski system construct; AP view **(A)** and lateral view **(B).**

were employed to link the rods. All-screws constructs extended the length of the affected vertebral segment.

So-called 360° procedures employed hybrid or screw constructs posteriorly and posterolateral bone graft in conjunction with anterior interbody fusion, predominantly using femoral rings (Fig. 9).

### Surgical Technique

A midline skin incision was used in all posterolateral procedures. The paraspinal muscles are mobilized laterally off the midline structures and ventrally to the intertransverse fascial ligament. Complete facet capsulectomies are then performed at the intervertebral levels to be incorporated into the fusion. Once adequate exposure is obtained, decompression or discectomy is performed, as indicated. Preparation for placement of the instrumentation system is then undertaken.

For pedicle screw placement, the central axis of the pedicle is identified and then drilled in the optimal trajectory. Drains are placed and the skin is closed in layers. When 360° procedures are performed, sequencing of the anterior and posterior procedures varies.

### Postoperative Protocol

Patients were ambulated on the first postoperative day. Average postoperative hospital stay after the earliest 54 procedures with all-hooks fixation was 7 days.

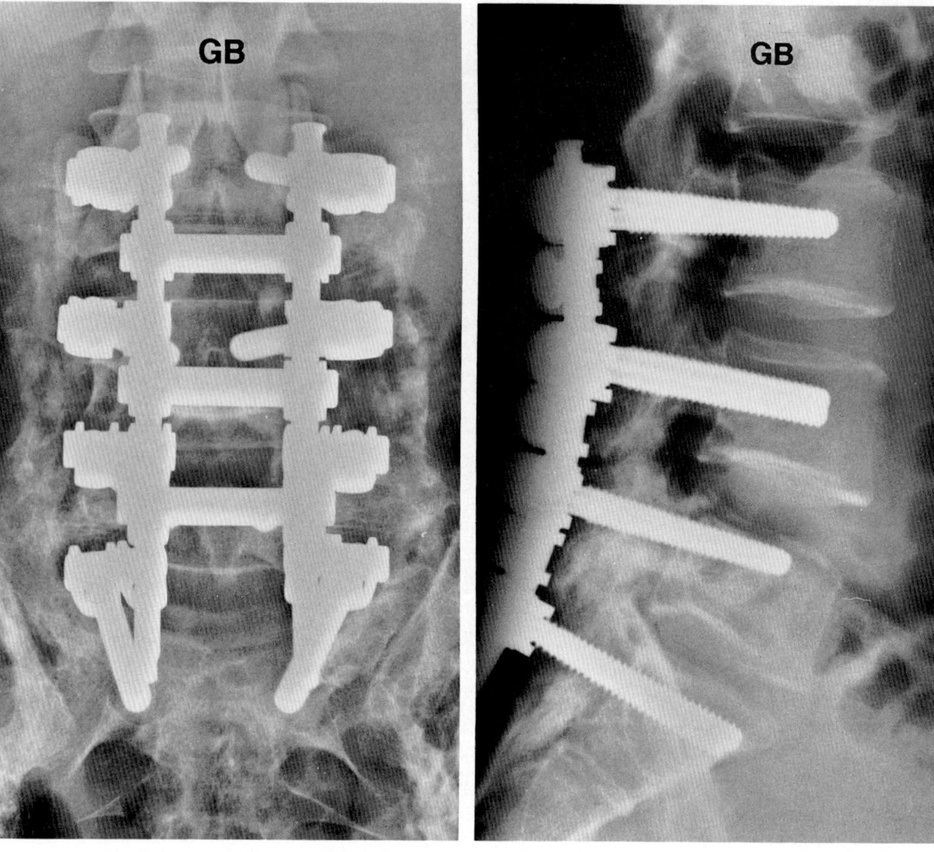

**FIG. 7.** Posterolateral three-level spinal fusion using an offset screw Rogozinski system construct; AP view **(A)** and lateral view **(B)**.

Hospitalization time has diminished with implantation of more rigid constructs, and averaged 4 days in 1992 for all patients at that time having either all-screws constructs or 360° procedures. No orthotic devices were employed postoperatively for patients with more rigid fixation types.

Fusion outcome was determined by serial radiographic examination. Anteroposterior, lateral, and stress films are taken at 6 weeks, 3 months, 6 months, 12 months, and annually thereafter. Radiographic criteria for solid union include examination for all of the following: (a) presence of bone from the tip of the process to the lateral border of the lamina; (b) bone continuous between processes; (c) trabeculation of bone across operative levels, (d) loss of cortical margins of the lamina and transverse processes; (e) facet fusion; and (f) no implant loosening (no "windshield wipering"). Minimal criteria for solid union are trabeculation of bone across all operative levels, absence of motion on stress views, and intact fixation.

## RESULTS

The 139 patients represented in this report were followed to the end of December, 1994. One patient had died of multiple myeloma within 10 months of surgery; how-

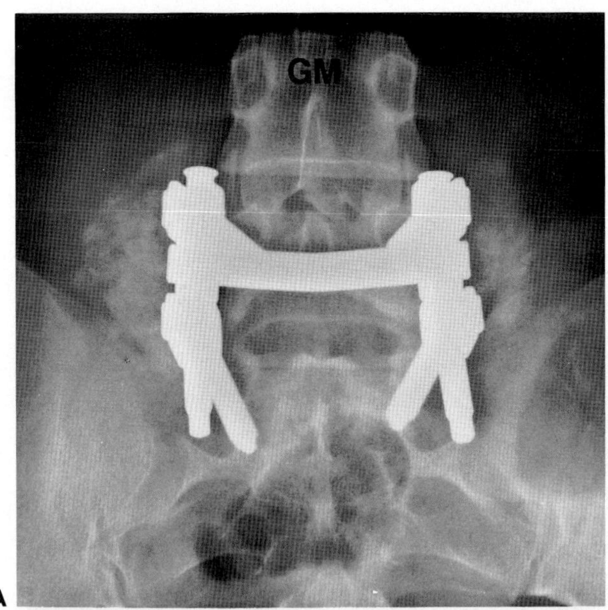



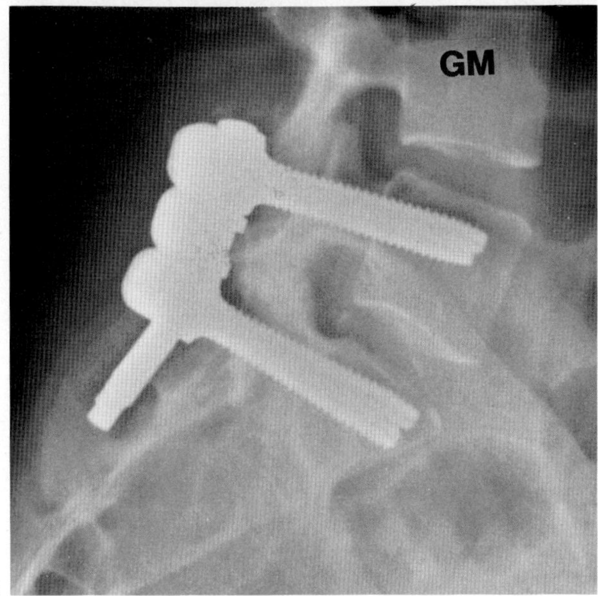



**FIG. 8.** Posterolateral one-level spinal fusion using a direct screw Rogozinski system construct; AP view **(A)** and lateral view **(B).**

ever, the radiographic appearance of the graft and the clinical result were consistent with a successful fusion. Two additional patients had died of cardiovascular disease by the end of the follow-up period, albeit several years after their surgery, and therefore their fusion result is included in tabulations.

## Overall

Fusion rates among the various groups are shown in Table 1. Patients having the 360° procedure showed the highest fusion rates overall, with all-screws, hybrids, and

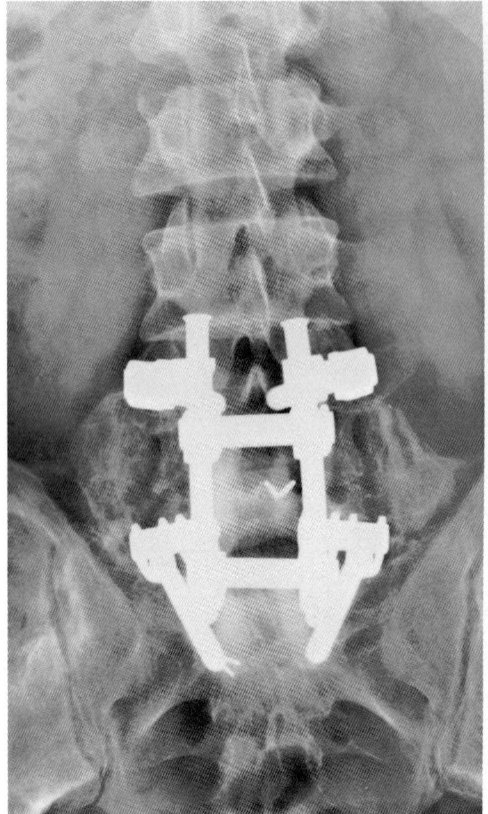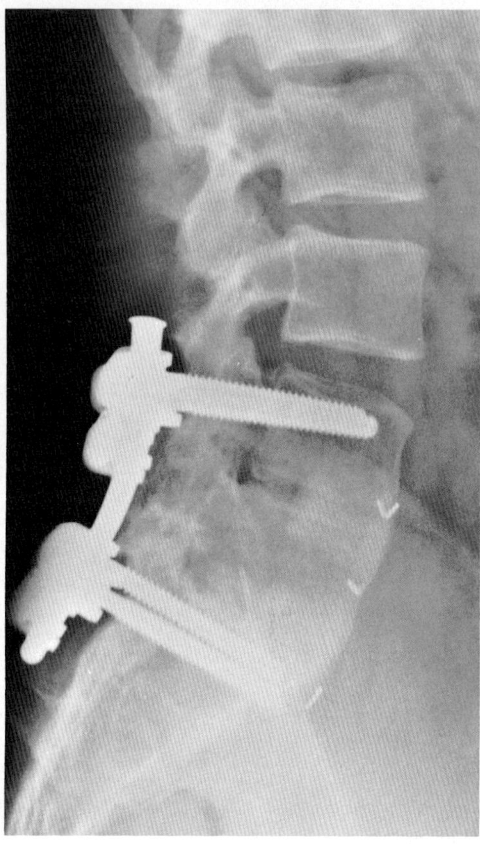

**FIG. 9.** A 360° fusion (posterolateral fusion and anterior interbody fusion with femoral rings) with an offset screw Rogozinski system construct posteriorly; AP view **(A)** and lateral view **(B)**.

all-hooks procedures following in descending order of fusion success. Complications occurring among all study patients are listed in Table 2.

## All-Hooks

Among this group, involving 51 patients in 54 procedures performed between 1988 and 1990, the average age was 38.8 years at the time of surgery (range 22–63 years). There were 43 men and 8 women.

After 54 procedures, 29 (54%) achieved solid union (Table 1); 25 (46%) resulted in

**TABLE 1.** *Results of fusion in 150 procedures, by construct type*

| Type (n) | Fusion (n/%) | Nonunion (n/%) |
| --- | --- | --- |
| All-hooks (54) | 29/54% | 25/46% |
| Hybrids (hooks and screws) (19) | 15/79% | 4/21% |
| All-screws (60) | 51/85% | 9/15% |
| Combined anteroposterior (360°) (17) | 16/94% | 1/6% |

**TABLE 2** *Complications*

| Complication | Number of patients |
|---|:---:|
| Posterolateral hooks (54 procedures) | |
| Persistent pain/narcotic pain meds | 2 |
| Deep vein thrombosis | 1 |
| Pseudarthrosis | 25 |
| Adjacent level DDD | 2 |
| Device coupling | 1 |
| Seroma I and D | 2 |
| Neuropraxia | 1 |
| Device removal | 1 |
| Radiculopathy | 1 |
| Posterolateral hybrids (19 procedures) | |
| Compartment syndrome, left leg | 1 |
| Pseudarthrosis | 4 |
| Posterolateral screws (60 procedures) | |
| Deep infection | 2 |
| Deep infection, graft site | 1 |
| Persistent pain | 3 |
| Pseudarthrosis | 9 |
| Adjacent level DDD | 1 |
| Seroma I and D | 4 |
| Neurologic sequelae (foot drop) | 2 |
| Device removal | 1 |
| Dural tear, no sequelae | 1 |
| 360° procedures | |
| Compartment syndrome, embolectomy | 1 |
| Pseudarthrosis | 1 |
| Deep infection | 1 |

nonunion. Complications included graft resorption or pseudarthrosis in 25 (46%); seroma requiring incision and drainage in two (4%); deep vein thrombosis (occurring 2 weeks postoperatively) in one (2%); and neuropraxia in one (2%). Persistent radiculopathy and back pain necessitated implantation of a morphine pump in three, and a pump was recommended in another. One had hardware removal at another center. No fixation failures occurred.

## Hybrid

Of the 19 patients, five were women and 14 were men. Average age was 36 years (range 22–54 years). Solid union was present in 15 (79%); nonunion occurred in four (21%). Compartment syndrome occurred in one patient after surgery; fasciotomy was performed on the left leg, with excellent return of function. Fixation failure occurred in one patient in whom there was uncoupling of a hook from a too-short rod.

## All-Screws

The average patient age at time of surgery was 38.6 years (21–59). There were 38 men and 22 women. After 60 procedures involving 60 patients, 51 (85%) resulted in solid union (Table 1). This group included the patient who died of multiple myeloma 10 months postoperatively but reported significant pain improvement of her back and legs; fusion was radiographically solid. There were no fixation failures. Complications included graft resorption or pseudarthrosis in nine (15%), deep wound infection requiring prolonged intravenous antibiotics in two (3%), seroma requiring incision and drainage in four (7%), dural tear with no neurologic sequelae in one (2%), and continuing back and/or leg pain in three (5%). One patient with preexisting foot drop experienced additional impairment in weakness one grade below the operative level. One patient experienced postoperative right foot and leg muscle weakness after embolectomy and fasciotomy of his leg. He was fitted with an ankle–foot orthosis.

### 360° Fusion

Average age in this group of 17 procedures was 40 years (range 31–55). Of the 17 procedures, 16 (94%) resulted in solid union. One patient was found to have resorption of graft at L3–L4 both anteriorly and posteriorly at the 2-year follow-up visit.

### Reoperation

From 1992 to 1994, a total of 16 patients in the series underwent reoperation for suspected pseudarthrosis and ongoing pain. Two had reoperation at other centers with removal of hardware. Fourteen had reoperation in our center (Table 3). Pseudarthrosis was evident at the time of surgical exploration in eight patients who subsequently had 360° fusion with posterior instrumentation. All went on to have solid union. Eight of the 16 reoperations were explorations of suspected pseudarthroses and posterior augmentation of the primary fusion. One of these was found to have solid fusion at reoperation. Subsequently, all but two of the patients having reexploration/posterior augmentation procedures went on to have solid union.

## DISCUSSION

### Biomechanical Considerations

From a clinical standpoint, an instrumentation system must provide adequate stability until fusion is achieved, at which time the load is transferred successfully to

**TABLE 3.** *Reoperations within study period[a]*

| Procedure 1 | Fusion result | Procedure 2 | Fusion result |
| --- | --- | --- | --- |
| Female, hooks | Pseudarthrosis | Hooks | Solid |
| Male, hooks | Pain but solid | Augment w hooks | Solid |
| Male, hooks | Pseudarthrosis | Screws | Solid |
| Male, hooks | Pseudarthrosis | 360° hooks | Solid |
| Male, hooks | Pseudarthrosis | Hooks | Nonunion |
| Female, hooks | Pseudarthrosis | Screws | Solid |
| Male, hooks | Pseudarthrosis | 360° hooks | Solid |
| Male, hooks | Pseudarthrosis | Hybrid | Nonunion |
| Male, hooks | Pseudarthrosis | Hooks (sandwich) | Solid |
| Male, hooks | Pseudarthrosis | 360° screws | Solid |
| Male, hooks | Pain but solid | Augment 360° hooks | Solid |
| Male, hooks | Pseudarthrosis | 360° hooks | Solid |
| Male, hooks | Pseudarthrosis | Screws | Solid |
| Male, hybrid | Pseudarthrosis | Screws | Solid |

[a] Study period from February 11, 1988 to March 26, 1992.

the fusion rather than the implant (6). Systems that provide the necessary support for this load transfer have been widely reported in the literature (8,9,11,22,23,26,28,29). This study shows the benefits of a more rigid fixation system in enhancing fusion and minimizing complications. However, excessive rigidity likewise has theoretical disadvantages. The question remains: Just how much rigidity is "enough," and what are the biomechanical features of an instrumentation system that enhance fusion?

The superior rigidity of pedicle screw systems over laminar hook or wire systems has been presented by earlier investigators and is suggested by the results of this paper (16,19,20,28). As development of various instrumentation systems has advanced, an improved end point (solid fusion) has occurred with incremental changes in bone–instrument attachments. Thus, hooks have produced better results than wire and, in turn, screws or bolts have produced better results than hooks (28). Semi-rigid systems have been defined as those that produce a nonrigid connection of bone attachment to longitudinal element (17,28). By this criterion, the hook–rod system described herein falls within that group. Motion of the lamina within the hook on flexion–extension, leading to failure to provide additional stability on rotation, results in inadequate immobilization and the disappointing fusion results in this group.

Transpedicular screw attachment, with a rigid connection between screw and longitudinal element, provides the support necessary to improve the clinical end point (fusion rate), as reflected in the rigid fixation group in this study. Choice of adequately large screw diameter (17) coupled with appropriate rod diameter (6.35-mm rods rather than 4.76-mm rods) (5) produces the desired $k_i/k_v$ ratio to achieve optimal load sharing between the implant and the spine. Achieving this balance of sufficient rigidity while avoiding the effects of excessive stiffness is the test of an effective system.

A system that incorporates cross-connection of longitudinal elements is more likely to possess the inherent rigidity to provide improved three-column support, especially in torsion. By mitigating those forces that produce shearing and other stress effects on pedicle screws, resultant screw pull-out, bending, and breakage are minimized. Johnston and co-workers (7) discuss "crosslinking" of longitudinal elements to effect rigidity, and they and others quantified the in vitro rigidity of systems employing such crosslinkages (1,2,7).

### Biomechanical Comparisons with Other Systems

The degree of rigidity of spinal instrumentation systems varies by product. In 1993, Cunningham et al. (4) published testing data showing the compressive stiffness of the Rogozinski system compared with other common spinal systems. The stiffness of the Rogozinski system was 70.4 kN/m, whereas the stiffness of TSRH, CD, and Isola systems was noticeably higher—131.1 kN/m, 136.9 kN/m, and 153.2 kN/m, respectively. In this study, the Rogozinski system was tested in its most modular form (screws offset from the rod) instead of its simple form (screws directly attached to the rod).

The stiffness of the Rogozinski system can vary, depending on the configuration of the construct. Testing in the manufacturer's laboratory has shown the offset screw constructs to have a compressive stiffness of 87.6 kN/m, whereas the direct screw constructs have a stiffness of 127.4 kN/m in compression, a 45% increase. The difference in the manufacturer's offset screw test data from the results of Cunning-

**TABLE 4.** *Results of posterolateral fusion by type of instrumentation*

|  | All-hooks (%) | All-screws (%) |
|---|---|---|
| Number | 54 | 60 |
| Graft type |  |  |
|   Autologous | 50 | 100 |
|   Banked* | 50 | 0 |
| Levels |  |  |
|   1 level | 28 | 50 |
|   2 or more | 72 | 50 |
| Previous surgery | 43 | 33 |
| Smokers |  |  |
|   Pre-op only | 69 | 25 |
|   Pre- and post-op | 50 | 12 |
| Internal bone stimulation | 9 | 72 |
| Solid fusion (*n*/%)** | 29/54 | 51/85 |

* Freeze-dried or cadaveric.
** Difference between all-hooks and all-screws $p = 0.00064$ based on the two-tailed Fisher's Exact Test.

ham et al. is produced by a slightly different test protocol. However, the important finding is the percent difference in stiffness between the two constructs (offset versus direct or in-line screws).

## Clinical Results

The results of this study support observations by earlier investigators of the superiority of a rigid system employing transpedicular pedicle screws rigidly attached to longitudinal elements over systems with nonrigid connection of components. Fusion rates are dramatically higher in the rigid fixation group.

It should be noted that a number of patient and treatment variables must be weighed in the determination of fusion success or failure. Table 4 shows a comparison of all-screws and all-hooks patient variables and results thereof. More patients receiving all-hooks fixation also were smokers and underwent repeat and multilevel back surgery. In addition, far fewer patients in the all-hooks group received the benefits of internal bone stimulation. Banked bone graft rather than autologous graft was used in a number of the earliest all-hooks procedures (Table 5), which we believe contributed to disappointing fusion rates in this group. As our understanding of the superior results from using autologous graft advanced, we abandoned the use of banked graft altogether.

The obvious factor of less surgeon experience must be considered in the earlier groups. Varying results among all groups point to the importance of careful patient selection and the imperative for highly experienced surgeons to perform these high-risk surgeries. Lee (13) has coined the term ''surgeon factor'' to document the obvious improvement in patient outcome when surgeons have had a sufficient learning curve.

Further improvements in fusion rates have been attributed to incorporation of anterior fusion with posterior instrumentation and fusion. This technique provides optimal three-column load-sharing, and investigators using the 360° fusion have reported the highest fusion rates of all techniques (10). Not all patients are appropriate candidates for this highly complex and invasive surgery, however. Our results using

**TABLE 5.** *Results of autologous versus banked bone graft*

| Graft type[a] | Number of patients | Number/% fused |
|---|---|---|
| Autologous + banked bone graft | 27 | 12/44 |
| Autologous alone | 27 | 17/63 |

[a] Graft with instrumented (hooks only) posterolateral fusion in all cases. Use of banked bone was abandoned in posterolateral fusions employing other construct types after August, 1990.

the 360° technique, compared with results in posterior fusions alone, are shown in Table 6.

Surgeons may anticipate the occurrence of increased adjacent level degeneration after spine instrumentation because of the resultant altered spinal biomechanics. However, fear of increased abnormal stress transfer must be weighed against maximizing the rate of fusion, which is still the primary goal of spinal fusion with instrumentation. In our experience with patients through the first 7 years of surgery, adjacent segment degeneration has not been a predictable outcome, although follow-up for its occurrence continues.

Postoperative smoking has been identified as a risk factor for pseudarthrosis within this series. Although smoking cessation is a prerequisite to surgery, some patients resume the habit postoperatively, with the effect that they have much lower fusion rates than nonsmokers and patients who permanently cease smoking before their surgery. Postoperative smokers undergoing more rigid fixations achieved solid union in only 77% of cases, whereas nonsmokers and preoperative-only smokers had a significantly higher fusion rate of 92%. Postoperative smokers in the least rigid (all-hooks) fixation group achieved solid union in only 48% of cases, with nonsmokers and preoperative-only smokers having a fusion rate of 67%. We have concluded from examining the patient population from the perspective of smoking that permanent smoking cessation is absolutely crucial to a successful outcome, but that higher levels of construct rigidity contribute to successful fusion regardless of smoking status.

Outcome in terms of pain levels and return to work within the first year after surgery have been studied in this patient series. Overall, 63% reported pain improvement (patient-reported levels by analogue scale from 0 to 10) from preoperatively to postoperatively. Rates of return to work were modest, as can be expected in patients requiring spinal arthrodesis surgery, many of whom (90%) are laborers receiving

**TABLE 6.** *Results of posterolateral versus 360° procedures, 1988 to 1992[a]*

| | Posterolateral | 360° |
|---|---|---|
| Number | 114 | 17 |
| Construct type (*n*) | | |
|   Hooks | 54 | 4 |
|   Screws | 60 | 13 |
| Solid union (%) | | |
|   Hooks | 54 | 100 |
|   Screws | 85 | 92 |
| Nonunion (*n*/%) | | |
|   Hooks | 25/44 | 0 |
|   Screws | 9/15 | 1/8 |

[a] Instrumentation, either all-hooks or all-screws, was applied posteriorly in all techniques. 360° procedures include use of banked bone plugs anteriorly.

Workers' Compensation. By the end of the first postoperative year, 24% were working at full duties, 18% at modified duties, 33% seeking work, and 20% unable to work because of pain, complications, or unrelated additional pathology. (Work status in the remainder is unknown or unrecorded.) Many patients seeking work were hampered in their search by lack of education and skills appropriate for the job market. However, a significant finding was that, of patients reporting 50% or more improvement in their level of pain from pre- to postoperatively, more than 60% had returned to work by the end of the first year.

Our study supports the conclusion that many systems, such as the Rogozinski system, now in use for instrumentation of lumbar spinal fusion possess sufficient strength and rigidity to support arthrodesis. We believe that the ability of the system to allow modulation of rigidity in the face of various clinical scenarios distinguishes the Rogozinski system from many others.

Regardless of the instrumentation used, surgical outcome is enhanced by careful patient selection, surgeon experience, and use of more rigid constructs. Ultimately, no instrumentation system is a replacement for good surgical judgment and impeccable surgical technique.

## REFERENCES


1. Abumi K, Panjabi M, Duranceau J. Biomechanical evaluation of spinal fixation devices: Part III. Stability provided by six spinal fixation devices and interbody bone graft. *Spine* 1989;14:1249–55.
2. Boos N, Marchesi D, Aebi M. Survivorship analysis of pedicular fixation systems in the treatment of degenerative disorders of the lumbar spine: a comparison of Cotrel-Dubousset instrumentation and the AO Internal Fixator. *J Spinal Dis* 1992;5:405–9.
3. Cotrell Y, Dubousset J. The use of pedicle screws and universal instrumentation for spinal fixation. Presented at the AO Trauma Course, Davos, Switzerland, December 1985.
4. Cunningham BW, Sefter JC, Shono Y, McAfee PC. Static and cyclical biomechanical analysis of pedicle screw spinal constructs. *Spine* 1993;18:1677.
5. Duffield RC, Carson WL, Chen L, Voth B. Longitudinal element size effect on load sharing, internal loads, and fatigue life of tri-level spinal implant constructs. *Spine* 1993;18:1697–703.
6. Gurr K, McAfee P. Cotrel-Dubousset instrumentation in adults: a preliminary report. *Spine* 1988;13:510–20.
7. Johnston CE, Ashman RB, Baird AM, Allard MS. Effect of spinal construct stiffness on early fusion mass incorporation: experimental study. *Spine* 1990;13:908.
8. Kaneda K, Satoh S, Nohara Y, Oguma T. Distraction rod instrumentation with posterolateral fusion in isthmic spondylolisthesis: 53 cases followed for 18–89 months. *Spine* 1985;10:383.
9. Knodt TH, Larrick R. Distraction fusion of the lumbar spine. *Ohio State Med J* 1964;62:140.
10. Kozak JA, O'Brien JP. Simultaneous combined anterior and posterior fusion: an independent analysis of a treatment for the disabled low-back pain patient. *Spine* 1990;15:322–8.
11. Krag MH. Lumbosacral fixation with the Vermont Spinal Fixator. In: Lin PM, Gill K, eds. *Lumbar interbody fusion: principles and techniques of spine surgery.* Rockville, MD: Aspen Publishers, 1988:251–60.
12. Krag MH, Beynnon BD, Pope MH, Frymoyer JW, Haugh LD, Weaver DL. An internal fixator for posterior application to short segments of the thoracic, lumbar, or lumbosacral spine: design and testing. *Clin Orthop* 1986;203:75.
13. Lee CK. Outcomes of solid spinal fusion: The surgeon's factor. Presented at the 8th Annual Meeting of the North American Spine Society, San Diego, CA, October 14, 1993.
14. Luque E. Interpeduncular segmental fixation. *Clin Orthop* 1986;203:54.
15. Luque E. The anatomic basis and development of segmental spinal instrumentation. *Spine* 1982;7.
16. Luque ER, Rapp GF: A new semi-rigid method for interpedicular fixation of the spine. *Orthopedics* 1988;11:1445–50.
17. McAfee PC, Farey ID, Sutterlin CE, Gurr KR, Warden KE, Cunningham BW. Device-related osteoporosis with spinal instrumentation. *Spine* 1989;14:9.
18. Olerud S, Karlstrom G, Sjostrom L. Transpedicular fixation of the thoracolumbar vertebral fracture. *Clin Orthop* 1988;227:44.

19. Panjabi MM. Biomechanical evaluation of spinal fixation devices: Part I. A conceptual framework. *Spine* 1988;13:1129–34.
20. Panjabi MM. Part II. Stability provided by eight internal fixation devices. *Spine* 1988;13:1135.
21. Rogozinski C, Rogozinski A. The Rogozinski spinal rod system: a new internal fixation of the spine. In: Arnold DM, Lonstein JE, eds. *Spine: state of the art reviews. Pedicle fixation of the lumbar spine.* Philadelphia: Hanley & Belfus, 1992:107.
22. Rogozinski C, Rogozinski A. The Rogozinski spinal rod system for fixation of the lumbosacral spine. In: Hitchon P, Rengachary S, Traynelis V, eds. *Techniques of spinal fusion and stabilization.* New York: Thieme Medical Publishers, 1995:362–72.
23. Roy-Camille R. Internal fixation of the lumbar spine. *Clin Orthop* 1986;203:7.
24. Roy-Camille R, Saillant G, Mazel C. Internal fixation of the lumbar spine with pedicle screw plating. *Clin Orthop* 1986;203:7.
25. Selby D. Internal fixation with Knodt's rods. *Clin Orthop* 1986;203:179.
26. Steffee A. Segmental spine plates with pedicle screw fixation. *Clin Orthop* 1986;203:45.
27. Steffee AD, Biscup RS, Sitkowski DJ. Segmental spine plates with pedicle screw fixation: a new internal fixation device for disorders of the lumbar and thoracolumbar spine. *Clin Orthop* 1986;203:45.
28. Zdeblick TA. A prospective, randomized study of lumbar fusion: preliminary results. *Spine* 1993;18:983.
29. Zielke K, Strempel AV. Posterior lateral distraction spondylodesis using the twofold sacral bar. *Clin Orthop* 1986;203:1151.
30. Zucherman J, Hsu K, White A, Wynne G. Early results of spinal fusion using Variable Spine Plating system. *Spine* 1988;13:570.

*Instrumented Fusion of the Degenerative Lumbar Spine: State of the Art, Questions, and Controversies,* edited by M. Szpalski, R. Gunzburg, D. M. Spengler, and A. Nachemson. Lippincott–Raven Publishers, Philadelphia © 1996.

# 15

# Louis' System For Lumbosacral Fusion

R. Louis and C. Louis

*Service d'Orthopedie et Chirurgie Vertébrale, Hôpital de La Conception, 13005 Marseille, France*

Our osteosynthesis method is based on the Roy-Camille pedicular screw principle (7). We created our own method in 1971, involving special features in terms of material and techniques. Instead of plates with holes at 13-mm intervals, we chose plates with holes at short intervals, separated by a 9-mm distance, so that we could always find a screw hole located directly over the pedicular site, regardless of the size of the patient.

For the L5–S1 region, we designed a so-called "butterfly" plate, which is particularly well adapted to the lumbosacral junction. Oblique screwing directed toward the sacral alae was designed and used for all lumbosacral osteosynthesis procedures, to minimize the risk for contact with a sacral root. This was followed by development of a series of plates for anterior vertebral osteosynthesis, with a curved plate for the thoracic spine, the same straight plates as in the case of posterior osteosynthesis for the thoracolumbar spine, and specific plates for repair of the odontoid process, for C1–C2 anterior arthrodesis, and for anterior osteosynthesis of the lower part of the cervical spine.

We also designed reduction equipment, a reducing device for shortening of the spine after vertebral osteotomy and a reducing set for reduction of spondylolisthesis via an anterior approach. Peroperative reduction of more severe vertebral deformities is obtained by the application of three forces under vertebral traction, one cephalic, the second podal, and the third posterior to the convexity of the deformity.

In contrast to the technique described by the majority of authors, arthrodesis associated with vertebral osteosynthesis is not intertransverse but rather is intra-articular posteriorly and intersomatic anteriorly. Posterior intra-articular arthrodesis usually does not require any extrafocal graft material, because corticocancellous shavings taken from one or more spinous processes are used.

The stainless steel plates can be modeled during the surgical procedure using three-tip forceps to adapt them to any curvature whatsoever. The plates also can be cut with large cutting forceps in such a way as to avoid leaving empty screw holes at the extremities of the montage.

*175*

This method of application of posterior vertebral osteosynthesis avoids any interference with the neurovascular bundles of the spinal muscles responsible for maintaining the trunk in an erect position. The majority of methods that use, starting from the midline, intertransverse grafts and insertion of material with pedicular screwing to the outside of the zygapophyseal joints, very often cause unavoidable damage to these neurovascular bundles, which is a surgical disaster when the importance of these muscular structures is considered.

Finally, the 20-year experience with our method offers a guarantee of reliability.

## LUMBOSACRAL SPINE

Like other vertebral sectors, the lumbosacral spine can be treated by posterior osteosynthesis, anterior osteosynthesis, or a combination of the two.

### Posterior Lumbosacral Osteosynthesis

Screws 5.5 mm in diameter with a round, hexagonal head are used for this region. A 3.2–mm-diameter drill bit is used to prepare the screw holes. We prefer to use a hand drill so as to avoid irremedial lesions should the bit run off-track with a power drill that cannot stop instantaneously (Fig. 1).

The point of penetration in lumbar pedicles is the crossing point between a vertical line running through the sagittal portion of the joint line covering the pedicle, a horizontal line passing 1 mm above the lower extremity of the facet, and a third curved line traced 4 mm upward and medial to the pars interarticularis notch. However, identification of the vertical line varies according to the anatomic shape of the posterior joints, which may vary the extent to which they are sagittal or frontal. Therefore, three types of vertical line can be described. When the joint space has a square shape, with a frontal medial part and a sagittal lateral part, the vertical line passes through the most lateral part of the joint interspace of the posterior joint. When the posterior joint has a frontal joint interspace, the vertical line should pass through the junction of the middle third and lateral third of the joint. When the disposition of the posterior joint is very sagittal, the vertical line should pass 2–3 mm lateral to the external part of this joint interspace. In any event, an anteroposterior

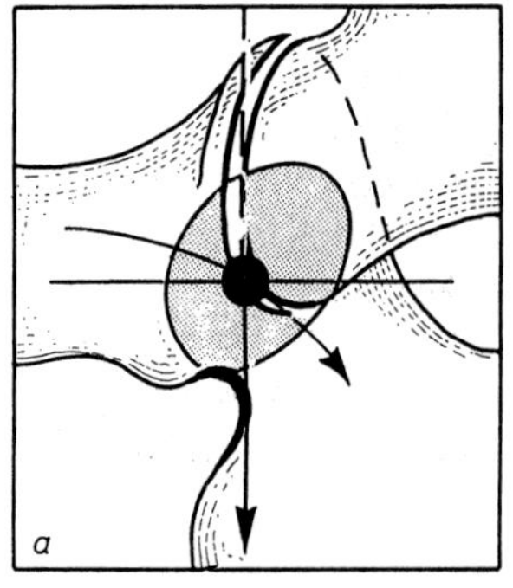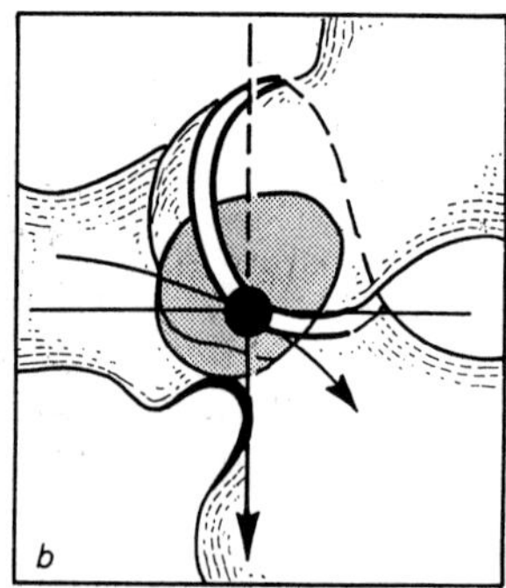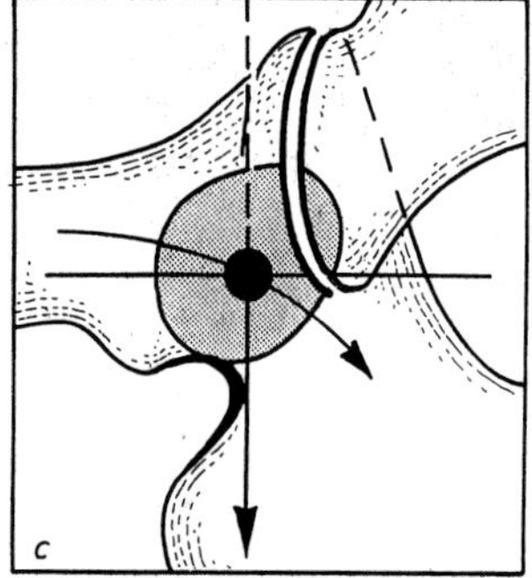

**FIG. 1.** Variation in projection of posterior joints in relation to pedicle.

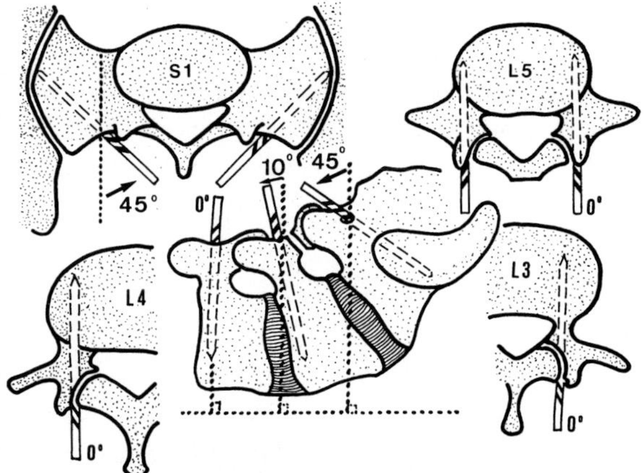



**Fig. 2.** Orientation of drilling and screwing for lumbar and sacral screws.

x-ray of the patient always shows pre- and perioperatively the position of the joint interspace in relation to the projection of the pedicle (Fig. 2).

For L5–S1 osteosynthesis, butterfly-shaped plates are available, i.e., imitating the morphology of the posterior arch, in a single block with four screw holes, the two upper holes being transversely elongated for the two pedicular screws of L5 and the two lower holes directed obliquely at 45° outwards and caudally to enable fixation in the sacral alae. These plates are available in three sizes, large, medium, and small, on the basis of the interpedicular distance of L5. Regardless of the plate model, sacral screw holes have been studied on the basis of anatomic data in such a way as to enable the positioning of sacral screws always at a distance from S1 or S2 spinal nerves (see Fig. 2).

Installation of a "butterfly" plate starts by use of the drill bit to make the two L5 pedicular holes after having shortened the tip of the overlaying facet (Fig. 3). A bayonet-shaped pedicular landmark pin is positioned in the drill holes, and the interpedicular distance enables choice of the type of plate to be used. The plate selected is slid along the two pedicular landmark pins and held by the operative assistant in such a way that the landmark pin remains clearly in the middle of the plate screw hole. Each landmark pin is removed in turn and is replaced by a screw held on the tip of the screwdriver. Drill holes for the sacrum are made directly through the holes of the plate and screws are positioned in the same way. Penetration of the drill bit into bone should be 1 cm only, as the screws are self-tapping.

For osteosynthesis extending from L4 or L3 to the sacrum, paired and symmetrical plates are used, each having an upper screw hole for sagittal pedicular screwing in L3 or L4 and two lower holes for oblique screwing in the sacral alae. The middle portion of these plates has closely spaced screw holes, four for the L4–S1 plate and eight for the L3–S1 plate, to enable precise screwing of intermediate pedicles (Fig. 4).

When this osteosynthesis is used provisionally for pars reconstruction in bilateral spondylolysis, the two defects are first prepared by freeing them of all fibrous and cartilaginous tissue, and cancellous bone shavings obtained from two spinous processes are inserted. The plate is then removed 4 months after the first stage in individuals who are in a period of growth and 2 months later for other patients. For permanent arthrodesis in bilateral spondylolysis, it is essential not only to graft the two pars defects but also to prepare L5–S1 posterior joints by resection of their

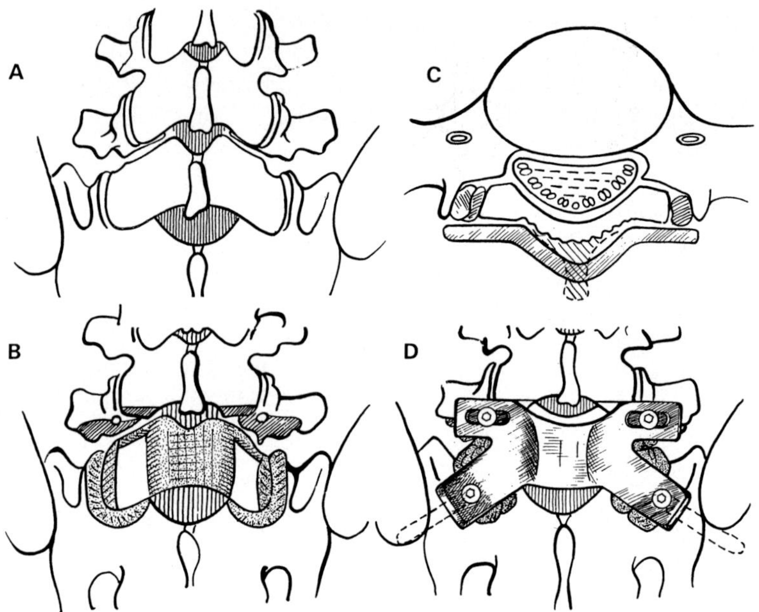

**FIG. 3. A,B:** Scraping of defect regions and of posterior joint interspaces for insertion of corticocancellous bone shavings, usually obtained from two spinous processes. **C,D:** Installation of "butterfly" screwed plate.

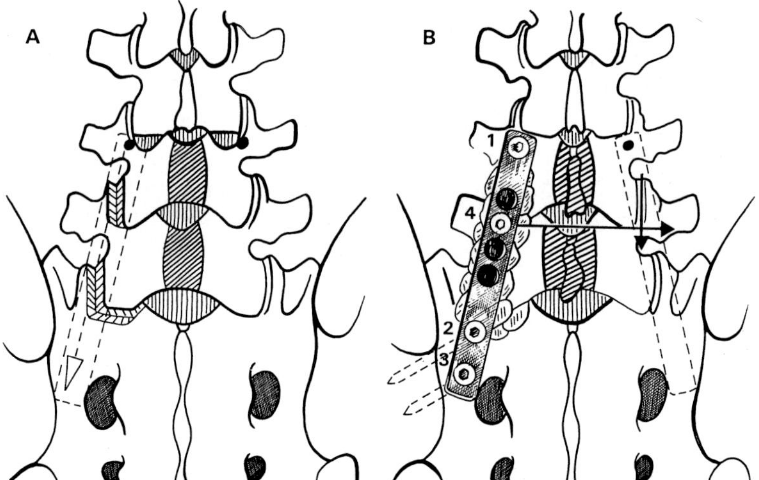

**FIG. 4. A:** Technique for installation of two screwed lumbosacral plates from L4 to S1. Capsule and cartilage of L4–L5 and L5–S1 posterior joint interspaces excised, with insertion of corticocancellous bone shavings obtained from two spinous processes. **B:** Installation of plates starts with L4 upper pedicular screw hole, then first sacral screw, followed by second and finally the intermediate screw for L5 pedicle using the contra-lateral pedicular landmark. Image intensification confirmation is essential.

capsules and their cartilaginous plates accessible in the sagittal portion. Bone shavings from the spinous processes are then packed into the scraped joint interspaces and into the zygapophysolaminar interspace underlying the facet joint. In our experience, it is of no value to graft outside the posterior joints.

For L4–S1 or L3–S1 lumbosacral plates, the procedure begins by positioning the upper screw, followed by alignment of the plate along the middle of the posterior joints, i.e., slightly divergent towards the sacrum. The first sacral screw is then inserted after a drill hole has been made through the plate, the second sacral screw then being positioned. Intermediate pedicular holes are identified in relation to the opposite side by choosing the screw hole that best corresponds. Screw lengths in the average adult are 45 mm for pedicles, 45 mm for the first sacral screw, and 35 mm for the second sacral screw.

Lumbosacral fusion via a posterior approach requires wearing of a lumbar-reinforced corset for 4 months. We have added two rules to our protocol to avoid postoperative low back pain:

1. Lumbosacral plates should be inserted with the patient in a position of 30° of flexion of the thighs in relation to the trunk.
2. For the first 2 postoperative months, the patient should avoid the natural sitting

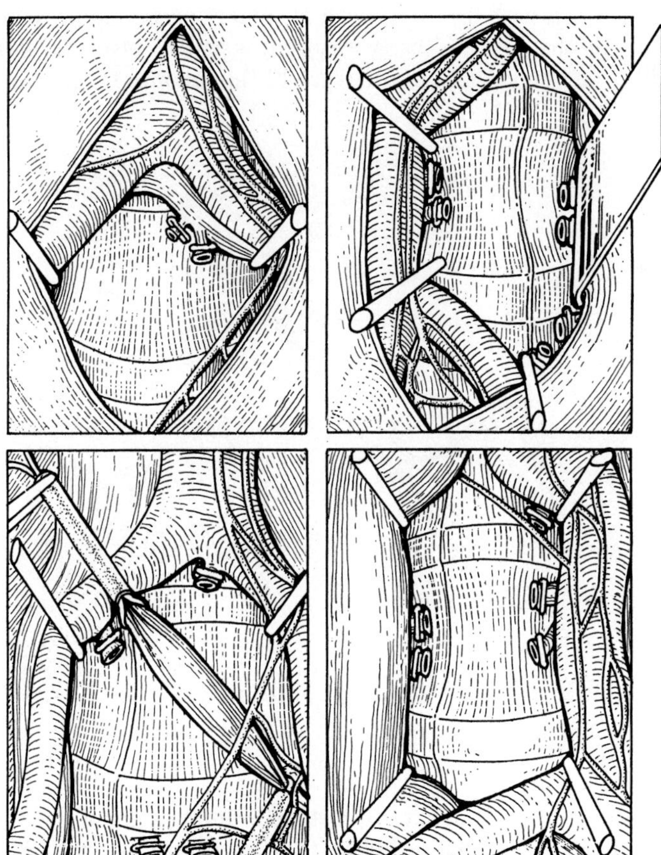

**FIG. 5.** Various maneuvers for mobilization of the prevertebral great vessels for exposure of the last three lumbar discs before lumbosacral fusion.

position, i.e., should keep one thigh along a line extending from the torso, with the knee in 90° flexion, while the other lower limb is in the natural sitting position. This position avoids automatic flexion of the lumbosacral spine in sitting position and thus avoids excessive traction on lumbosacral screws.

Image intensification should be used during each surgical procedure for identification, if necessary, of pedicles using temporary Kirschner pins inserted at the point selected on pedicles, and for assessment of the montage at the end of the procedure.

### Anterior Osteosynthesis of the Lumbosacral Spine

Two techniques are available, particularly for spondylolisthesis surgery.

When perioperative vertebral traction in slight lordosis enables satisfactory reduction of L4–L5 or L5–S1 spondylolisthesis, a fibular peg is used. A 5- to 6-cm segment of fibular shaft obtained during the surgery is positioned through the vertebral bodies, passing through the olisthesic intervertebral disc. To insert this graft, a transperitoneal approach is used, with exposure of the disc above the olisthesic disc. A Kirschner pin is inserted in the midline at an angle of 45° in relation to the anterior aspect of the vertebral body, for a distance of 6 cm along the axis of the vertebral bodies and of the body of the sacrum, and under image intensification. Once the proper position of the pin has been ensured, a tap is inserted along it that will produce a tunnel corresponding to the track of the pin and for the same length. The

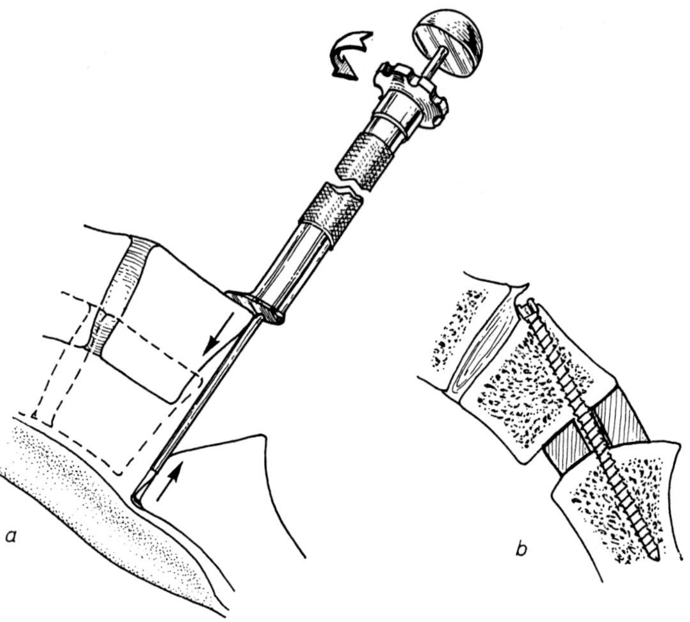


**FIG. 6. a:** Anteroposterior reduction of olisthesic vertebra using our reduction device supported on the posterior edge of the sacral plate and the anterior aspect of L5. The screwing mechanism enables control of reduction under image intensification. **b:** Fixation involves a long 7.5-mm-diameter transcorporeal axial screw. Intersomatic fusion is acquired by four fragments of fibular shaft arranged vertically around the axial screw.

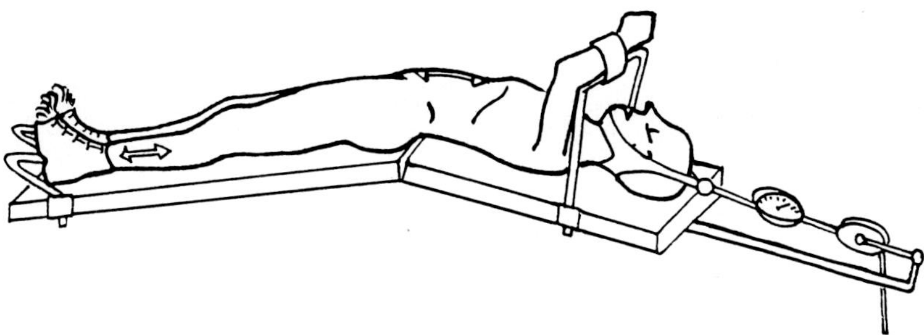

**FIG. 7.** Vertebral traction for perioperative reduction in different types of vertebral deformity.

fibular graft is then inserted with slight force through the prepared tunnel, simultaneously resulting in osteosynthesis and autogenous bone grafting (Fig. 5).

The second type of osteosynthesis used is complementary to reduction of severe spondylolisthesis via an anterior approach, in cases where perioperative lordotic vertebral traction is insufficient to obtain adequate reduction. This technique involves instrumental reduction by excision of the olisthesic disc as far as the anterior surface of the dural sac, via a transperitoneal approach. A system of elevators with angulations ranging from 90° to 180° enables lifting of the olisthesic vertebral body above the sacrum, followed by insertion of our reducing device (Fig. 6) through the emptied and widened intervertebral space, its axial portion then being hooked onto the posterior edge of the sacral plate and its peripheral portion onto the anterior surface of the olisthesic vertebral body. Screwing of the two parts of the reducing device enables the L5 vertebral body to be pushed backwards until alignment with the sacrum is obtained under image intensification. This reduction is held in place by a large axial transcorporeal screw inserted from the inferior edge of the above disc along the midline, through the body of L5, the L5–S1 intervertebral space, and the body of the sacrum, for a distance of 6–7 cm. Four fragments of fibular diaphysis are inserted into the vertebral interspace on either side of the central screw.

### Combined Approach to the Lumbosacral Spine

When spondylolisthesis is treated via an anterior approach, the montage is always completed 8 days later by posterior lumbosacral osteosynthesis. After reduction of severe spondylolisthesis, it is preferable to fit the patient with a lumbosacral plaster cast for 4 months.

## SPECIAL ASPECTS

### Perioperative Vertebral Traction

When a kyphotic deformity of the spine is present, vertebral traction is applied perioperatively using a leather helmet fitted to the head and attached to a cradle fitted to the operating table by a pulley block and a dynamometer. The patient's feet are placed in surgical shoes attached to the caudal end of the table. Finally, the table is angulated as required under the summit of the kyphosis requiring reduction (Fig.

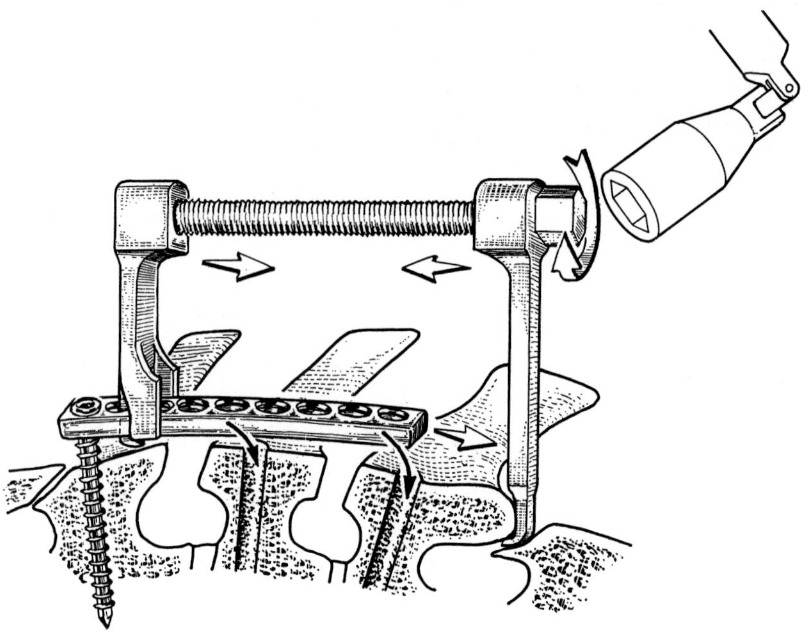

**FIG. 8.** Vertebral compression system for osteosynthesis after vertebral osteotomy. The screw plate is fixed at one extremity while the compressor draws the plate toward the other extremity of the spine.

7). The three forces are increased during the procedure, traction not exceeding 5 kg for the cervical spine and 10–15 kg for the thoracic or lumbosacral spine. Posterior angulation of the table is increased until an almost anatomic vertebral curvature is obtained. This method avoids dangerous maneuvers and obviates the need for equipment to be accompanied by an incorporated vertebral reduction system, making it lighter, less voluminous, and far less expensive.

### Compression or Distraction Device for Posterior Screwed Plates

Ancillary instruments have been developed, consisting of a pair of reducing devices for the application of tension, particularly during compression, to screwed plates when reduction of kyphosis after vertebral osteotomy is desired. The two osteosynthesis plates are screwed at their upper extremity and the compression apparatus is installed such that the cranial hook is fixed to one screw hole of the plate and the caudal hook to the lower edge of a lamina. Screwing of the two hooks of the compressor causes the lower extremity of the plate to slide along the spine and thus brings the lower screw hole of the plate to the level of the pedicle selected for osteosynthesis. Screws are then inserted directly through the plate under tension. This device is used, in addition to vertebral traction, in other deformities to avoid incorporation of a reduction system into osteosynthesis material (Fig. 8).

### Possible Complications

When cobalt–chrome screws were used, up to 13% of patients experienced one or two broken, twisted, or partially expelled screws. Since 1985, we have carefully studied and experimentally evaluated a new range of stainless steel screws with design and measurements particularly specific to the structure of vertebral bone. At present we see virtually no screw problems in our patients. Complications that may accompany pedicular screwing include damage to a spinal nerve in a foramen, in the vertebral canal, or outside the pedicle. To avoid such complications, very careful attention must be paid to using the points of penetration described, and surgeons beginning to use the technique must use Kirschner pins for provisional identification of pedicle tracts by superficial introduction at the points of penetration selected with perioperative image intensification. Finally, it is important an assistant to touch the lower or upper limb on the side of osteosynthesis during the procedure so that pedicular penetration can be stopped immediately if any spastic movement is felt.

If a patient experiences severe nerve root pain after recovery from anesthesia, or any signs of neurologic deficit, it is absolutely essential to rapidly remove the screw, either under local anesthesia via a small side incision over the head of the screw considered to be responsible or directly with general anesthesia. Complications associated with anterior screws may also be caused by poor screw position, and therefore great importance is attached to performance of procedures in a strict supine position for anterior approaches so as to be always completely aware of the orientation of screws in relation to the midline sagittal plane. Surgery in the lateral position has the potential for much greater error positioning of screws. Similarly, anterior osteosynthesis must avoid any damage to vital structures caused by screw loosening. It is therefore absolutely contraindicated to place osteosynthesis material behind the great vessels.

### Consolidation

With our technique of osteosynthesis by screwed plates and fusion of posterior joints, in the lumbosacral region of a series of 500 patients analyzed, a fusion rate of 94.7% was obtained for posterior approach only and 100% for combined approaches. Anterior osteosynthesis using a fibula has invariably obtained excellent results, virtually free of nonunion and of loosening.

### Absence of Interference with Vertebral Blood and Nerve Supply

Our posterior osteosynthesis technique, involving the insertion of screwed plates along the posterior joints without passing beyond the lateral edge of the pars, avoids damage to the metameric neurovascular bundles of erector spinae muscles, both in exposing lesions and in osteosynthesis fixation. These bundles are in actual contact with the pars, forming the notch that limits each pars. Techniques that involve laying bare the area beyond this pars notch and which, in addition, involve insertion of large intertransverse grafts and of large amounts of osteosynthesis material beyond the facets, considerably threaten the blood and nerve supply of muscles that are particularly important in supporting the erect position. Many painful postoperative syndromes described as being due to epineuritis or other reasons are in fact related to ischemia and denervation of the erector spinae muscles, which then become relatively incapable of allowing bipedal ambulation without pain. Similarly, our combined approaches for extended vertebral excision for malignant tumor enable us to avoid sectioning of the radiculomedullary arteries. Vertebral excision via the pos-

terior approach only routinely requires coagulation or clipping of two to four radiculomedullary arteries, thus exposing the patient to postoperative neurologic compromise.

## REFERENCES

1. An HS, Cotler JM. *Spinal instrumentation.* Baltimore: Williams & Wilkins, 1992.
2. Louis R. *Surgery of the spine. Surgical anatomy and operative approaches.* Berlin, Heidelberg, New York: Springer-Verlag, 1982.
3. Louis R. Lumbo-sacral fusion by internal fixation. *Clin Orthop Relat Res* 1983;203:18–33.
4. Louis R. Spinal stability as defined by our three column spine concept. *Anat Clin* 1985;7:33–42.
5. Louis R, Maresca C. Les arthrodeses stables de la charnière lombo-sacrée. *Rev Chir Orthop* 1976; 62(suppl II):70–9.
6. Louis R, Maresca C, Bel P. Les fractures instables, la réduction orthopédique. *Rev Chir Orthop* 1977;65:449–51.
7. Roy-Camille R. Ostéosynthèse du rachis dorsal, lombaire et lombo-sacré par plaques métalliques vissées dans les pédicules vertébraux et les apophyses articulaires. *Presse Med* 1970;78:1447.

*Instrumented Fusion of the Degenerative
Lumbar Spine: State of the Art, Questions,
and Controversies*, edited by M. Szpalski,
R. Gunzburg, D. M. Spengler, and
A. Nachemson. Lippincott–Raven
Publishers, Philadelphia © 1996.

# 16

# DDS: The Marburg Experience

M. Pfeiffer, P. Griss, and *V. K. Goel

*Department of Orthopaedic Surgery, Philipps University, D-35033 Marburg,
Germany; and *Department of Biomedical Engineering, University of Iowa,
Iowa City, Iowa 52242*

Posterior lumbar spinal fusion is a well-established procedure for pain relief in cases of spinal instability and degenerative disc disease. Much concern has recently been raised about the rigidity of posterior fusion systems often utilized for the procedure. It has been proved that stress shielding-induced osteopenia and bone graft resorption may occur after instrumentation. Excessively rigid instrumentation also leads to compensatory hypermobility at adjacent segments, probably due to damage inflicted to these segments during (not after) the bony fusion process. Less rigid systems could be the solution to these problems.

The new, versatile DDS (Dorsal Dynamic Spondylodesis) system combines a self-tapping, full-titanium, tapered 6.5-mm screw connected with either titanium rods or cables for either rigid or "semi-rigid" transpedicular fixation (Fig. 1). Rods or cables can be tilted within the slotted screw head up to 30° in the sagittal plane using a half-ball-in-socket fixture for three-dimensional alignment (Fig. 2). Unlike other systems, no additional parts have to be aligned on the rod. Therefore, less "fiddling" is necessary, and the ultimate bending strength at the screw–rod interface for the same torque of the locking nut has shown to be higher than in a construct with a full-ball fixture. The locking nut is accessible via the same direction as the insertion portal without additional soft-tissue removal. In its semi-rigid version, the flexible titanium cable is snugly inserted instead of the rods. It is especially suitable for situations with steep lumbosacral angles or differently located insertion portals on the vertebrae to be fused (e.g., due to malformation or previous instrumentation). There are no outriggers or plates to damage the soft tissue or increase operation time (a common occurence in bulkier systems). Compared, for example, to the AO fixator, the transverse diameter of the device at the rod–screw junction is 19% less, and is 44% less than with the VSP system. The DDS rods/cables are 29% and 69% narrower than the AO rods and the VSP plates, respectively. Shaping of the rods is seldom necessary, and the material properties of the rods therefore remain unchanged. The system comes with easy to handle instruments, e.g., allowing reaming of the insertion portal and partial facetectomy at the same time.

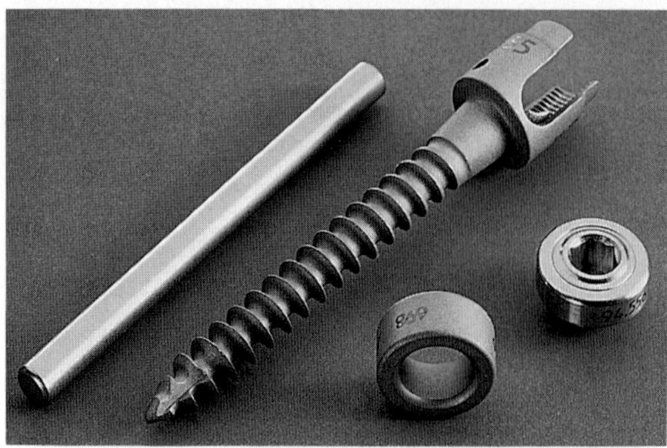

**FIG. 1.** The DDS screw with a short rod, the locking nut, and an optional washer for increasing the screw offset. Note the tapered shape and the reinforced conical neck.

The DDS system is the first pedicle screw implant ever tested comprehensively for fatigue over 5,000,000 cycles of bending compression. The testing protocol has been adopted by commissions for the development of ASTM and FDA standards. With an axial stiffness of 929.2 N/mm (for rod use) a bilateral one-segment DDS construct, tested without anterior column support, ranges in the lower field of commercially available systems, thus preventing overly rigid instrumentation.

The purpose of the semi-rigid fusion is to provide adequate stabilization to promote bony union without inducing the above-mentioned adverse effects and to reduce screw stresses for prevention of screw breakage. In vitro, the semi-rigid instrumentation significantly reduces the motion of the transfixed vertebrae in all primary motion planes from 42.5 to 84.8%, compared to intact. Bilateral rod fusion significantly reduces the motion of the transfixed vertebrae in all primary motion planes from 67.1 to 86.9%. The smallest differences between the bilateral rod and the semi-rigid system are found for lateral bending, which can be explained by the loading mode, location of the instantaneous center of rotation, and biomechanical characteristics. The calculated axial/tension stiffness of the cable amounts to 76% of the rod, whereas its bending/torsion stiffness is 3%. In theory, therefore, unilateral cable instrumentation should be used only in combination with rod instrumentation on the opposite side. Unilateral rod instrumentation is possible and gives less overall stabilization than bilateral cable instrumentation. The former has already proved to work in clinical practice. The cables may also be used in facetectomy, which is not advisable for pure "tension-band systems" such as the Graf implant.

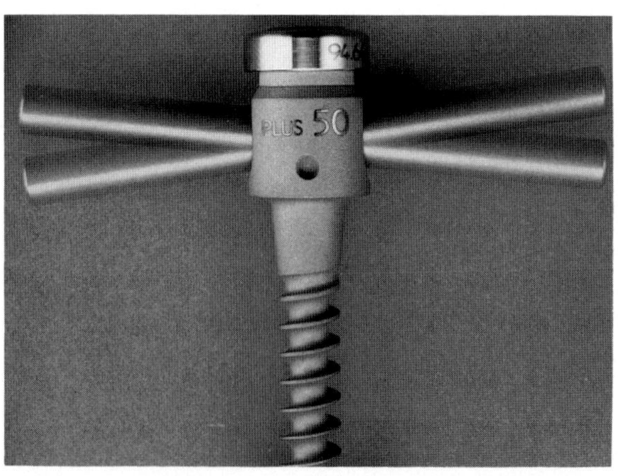

**FIG. 2.** This superimposed picture depicts two possible rod positions. The angle can be infinitely variable, adjusted within a 30° range.

## INDICATIONS (THE MARBURG CONCEPT)

In our department, the DDS system is presently used for greater than 1° spondylolisthesis at L5–S1, instability above L5, and multilevel instabilities (independent of their Meyerding grade), scoliosis/kyphosis (with hook assortment available), tumors, and spondylitis (extrafocally). It has not replaced uninstrumented fusion but has narrowed the indication for a Wiltse (PLF) technique to low-grade olisthesis at L5–S1 and for an O'Brien (ALIF) procedure to instabilities with isolated anterior pathology above L5. Postoperative bracing can therefore be reduced. Circumferential fusion is reserved for cases with spondyloptosis at L5–S1 or complete loss of anterior column support. In general, a posterior short segment instrumentation alone in the latter case will fail, independent of the type of implant, due to lack of load sharing and material fatigue.

## BIOMECHANICS: PURE CONSTRUCT TESTING

### Materials and Methods

A lot of controversy has been sparked about the use of pedicle screw systems in the United States during the last 2 years because of mechanical implant failure. FDA regulations now under way demand the development of testing protocols for measurement of mechanical properties of spinal implants. ASTM standards and ISO standards are currently devised based on the research of Chang et al. (2), Cunningham et al. (4), and the work partly presented here. The device tested was the first ever to undergo the henceforth recommended series of up to 5 million-cycles bending tests.

More than 200 pure construct tests (without involvement of human tissue) have been performed on the DDS pedicle screw–rod system. They involved semi-static axial compression (AS), semi-static bending compression (BS), semi-static axial torsion (TS), and cyclic bending compression (BC) tests in polyethylene blocks, mounted as a "missing-element model" in a material tester. The bilateral cable implant was tested with a fulcrum between the plastic blocks, resulting in mainly tensile loads (BT) on the implant.

Basic construct properties such as stiffness, flexibility, load to failure, and S–N curve were determined. Loosening torque of the screw nut after standardized tightening was measured without and after loading procedures. Each implant was used only once. Failure modes were described and the role of stress raisers evaluated.

### Results

The safety of the screw–rod or screw–cable interface is dependent on the nut tightening torque. A torque meter with ratchet design comes with the instrumentation sets. The half-ball-in-socket fixture proved to be superior to a full-ball-in-socket fixture as used, e.g., in the Diapason system. The gripping force of the screw head at comparable torque was worst for the full-ball, best for the half-ball–rod combination. Tightening beyond 15 Nm gives no significant improvement of the rod grip and should therefore be avoided. The achieved values at 15 Nm torque by far exceed the values that can be expected in a clinical case. The superiority of the half-ball over the full-ball was also obvious in quasi-static bending compression tests.

The bilateral rod implant reached stiffness values in the lower range of other commercially available and clinically used constructs (Table 1). $F_{max}$ for 5 million cycles without failure was 250 N (equal to 8 Nm) (Fig. 3). During the static tests, no breakage could be provoked. In cyclic testing, mechanical failure occurred as expected at the screw–rod interface, except for the two highest load settings. There was no rod comminution.

### Significance of Findings

The testing protocol as performed is a rigorous method for evaluating material properties of the construct and can be recommended for the future. However, it is expensive, time-consuming (at 7 Hz, 5 million cycles take about a week of testing for a single specimen), and it does not predict the in vivo behavior of the device in the standard load-sharing case. It must be borne in mind that increasing stiffness is not necessarily a precondition for sufficient spinal fusion. The endurance limit of the DDS implant allows enough time for load transfer from the implant to the consolidating graft material at clinically relevant bending moments (18).

## BIOMECHANICS: SCREW TESTING

### Materials and Methods

Purely axial pullout tests for DDS screws from 26 isolated lumbar vertebral bodies were done using an MTS machine. The specimens had not been screened for exclusion of osteopenia. They were secured in an adjustable, custom-made clamp fixture. Pull-out tests were attempted on both left and right pedicles of each specimen, and maximal pedicle screw pull-out forces were recorded for insertion up to, but not through, the anterior cortex. Even though axial pull-out is rarely a clinical failure mode, it allows assessment of the efficacy of screw purchase in general and comparisons to the literature that has focused on this type of testing.

In addition, torque-to-failure tests were done, comparing DDS to Steffee (VSP) screws on corresponding sides of vertebral bodies. The torque was measured via a calibrated electronic wrench and the maximal values recorded.

Measurement of bone mineral density (BMD) by means of DXA, in addition to macroscopic and SEM histologic analysis, microradiography, and EDAX, were performed post test to assist in the interpretation of the data.

### Results

Post-test visual inspection of the pedicle screws revealed that all of the screws had remained intact, with no macroscopic signs of thread damage. The mean $F_{max}$ was

**TABLE 1.** *Quasi-static test results of the DDS implant*

| Test | AC | BC | TS | BT |
| --- | --- | --- | --- | --- |
| Ultimate strength | 1403.20 N | 24.38 Nm | 42.30 Nm | 3,432.50 N |
| Ultimate displacement | 2.69 mm | 20.86 mm | 38.00° | 12.37 mm |
| Elastic displacement | 1.87 mm | 6.27 mm | 8.88° | 4.20 mm |
| Stiffness | 929.20 N/mm | 3.07 Nm/mm | 2.58 Nm/° | 114.83 N/mm |

818.5 N. Linear regression analysis of $F_{max}$ with transversal bone mineral density (BMD) in the scanned region of interest (ROI) revealed a highly significant correlation ($r = 0.8011$; $p \leq 0.01$). The absolute BMD values obtained here are not comparable to those obtained in living persons. However, severely osteoporotic vertebrae should be excluded from standard tests of pull-out strengths because they ought to be excluded from clinical application of pedicle screws.

When the highly osteoporotic vertebral bodies (with an ROI BMD below the 25th percentile of all measured vertebrae) were removed from the statistical analysis, mean $F_{max}$ was 916.4 N. The highest measured single value was 1,637.5 N. The values were independent of whether the pedicle was tested first or second in a particular vertebral body: mean $F_{max}$ = 920.8 N and 912.0 N, respectively. The average torque-to-failure for DDS screws was 3.04 Nm and for 7-mm Steffee screws was 1.94 Nm ($p \leq 0.005$; $n = 28$).

### Significance of Findings

If the results are to be compared with other commercially available screws, only studies with sufficient data about the experimental setting should be used. In our

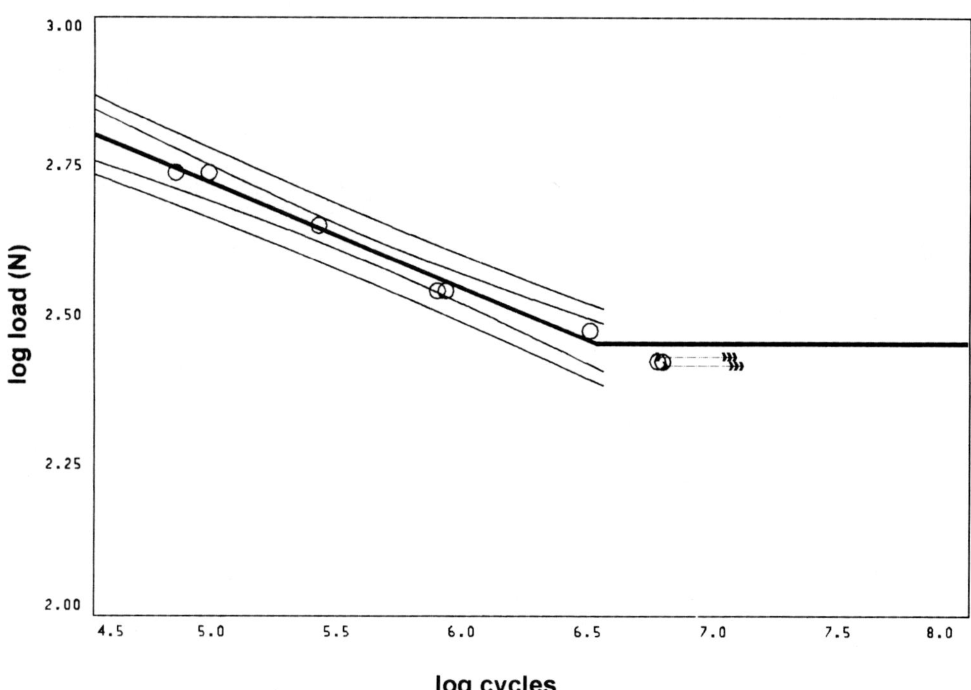

**FIG. 3.** S–N (or Woehler) diagram. The endurance of the specimen is plotted against the bending load (log–log plot). The test does not represent a clinical situation but a worst-case simulation with pure construct loading (no load sharing). The linear regression (*bold line*) and the 95% confidence intervals for individual and mean values are plotted above and below the regression. The endurance limit load equals 8 Nm bending moment.

standard protocol for pull-out tests in vertebral bodies the following variables were controlled:

Screws: material, inner and outer diameters, length, pitch and type of thread, tapping method, order, depth, and direction of insertion, and definition of anterior cortical purchase, e.g., by insertion torque.

Jig: exact three-dimensional alignment, prevention of vertebral tilt, quasi-static loading, load displacement sampling rate.

Vertebrae: e.g., lumbar, fresh, humid, known BMD, no resin embedding.

Post-test evaluation: macroscopic and microscopic, screw wear, debris, intrusion artifacts (EDAX).

Not all variables can be discussed here in detail but are to be published elsewhere (16). This work, in times of increasing importance of material properties of spinal implants, should be also taken as a plea for test standardization to enhance compatibility of results from different studies.

The DDS screw achieved pull-out values superior to those of several other commercially available screws of similar diameter (Table 2). Its torque-to-failure significantly exceeded the values of the screw with the highest pull-out forces mentioned in the literature.

## BIOMECHANICS: IN VITRO TESTING

In vitro evaluation of spinal devices is only one avenue to accomplish stabilization-related studies. Basically, two different approaches have been used in the past to evaluate the in situ performance of a device. The first is measurement of the overall stability provided by the device in stabilizing an injured area within the spine, based on the overall load displacement behavior of the entire specimen. Those studies have shown that the degree of stabilization imparted by different implants can vary among devices. Measurement of the precise changes in rotational motion characteristics across destabilized, instrumented, and adjacent segments is a relatively new approach to evaluate the performance of a fixation device (6).

**TABLE 2.** *Quasi-static pull-out forces of pedicle screws in nonembedded human lumbar vertebrae at 80–100% insertion with caudal/cranial angulation/excluded*

| Reference | Screws tested | Inner/outer diameter/ pitch (mm) | Direction | Fixation technique | Average force (N) | Remarks |
|---|---|---|---|---|---|---|
| Zindrick et al. (21) | Steffee (old) | 6.5/3.0/2.75 (V-type thread) | Axial | No details | 903 | At "visible motion" |
| Moran et al. (15) | Steffee | 7.0/6.0/3.0 (buttress thread) | Axial | No details | 628 (calculated from fig.) | Higher values if angulation ignored |
| Skinner et al. (19) | Steffee (old) | 6.5/3.0/2.75 (V-type thread) | Semi-axial | No details | 697 | Steffee was strongest, compared to AO, Schanz, RC |
| Pfeiffer et al. (16) | DDS | Maximum 6.5/4.6/3.0 (tapered) | Axial | Vise fixation | 916 | Above 1,000 N, endplates yield |

## Materials and Methods

Fresh human lumbar spine specimens (L1–sacrum) were freed of excessive soft tissue and pelvis, leaving intact all except the iliolumbar ligaments. The specimens were immediately sealed in double plastic bags and frozen at −20°C. The spines were x-rayed and their radiologic appearance examined. Only spines without signs of malignant tumors, spondylitis, fractures, or spontaneous fusion were selected. The degree of degeneration was graded. The L3–L4 level was oriented horizontally. The sacrum was then plotted in a plastic padding base. L1 was then connected to a square aluminum loading frame. The rods extended outside of the loading frame for attachment of loading rods and weights. The specimen was removed from the holding fixture and the loading frame filled with plastic padding. During the entire procedure the specimen was kept frozen.

A total of 18 LEDs were attached to the transverse and spinous processes of L2–L5 and to the base plate and loading frame, making three LEDs at each level. The LEDs were hooked up to the CPU of a SELSPOT-II system.

The completely thawed specimen was mounted in a testing frame, the LEDs facing the two stereophotogrammetric video cameras of a previously calibrated SELSPOT system. The three-dimensional load displacement characteristics of all vertebrae were then measured for stepwise application of up to ±3 Nm in flexion–extension (FE), left and right lateral bending (LB), and left and right axial rotation (AR). Henceforth, the rotations in the same plane as the applied loads are called "primary" and the corresponding ones in the two other planes "coupled" motions.

The loads were incrementally applied as pure bending moments, via loading rods connected to the fixation rods of the loading frame. The corresponding displacement data of the vertebral bodies recorded at 0, 0.75, 1.5, 2.25, 3, and again 0 Nm.

Testing was repeated after bilateral removal of the inferior facets of L3 and L4 and left posterior nucleotomy at L3–L4–L5 to simulate clinically relevant instability at two levels. Five other specimens were stabilized with the semi-rigid system, consisting of six pedicle screws and two titanium cables. Five specimens were equipped with bilateral rods instead of cables. Three specimens obtained unilateral rod instrumentation. The screws were inserted level by level according to the method of Magerl (14). The longest possible screws were used without perforating the anterior cortex. As far as possible, the original position of the vertebrae was not altered, i.e., no major distraction or compression was induced. The torque moments of the locking nuts were recorded with an electronic torque wrench. SELSPOT testing was repeated after completed stabilization. The specimens then were subjected to 5,000 cycles of FE at 0.5 Hz under off-center axial loading and under displacement control with an initial peak load of ±3 Nm in a hydraulic materials testing MTS machine. SELSPOT testing was repeated after cycling. During all the steps, the specimen was kept moist by repeated spraying with saline. The cyclic testing was performed in a sealed chamber at 100% relative humidity.

The principles of rigid body mechanics were utilized to describe the motion of the vertebral bodies with respect to the position of the specimen at the start of the loading procedure, in terms of Bryant–Euler angles. The rotational values were normalized with respect to the intact state.

After all the connecting elements (rods or cables) were removed and the loosening torques of the locking nuts recorded, the connecting elements and nuts were checked for damage. The screws were manually checked for loosening in axial and craniocaudal–mediolateral direction. The vertebral bodies were then separated, dissecting the intervertebral disc and grading its degeneration according to Galante (5). The screws were then removed and checked for damage.


## Results

Evaluation of the degree of degeneration of the specimens, based on the radiologic and morphologic score, showed an even distribution among the two instrumentation groups. The intact specimens showed a motion behavior with about 35° FE, 30° LB, and 10° AR of total ROM in the primary motion planes at full load. There was no significant motion difference between the three operative groups before operation. Destabilization led to a significant increase of the average motion at the injured levels (compared to intact) of 162.9% FE, 25.7% LB, and 186.7% AR in the primary planes. Effects of the different instrumentation are presented in Tables 3 and 4.

Semi-rigid instrumentation significantly reduced the motion of the transfixed vertebrae in 18 of 18 possible combinations of primary motion planes and vertebrae. Unilateral rod instrumentation significantly reduced the motion of the transfixed vertebrae in 17 of 18 possible combinations of primary motion planes and vertebrae. Bilateral rod fusion significantly reduced the motion of the transfixed vertebrae in 18 of 18 possible combinations of primary motion planes and transfixed vertebrae. It showed throughout higher stabilization values than the two other methods. It was significantly more stable than the semi-rigid fixation in FE and AR. The unilateral rod fixation was significantly less stable than the semi-rigid fixation in LB and AR and showed throughout lower values than the two other methods. It was therefore the least stable fixation.

Both rod methods significantly increased the motion of the adjacent segment levels in two of 18 cases, whereas the semi-rigid method did so in only one case. The coupled motions (in planes other than loading plane) generally behaved more inconsistently, partly due to the one order of magnitude smaller motion amplitude compared to the primary motion planes. Possible trends are thus often obscured by higher scatter of the values. Nevertheless, the following observations proved to be statistically significant: Semi-rigid and unilateral rod fixation reduced the average motion of the transfixed vertebrae in 31 of 36 possible combinations of coupled motion planes and vertebrae; bilateral rod fixation reduced the average motion of the

**TABLE 3.** *Changes of motion after stabilization compared with intact state of some specimens*

| Primary motion plane fusion type | Reduction of motion at L3–4 and L4–5 | Increased motion at adjacent segment levels |
|---|---|---|
| FE/semi-rigid | L3–4 −79.6%; L4–5 −82.1% | None |
| FE/unilateral rod | L3–4 −59.6%; L4–5 n.s. | None |
| FE/bilateral rod | L3–4 −87.3%; L4–5 −86.9% | None |
| LB/semi-rigid | L3–4 −82.7%; L4–5 −84.8% | None |
| LB/unilateral rod | L3–4 −56.8%; L4–5 −64.7% | L1–2 15.2%; L2–3 8.9% |
| LB/bilateral rod | L3–4 −86.3%; L4–5 −85.5% | L1–2 6.9%; L2–3 4.5% |
| AR/semi-rigid | L3–4 −51.7%; L4–5 −42.5% | L2–3 20.8% |
| AR/unilateral rod | L3–4 −25.7%; L4–5 −46.9% | None |
| AR/bilateral rod | L3–4 −76.8%; L4–5 −67.1% | None |

**TABLE 4.** *Significance of differences between semi-rigid and rod instrumentations at levels and combinations as in Fig. 3*

| | Bilateral rod | Unilateral rod |
| --- | --- | --- |
| FE/semi-rigid | L3–4 $p \leq 0.001$; L4–5 $p \leq 0.001$ | L3–4 n.s.; L4–5 n.s. |
| LB/semi-rigid | L3–4 n.s.; L4–5 n.s. | L3–4 $p \leq 0.001$; L4–5 $p \leq 0.014$ |
| AR/semi-rigid | L3–4 $p \leq 0.002$; L4–5 $p \leq 0.006$ | L3–4 $p \leq 0.008$; L4–5 n.s. |

n.s., nonsignificant.

transfixed vertebrae in 32 of 36 possible combinations of coupled motion planes and vertebrae; the coupled motions at adjacent segment levels were not significantly increased by any spinal fusion method.

The cyclic loading of the specimens did not affect their performance at the postcyclic test. Detectable loosening occurred neither at the screw head (implant–implant) nor at the screw–bone interface. The postcyclic loosening torque of fixation nuts was reduced. The decrease of the locking nut torque was 31.5% for the rods and 50.8% for the cable. However, disassembling the implant did not reveal any loosening at the screw head or failure of the screw thread. In an (afterwards excluded) specimen which was finally subjected to a cyclic overload of $\pm 12$ Nm, the sacrum broke off in the plastic padding after about 100 cycles. The implant and the instrumented vertebrae remained unaffected.

## Significance of Results

The bilateral DDS rod system shows stabilization values of the same magnitude as other tested, well-established rigid devices (10). Semi-rigid devices at the moment are rarely used for the purpose of permanent lumbar fusion. Conceptually, the Graf tension band device (as well as other French developments based on the same principle) is more of an augmentation for degenerated facet joints (7). It fails to work biomechanically in cases of facetectomy (1). No comparable data are available for Luque's semi-rigid ISF (13) or the ISOLOCK system (9). Yoganandan et al. (20) have confirmed in their experiments that significantly increased mobility above and below the fusion area may occur. They attribute this to "excessively rigid" stabilization of an injured motion segment. Hypermobility can lead to accelerated degeneration of the affected motion segments and is therefore unfavorable. Hypermobility rarely occurred with the DDS system.

A "semi-rigid" system, however, must not be too flexible, because the risk of bony malunion may increase with high flexibility. However, the "ideal" rigidity of an implant has not yet been determined. The semi-rigid DDS system showed no excessive flexibility in our experimental setting and stabilized the segments significantly in FE, LB, and AR.

Unilateral rod fixation exhibited stabilization values similar to or exceeding unilateral Steffee (VSP) fixation (6). The latter has already proved to be as clinically effective as bilateral instrumentation (11).

The semi-rigid DDS fixation device provided stability values ranging between those of unilateral and bilateral rod instrumentation. With the additional advantage of reduced operation time and the possible reduction in stress shielding and adjacent hypermobility, the semi-rigid device will undergo a clinical trial.

## CLINICAL APPLICATION

### Materials and Methods

A retrospective clinical study comprising the first 50 consecutive rod-instrumented patients with lumbar instability was conducted with a minimal 1-year follow-up. Among them were 30% previously operated patients with failed-back syndrome. The male-female ratio was almost 50:50. There were 35 bilaterally (Fig. 4) and five unilaterally (Fig. 5) instrumented patients. In 10 patients, an additional ALIF was added to the posterior instrumentation. Indications were degenerative instabilities, spondylolisthesis with spondylolysis, postdiscectomy syndrome, and fractures. Tumor and spondylitis cases were excluded from the study.

The follow-up was based on clinical assessment via the Marburg Score questionnaire, which has shown its validity in comparison to the Oswestry Score and has a high test–retest reliability and internal consistency. The questionnaire evaluates the ability of patients to perform defined tasks and allows discrimination between leg and back pain. It consists of eight questions, each with a maximal score of 6 and a minimal score of 0. The higher the score, the better the situation of the patient. As is known also from the Oswestry Score, the preoperative score ($MS_{pre}$) has an impact on the follow-up score ($MS_{fu}$). The normalized score change can therefore be related to the preoperative score by the following formula (12), negative values indicating improvement.

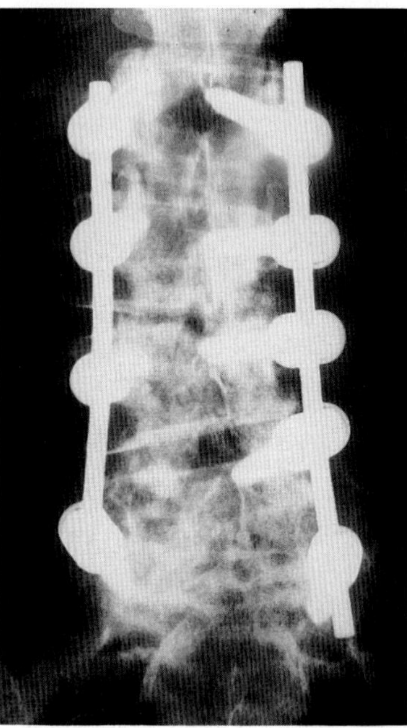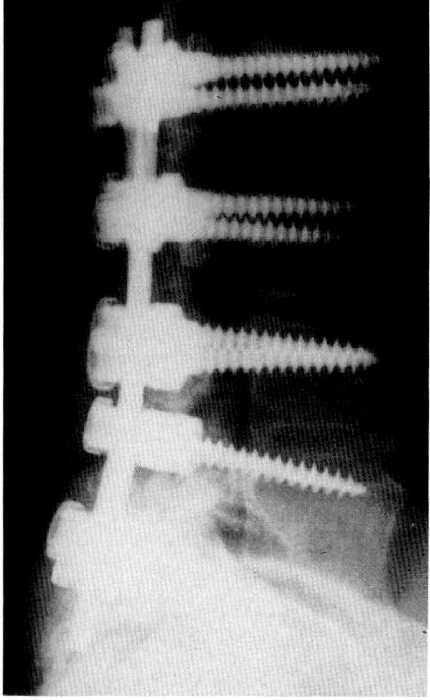

**FIG. 4.** Clinical example of a bilateral DDS instrumentation in an elderly multilevel instability patient with osteopenia. Note that the presacral vertebra required only one screw to facilitate straightening of a rotational instability. The screw is placed close to the endplate to obtain maximal purchase.

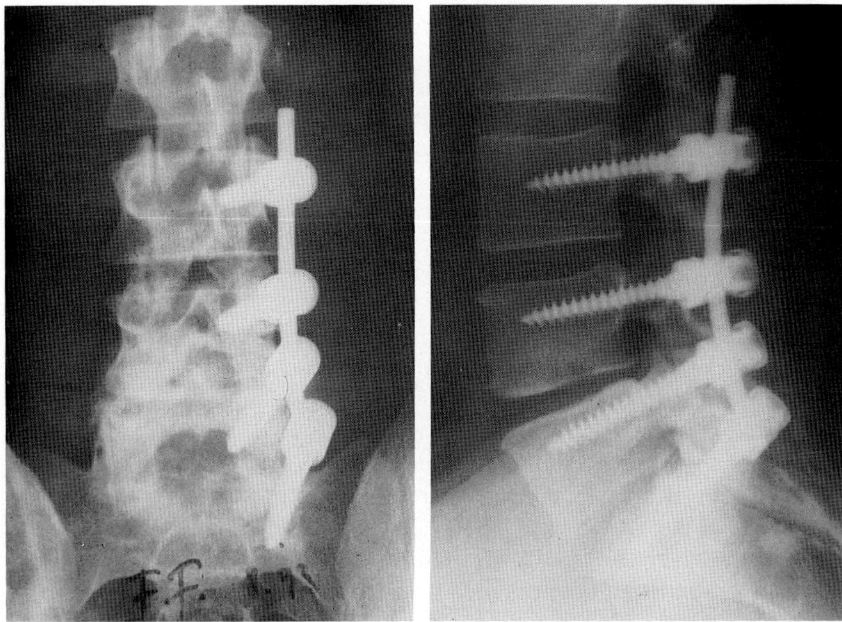

**FIG. 5.** A 40-year-old patient with failed back and arachnitis spinalis. Revision of the L3–L4 and L4/L5 root was done on the right side and the instability instrumented, together with the degenerated segment L5–S1. Note the restoration of physiologic lordosis by the steep angulation of the lower screws on the rod. Slight bending adjustment of the rod added to the effect.

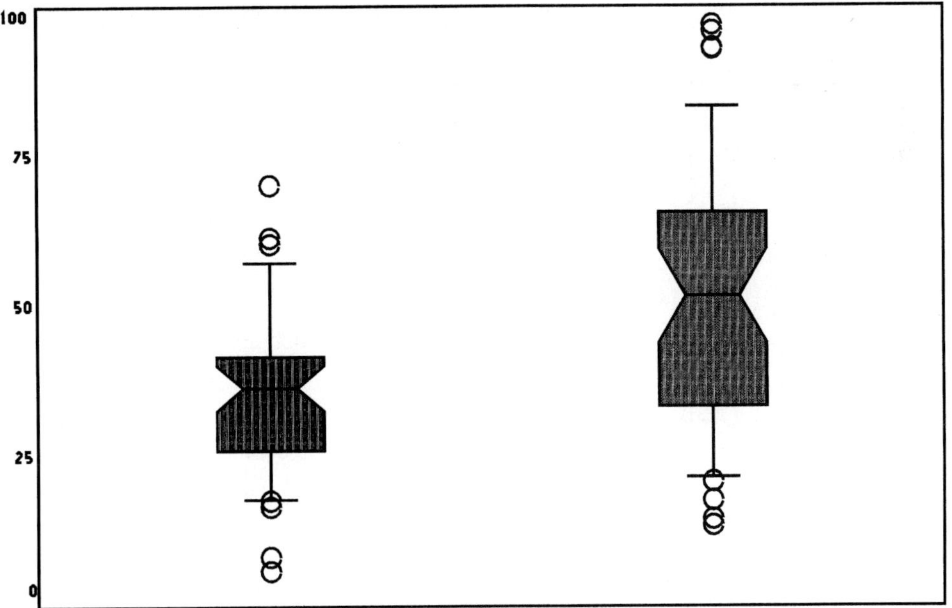

## Marburg Score pre- and postoperatively

**FIG. 6.** Box plots showing improvement of the normalized Marburg score toward follow-up. Lack of overlap of the notches indicates significance of the difference. Mean, 10th, 25th, 75th, and 90th percentile are depicted.

$$(MS_{pre} - MS_{fu}/MS_{pre}) \times 100 = \Delta MS$$

In addition, the average change of the intervertebral distance was measured by digitizing standard x-rays, pre-, postoperatively, and at follow-up, using a special technique that accounts for different magnification factors and possible tilting of the vertebrae.

### Results

The age of the patient was normally distributed between 24 and 80 years at time of surgery; the average follow-up time was 1.4 years. One patient was lost to follow-up by death. Complications included two infections, two pulmonary embolisms, one implant loosening, and two postoperative nerve lesions.

The questionnaires of 82% of the patients could be evaluated. There was a significant improvement of the normalized Marburg Score toward follow-up (Fig. 6). The calculated index change $\Delta MS$ was $-68.18\%$ on average. Patients operated on for the first time tended to have a better $\Delta MS$ than patients with previous spine surgery, but the difference was not significant. There was no outcome difference for the different preoperative diagnoses. Gender and presence of leg (radicular) pain was not a con-

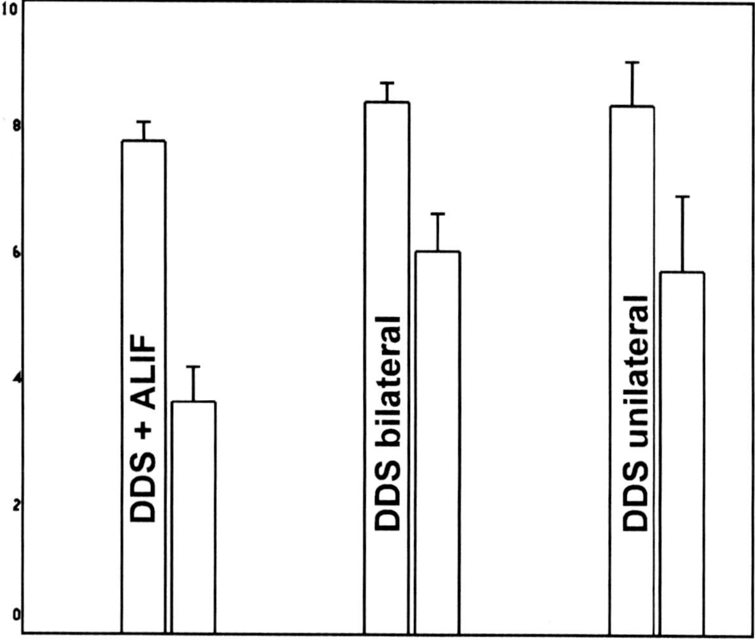


## Visual Pain Scale preop. vs. follow-up

**FIG. 7.** Visual Analogue Pain Scale change for the different operation techniques, reflecting results of the Marburg Score. It cannot be concluded that circumferential techniques are superior in every case. In our study, they were reserved for cases for anterior column support loss. Note the preoperative similarity and the similar values of uni- and bilateral instrumentation, which were used arbitrarily.

founding factor. Age of the patient and length of postoperative hospitalization were not correlated with the outcome.

The pain rating on a Visual Analog Scale (10 = maximal pain, 0 = no pain) was significantly improved at time of follow-up (Fig. 7). The difference was significantly correlated to ΔMS. Most patients obtained slight distraction intraoperatively. This average height loss was 6.9% for bilateral, 10.5% for unilateral, and 0.3% for circumferential fusion. For a comparable group of bilateral non-DDS instrumentation with a 3-mm threaded rod, the loss was 10.7%. ALIF alone yielded 0.5%. There was no significant correlation between an intervertebral height loss at follow-up, compared to the postoperative situation, and ΔMS. Therefore, slight height loss does not appear to have an impact on the outcome, at least as long as no pseudarthrosis occurs. No implant breakage occurred in our DDS study but breakage did occur in 9.2% of the non-DDS instrumented patients. None of the patients required revision because of pseudarthrosis.

A survey of the results of follow-up studies with a total of 214 patients from our department is shown in Fig. 8. We confirmed the results of other studies (3,11) showing that there was no significant difference in improvement between bi- and unilateral instrumented patients.

### Significance of Findings

The values from Fig. 8 cannot all be directly compared to each other because the particular indications were not the same for anterior, posterior, and circumferential

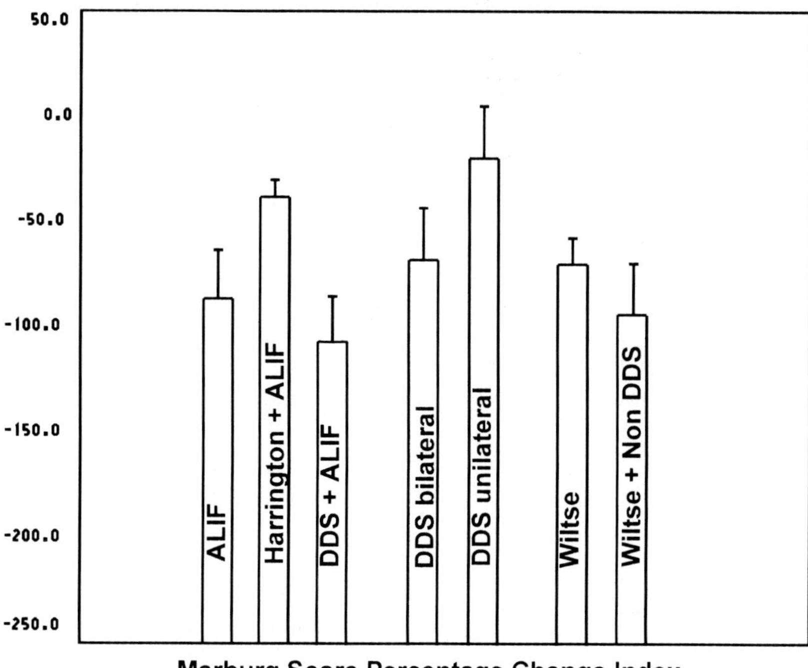


**FIG. 8.** Survey of results of different indication-based techniques in more than 200 patients.

procedures. For example, Harrington + ALIF was reserved for young patients with high-grade spondylolisthesis caused by spondylolysis, and DDS + ALIF was indicated only in cases of severe anterior column support loss. However, these values prove the usefulness of the Marburg concept (8,17) mentioned above for obtaining almost equally good clinical results for all of our indication-based fusion methods.

The intertransverse (Wiltse) fusion does not need to be added to the DDS instrumentation (as was done in non-DDS cases) and was replaced by merely posteromedial and articular bone grafting, which saves operation time and reduces blood loss. It still is justified in one-level, low-grade slip cases at the lumbosacral junction, for which it yields good results with low complication rates, even without pedicle screw use.

In general, obesity (especially in young patients), secondary gain (compensation claims), and patient satisfaction (which may be linked to psychological disturbances) were found to be confounding factors for the outcome.

To date, more than 150 patients have been operated on, including scoliosis cases. The semi-rigid cable has been used in scoliosis. In tumor cases, DDS has also been used for anterior reinforcement of vertebral body replacement. In addition to technical skill and a good implant, careful patient selection remains the key to successful spine surgery.

## REFERENCES


1. Angst M, Winter M, Lang MC. Dorsal tension band stabilization for the lumbar spine analyzed in vitro. [Abstract]. *J Biomech* 1993;26:817.
2. Chang KW, Dewei Z, McAfee PC, Warden KE, Farey ID, Gurr KR. A comparative biomechanical study of spinal fixation using the combination spinal rod-plate and transpedicular screw fixation system. *J Spinal Dis* 1988;1:257–66.
3. Cinotti G, Postacchini F. Unilateral versus bilateral pedicle fixation in patients undergoing single-level posterolateral fusion. [Abstract]. *Proc 22nd ISSLS Meeting,* Helsinki 1995;25.
4. Cunningham BW, Sefter JC, Shono Y, McAfee PC. Static and cyclical biomechanical analysis of pedicle screw spinal constructs. *Spine* 1993;18:1677–88.
5. Galante JO. Tensile properties of the human lumbar annulus fibrosus. *Acta Orthop Scand* 1967;100 (suppl):30–2.
6. Goel VK, Lim TH, Gwon J, et al. Effects of rigidity of an internal fixation device. A comprehensive biomechanical investigation. *Spine* 1991;16:S155–61.
7. Graf H. Instabilité vertébrale. Traitement a l'aide d'un système souple. *Rachis* 1992;4:123–37.
8. Griss P. Der Kreuzschmerz—operative Therapie. In: Springorum HW, Katthagen BD, eds. *Aktuelle Schwerpunkte der Orthopädie*. Stuttgart: Thieme, 1990:37–44.
9. Grob R, Grosskopf D. Spondylolisthesis by spondylosis—indications and results: data from a study out of 36 cases. *Actualités Vertébrales* 1993:5–7.
10. Gwon JK, Chen J, Lim TH, Han JS, Weinstein JN, Goel VK. In vitro comparative biomechanical analysis of transpedicular screw instrumentations in the lumbar region of the human spine. *J Spinal Dis* 1991;4:437–43.
11. Kabins MB, Weinstein JN, Spratt KF, et al. Isolated L4-L5 fusions using the variable screw placement system: unilateral versus bilateral. *J Spinal Dis* 1992;5:39–49.
12. Little DG, MacDonald D. The use of the percentage change in Oswestry Disability Index Score as an outcome measure in lumbar spinal surgery. *Spine* 1994;19:2139–43.
13. Luque ER, Rapp GF. A new semirigid method for interpedicular fixation of the spine. *Orthopedics* 1988;11:1445–50.
14. Magerl F. External skeletal fixation of the lower thoracic and the lumbar spine. In: Uhthoff HK, Stahl E, eds. *Current concepts of external fixation of fractures*. New York: Springer, 1982:353–66.
15. Moran JM, Berg WS, Berry JL, Geiger JM, Steffee AD. Transpedicular screw fixation. *J Orthop Res* 1989;7:107–14.
16. Pfeiffer M, Gilbertson LG, Goel VK, et al. Effect of specimen fixation method on pullout tests of pedicle screws. *Spine* [in press].
17. Pfeiffer M, Schuler P, Orth J, Griss P. Operative Therapie bei Kreuzschmerzen—Marburger Reper-

toire. In: Matzen KA, ed. *Wirbelsäulenchirurgie II—Operative Behandlung chronischer Kreuzschmerzen*. Stuttgart, New York: Thieme, 1992:265–76.
18. Rohlmann A, Bergmann G, Graichen F, Mayer HM. In vivo measurements of the loads of an internal spinal fixation device following stabilization of a lumbar fracture [Abstract]. *Trans 22nd ISSLS Meeting*, Helsinki, 1995;128.
19. Skinner R, Maybee J, Transfeldt E, Venter R, Chalmers W. Experimental pullout testing and comparison of variables in transpedicular screw fixation. A biomechanical study. *Spine* 1990;15:195–201.
20. Yoganandan N, Pintar F, Maiman DJ, et al. Kinematics of the lumbar spine following pedicle screw plate fixation. *Spine* 1993;18:504–12.
21. Zindrick MR, Wiltse LL, Widell EH, et al. A biomechanical study of intrapeduncular screw fixation in the lumbosacral spine. *Clin Orthop* 1986;203:99–112.

*Instrumented Fusion of the Degenerative Lumbar Spine: State of the Art, Questions, and Controversies,* edited by M. Šzpalski, R. Gunzburg, D. M. Spengler, and A. Nachemson. Lippincott–Raven Publishers, Philadelphia © 1996.

# 17

# CCD: Concepts and Strategy

N. Passuti, J. Delécrin, and S. Takahashi

*Nantes University, 44035 Nantes, France*

The CCD is a direct derivation of the Cotrel-Dubousset instrumentation, and is a segmental multilevel instrumentation that allows different correction maneuvers, including derotation of the rod, application of compression or distraction forces at different levels, and in situ bending of the rod. CCD instrumentation is used between the thoracolumbar level and the lumbosacral level for a variety of conditions, including trauma, tumors, degenerative lumbar spine, spondylolisthesis, and lumbar scoliosis.

In general, CCD 1 and 2 are very simple and versatile instrumentations that use open vertebral screws (diameters 5, 6, or 7 mm) open sacral screws, and regular screws for sacral or iliac fixation, associated with sacral Chopin blocks or specific connectors.

Lumbar fixation can also be performed with offset blade hooks that act as a supralaminar or an infralaminar "claw" to protect screws against dislodgement. Double-threaded screws are available for reduction of dysplasic spondylolisthesis. The rods are 6 mm in diameter and the DLT is used to construct a rectangular frame at the end of the operation. All of the implants can be easily removed if necessary.

The use of metallic instrumentation (stainless steel or titanium alloy) must be considered when the pathology requires a solid construct (rigid fixation) for a lumbar fusion, when correction of a displacement or a deformity is necessary, and to allow the patient to walk soon after surgery according to the stability of the construct.

## CONCEPT OF THE IMPLANTS

The basis of fixation is the pedicular screws that can be used between T12 and L5 according to well-known principles of anatomy. For segmental fixation, we recommend ending the construct with a bilateral claw. At the inferior level, we use a pediculoinfralaminar claw at the same vertebral level and accompanied by CD instrumentation. After more than 5 years and with long-term follow-up this appears to be a very safe and secure method of fixation. In more than 100 cases we have never observed breakage or dislodgement of this kind of fixation. At the superior level, the supralaminar hooks are placed one level above the vertebral screw, but with the CCD 2 we can use a specific implant that allows the fixation on the lamina of the

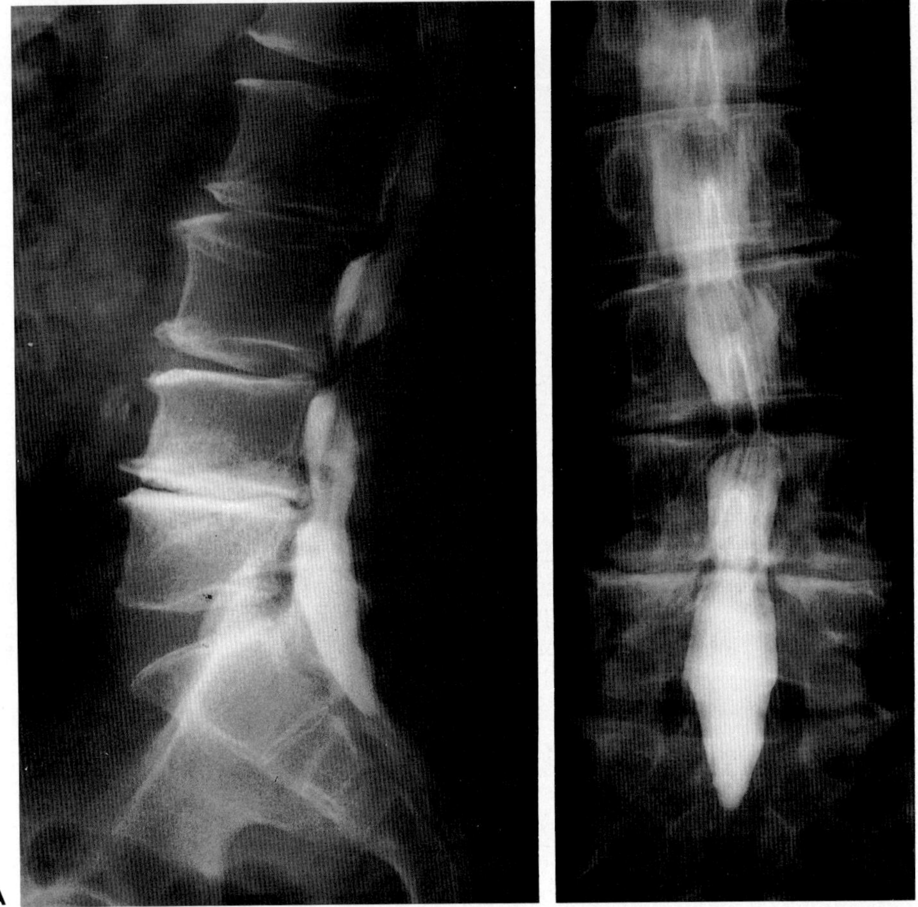

**FIG. 1. A:** Myelograms of a 64-year-old man who presented with very severe lumbar stenosis associated with degenerative scoliosis and a segmental lumbar kyphosis (severe lumbar pain in the standing position). There is lateral compression at three levels and a 15° scoliosis. **B:** Sagittal view confirms the complete stenosis and the lumbar kyphosis (L1–L4 = 0°).

same vertebra. When we use this system we must apply selective compression between the hook and the screw to increase the strength of vertebral fixation.

Sacral fixation remains a problem, but we have arrived at some solutions for different situations. For short lumbosacral constructs (L4–L5–S1) without important sagittal correction we use only an S1 sacral screw oriented toward the anterior part of S1. This provides a solid fixation, as demonstrated by Prof. Argenson (Nice, France). We recommend placing the screw guided by a lateral perioperative fluoroscopic view to obtain a perfect fixation. When we need solid sacral fixation for correction of a deformity or for reduction of a dysplasic spondylolisthesis, we increase the strength of the fixation by use of sacral Chopin blocks or the new Stephanie connector. The first screw is placed as previously described and the second screw, just below, is oriented laterally toward the lateral area of the sacrum to provide a divergent construct. The Chopin block is bulky, and in some cases we have observed dislodgement of the second screw, so we recommend use of the Stephanie connector, which is less bulky and is very easy to use when the rod has been placed.

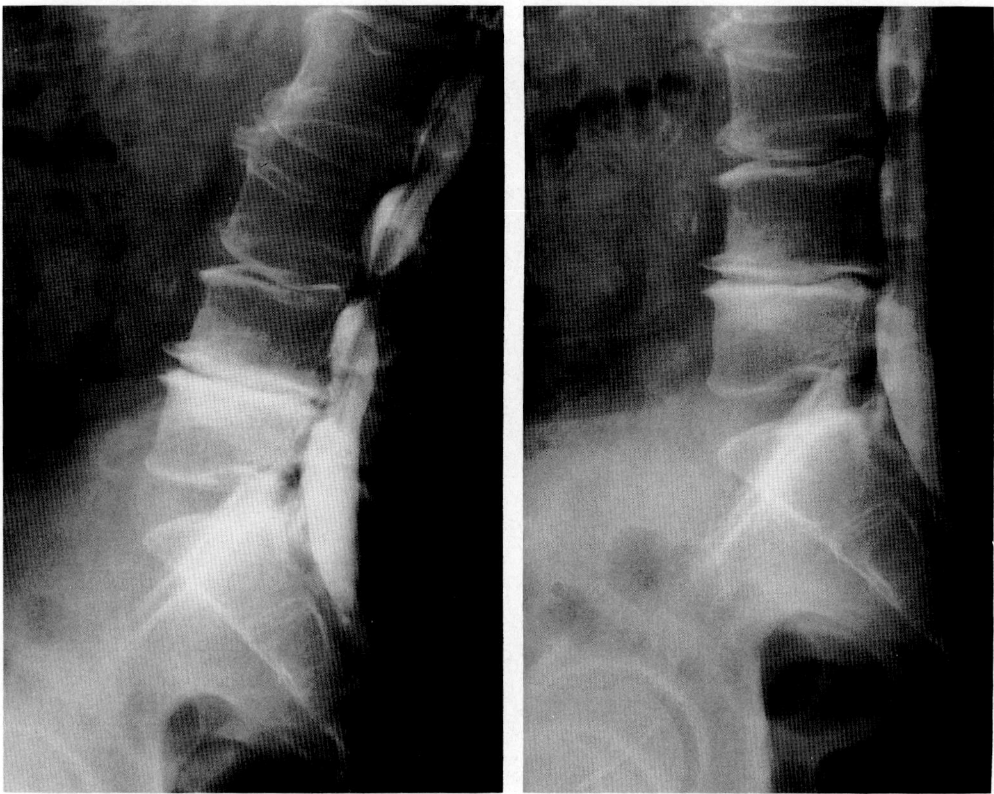

**FIG. 2. A, B:** Dynamic views of the same patient as in Fig. 1 delineate the instability in flexion–extension films.

For difficult cases such as surgical revision, severe spondylolisthesis, or inferior fixation of a long construct in a previously operated patient, we can increase the strength of the fixation by an iliac extension. We place a specific connector at the end of the rod and expose the posterior iliac crest to position a regular long screw (50–60 mm long) into the ilium. This achieves a solid sacroiliac fixation at three points, and 9 to 12 months later it is possible to remove the iliac screw and free the sacroiliac joint.

For very difficult surgical procedures, such as inferior fixation in spina bifida or multiple revision surgery, we use the iliosacral screw described many years ago by Jean Dubousset. A long, large-diameter screw is placed between the posterior iliac crest and the anterior area of the sacrum, and a specific connector allows fixation to the rod. This provides very solid fixation, particularly for correction of severe pelvic obliquity.

## STRATEGY FOR CORRECTION

The first point concerns the rod, which must be bent to restore the normal lumbosacral lordosis. The rod is placed into the implants with rod pushers. The CCD allows specific maneuvers, particularly with the special rod introducer: we can in-

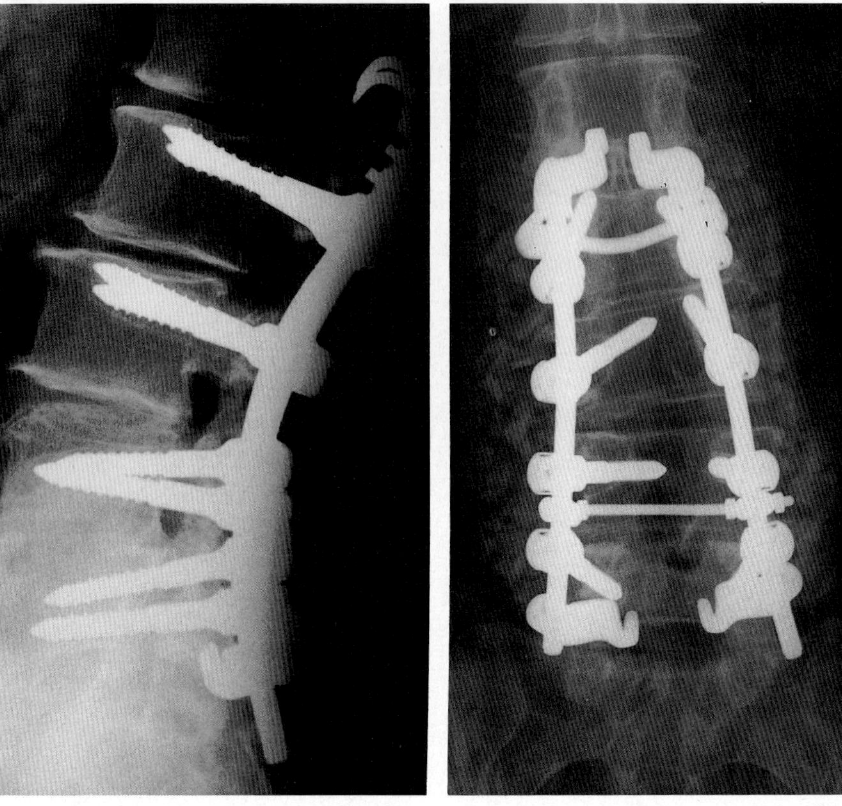

**FIG. 3. A, B:** Views after surgery in the same patient, showing a large and complete decompression with posterior osteotomies at levels L3, L4, and L5, segmental fixation with CCD between L1 and L5. Lumbar lordosis at L1–L5 = 30°.

troduce the rod into the screw and achieve, by a lever arm movement, a reorientation of the vertebra with moderate rotation of its axis. For difficult situations, the articulate rod introducer is used before positioning the plug.

Introduction of rod into the implants provides a beginning of segmental lordosis. After that, in situ bending with the Jackson benders between different levels can increase the lordosis by opening the anterior disc space. Selective compression between the different implants increases the regional lordosis by shortening the posterior column.

It is important to note that after each correction maneuver (in situ bending and segmental compression) it is necessary to further tighten the plug inside the screw, so that these successive maneuvers can obtain and restore regional lumbosacral lordosis. At the end of the operation we apply two DLTs (one superior and one inferior) with transverse compression to increase the pedicular fixation (three-point effect) and to provide a rectangular frame construct. Posterolateral fusion can be performed on the transverse processes for long-term stability.

## CONCEPTS FOR SPECIFIC INDICATIONS

### Degenerative Spine

For lumbar stenosis, a short construct is usually done between L4–L5–S1. We recommend, first, excision of posterior articular facets, implant fixation (screws in

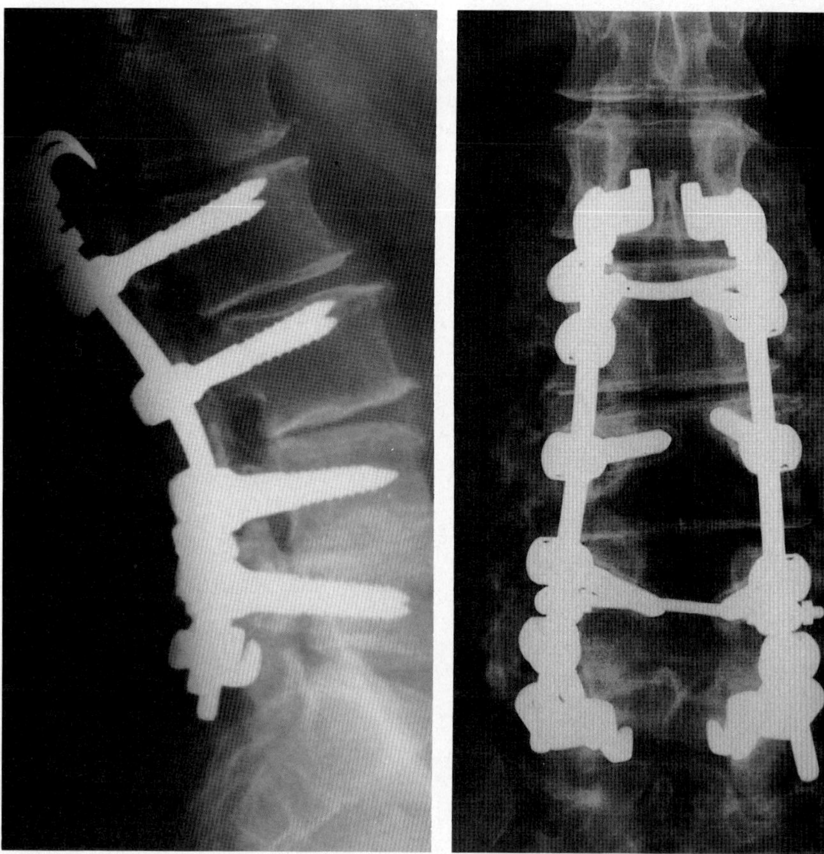

**FIG. 4. A, B:** Same patient at 2-year follow-up, with an excellent clinical result. X-rays confirm the posterolateral fusion and the lumbar lordosis is stable.

L4–L5 and S1), and fixation by two rods. After stabilization we perform large decompression with laminectomy and lateral release, thus decreasing the blood loss from the lateral decompression (posterolateral venules). For the short construct we do not need a superior supralaminar claw, and one sacral screw is sufficient.

A long construct is sometimes necessary for multilevel stenosis (very often decompression from L3 to L5). We recommend ending the instrumentation at the superior level with a pedicular supralaminar claw at one level above to stabilize the transitional zone. We have now more than 5 years of follow-up experience with decompression associated with segmental instrumentation. We have obtained very satisfactory results with good fusion and a high level of survival of the metallic implants without secondary osteoporotic problems (rigid instrumentation). Figures 1–4 show a 64-year-old male patient presenting with a severe lumbar stenosis associated with degenerative scoliosis and segmental lumbar kyphosis. This patient complained of severe pain in standing position.

In lumbar degenerative scoliosis, true secondary degenerative scoliosis is a common problem, and after a positive brace test we consider surgery. With CCD we can obtain segmental short correction of the lumbar curve without any instrumentation at the thoracic level.

The strategy for correction is first to perform complete, wide excision of the articular facets to increase the flexibility of the curve. We expose the transverse

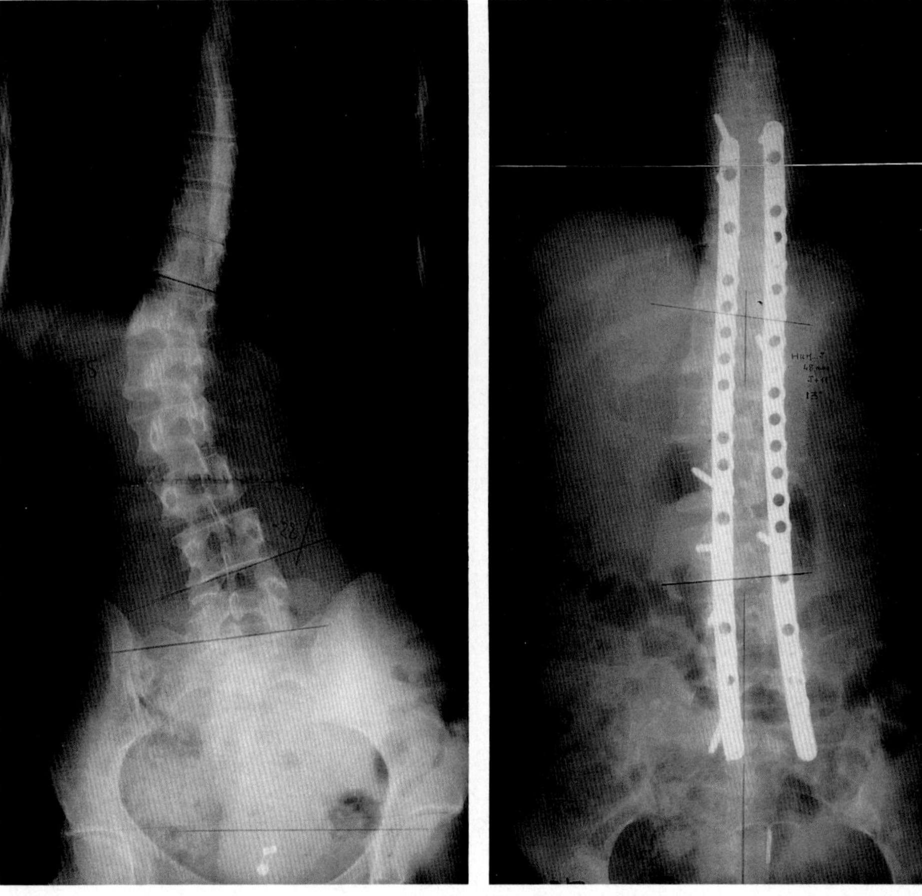

**FIG. 5.** Frontal view in standing position of a 55-year-old woman who presented with an idiopathic thoracolumbar curve (35° in 1975) and was operated on in 1987, with placement of a long plate with segmental screw fixation (T9–S1) and posterior fusion. **A:** Before surgery. **B:** After surgery.

processes and the isthmic area to prepare the screw fixation (most often L1 to L5). Then we apply the first rod on the convex side according to the spinal curve and next apply selective compression and derotation of the rod to obtain realignment of the lumbar spine in the frontal and sagittal planes with segmental lordosis. For this maneuver, the claw is very useful. After that, we place the second rod on the concave side with the different rod introducers to complete the segmental correction.

At the superior level, we recommend including the thoracolumbar junction (screws in L1 and supralaminar hooks in T12) to avoid a secondary segmental kyphosis. At the inferior level, when L5 is very deep between the iliac crests and the L5–S1 disc appears normal (height of the disc space on MRI), we stop in L5 to avoid sacral fixation. However, when L5–S1 is very degenerative we must include the sacrum with one open sacral screw and lumbosacral fusion.

## COMMENTS

A degenerative lumbar curve associated with a dynamic lumbar stenosis can be corrected in the same way as a degenerative lumbar curve. The most important point

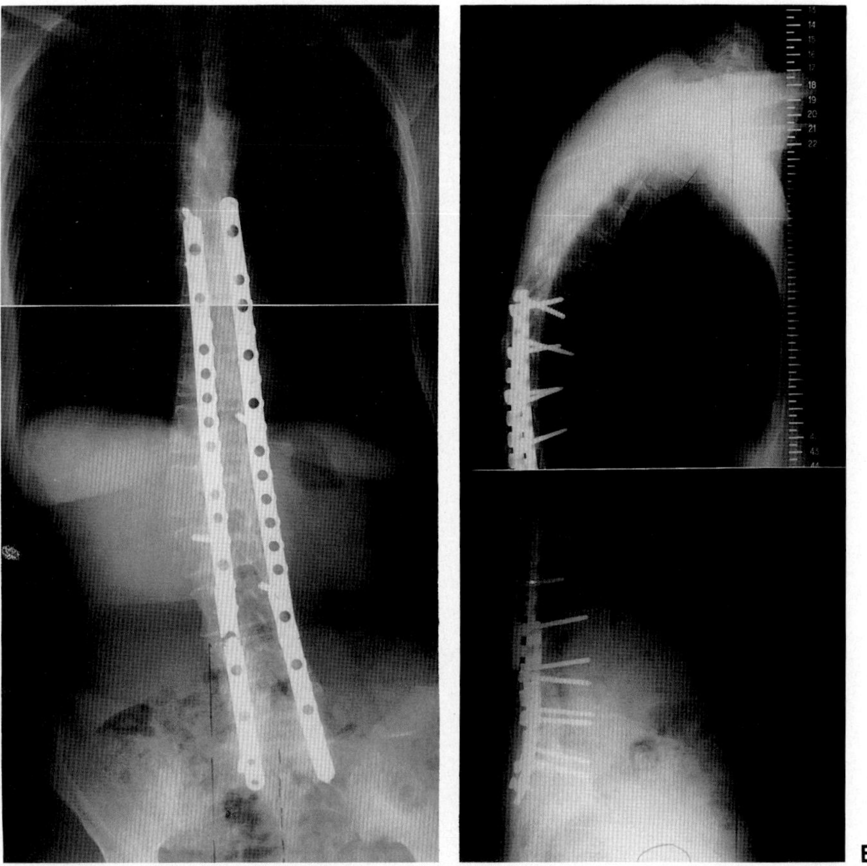

**FIG. 6. A, B:** In 1990 the same patient as in Fig. 5 presented with a nonunion and pseudarthrosis, with progressive frontal imbalance and lumbar kyphosis.

is to precisely determine before surgery the association between scoliosis and dynamic stenosis by dynamic electrophysiologic assessments and a dynamic myelogram. In such cases, the strategy is the same, with segmental correction of the curve without laminectomy. The three-dimensional correction of the curve provides recalibration of the canal with stabilization.

## CORRECTION OF DYSPLASIC SPONDYLOLISTHESIS

For grade 1, 2, or 3 spondylolisthesis without lumbosacral kyphosis, segmental fixation with pedicular screws and double sacral fixation is sufficient to obtain correction and stabilization of the unstable level with posterolateral fusion.

For grade 4 spondylolisthesis and spondyloptosis, a large and complete release of the L5 roots and solid sacral fixation (double sacral screws) is necessary, and sometimes an iliac extension when the kyphotic angle at L5–S1 is very severe. We used open screws in L4 and double-threaded screws in L5. After that, two short rods are fixed into the sacral area, and we push the two rods into L4 to obtain reduction of the lumbosacral kyphosis. Then we reduce the slippage of L5 by tightening open nuts on the double-threaded screws of L5 to obtain a spondylolisthesis of around

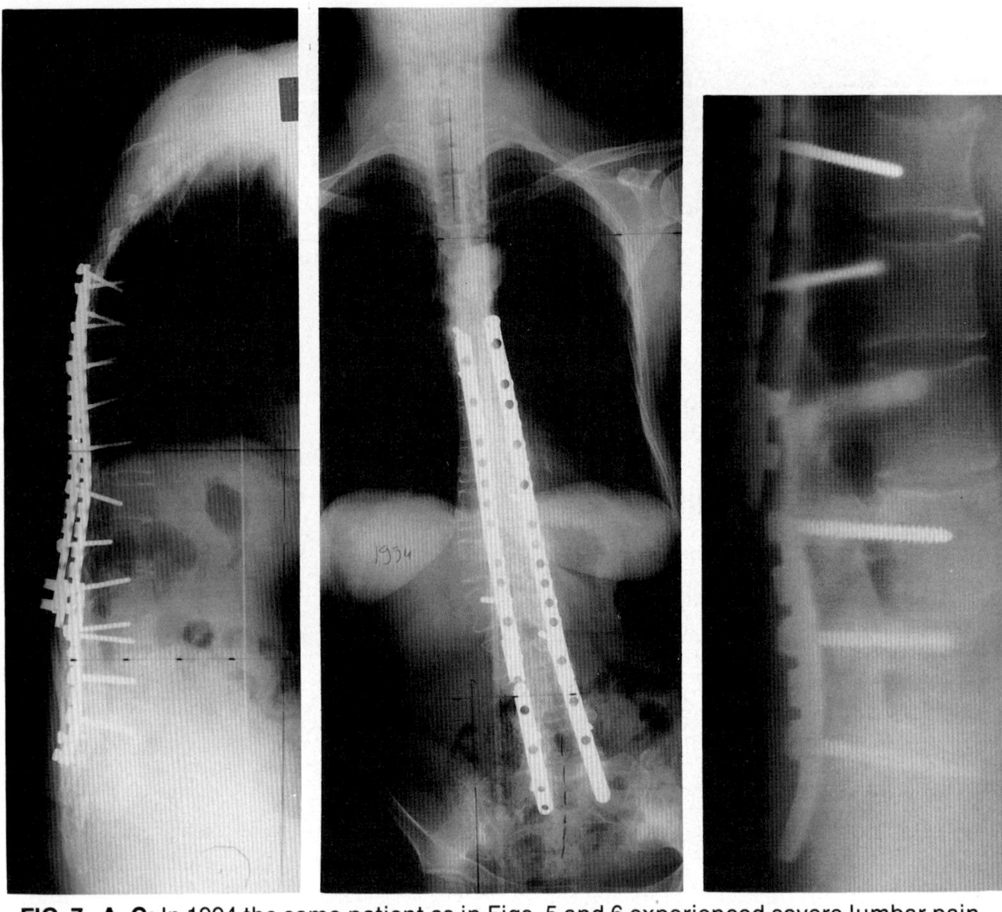

**FIG. 7. A–C:** In 1994 the same patient as in Figs. 5 and 6 experienced severe lumbar pain and also an increase of the frontal right imbalance and lumbar kyphosis, with breakage of the plate (tomogram).

grade 2. We complete the procedure by posterolateral fusion and sometimes by an anterior approach for intervertebral fusion. Figures 5–8 relate to a 55-year-old female patient presenting an idiopathic thoraco-lumbar curvature (35° in 1975) and operated on in 1987, using a long plate with segmental screw fixation (T9–S1) and posterior fusion.

## CORRECTION OF LUMBAR KYPHOSIS

This is a very difficult clinical situation. We perform a posterior release with segmental fixation (pedicular screws) when the two rods bent in normal lordosis shape are ready, and we recommend a posterior osteotomy by resection of the isthmic areas at two or three levels. Introduction of the rods allows stabilization of the lumbar spine and segmental correction of the kyphosis, with in situ bending and selective compression to restore normal lordosis. When the kyphosis is rigid, we use an anterior release (lombotomy) before the posterior correction.

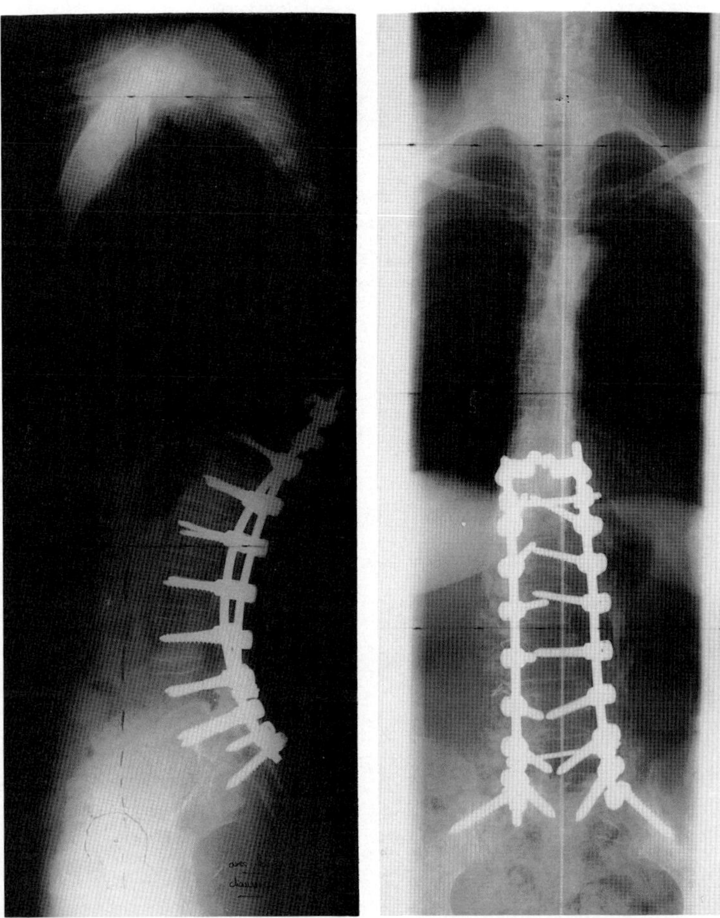

**FIG. 8. A, B:** Using a posterior approach, we performed a complete posterior release with osteotomies at three different levels (L2, L3, and L4) and segmental fixation with CCD (T11 to S1) (same patient as in Figs. 5–7). We used iliac extension to increase the inferior stability. X-rays in standing position show correction of the frontal translation and restoration of a segmental lordosis with sagittal balance (L1–L5 = 46°).

## CONCLUSION

The CCD is a segmental instrumentation well adapted to the lumbar spine. The strategy remains the most important aspect of the surgery, including indications, patient selection, levels of fixation, indication for frontal or sagittal correction, or three-dimensional correction by derotation. The use of rigid fixation in the lumbar and lumbosacral areas is recommended when a primary stable fixation or correction of a deformity is needed. Fusion can be performed by posterolateral arthrodesis, sometimes combined with an anterior approach and intercorporeal fusion.

*Instrumented Fusion of the Degenerative
Lumbar Spine: State of the Art, Questions,
and Controversies*, edited by M. Szpalski,
R. Gunzburg, D. M. Spengler, and
A. Nachemson. Lippincott–Raven
Publishers, Philadelphia © 1996.

# 18

# Surgical Treatment of Degenerative Lumbar Spinal Instability by SIR

P. Bartolozzi, M. Cassini, D. Pasquetto, and E. Boero

*Policlinico di Borgo-Roma, I-37134 Verona, Italy*

Chronic low back pain, sometimes associated with radiating radicular pain, is the most common manifestation of degenerative disorders of the lumbar spine. Because of its high degree of mobility and its function in supporting the physiologic load, the lumbar spine is particularly exposed to degenerative modifications due to uni- or multilevel instability, which are responsible for a container–content conflict secondary to stenosis of the spinal canal. In the same way, such manifestations may aggravate situations in which the spinal load axis is already altered, such as scoliosis or kyphosis in adolescents, with the possibility of worsening in adulthood.

Surgery is the last therapeutic option, after failure of the common conservative and orthotic measures, in the treatment of these disorders. The aim of the operative procedure is to stabilize the unstable spinal units, combined with decompression of the nerve structures when necessary.

## MATERIALS AND METHODS

In degenerative disorders involving instability of the lumbar spine, after neurolysis, as necessary, we perform an instrumented posterior fusion with SIR. In selected cases the latter is combined with a posterior lumbar interbody fusion (PLIF) with the aid of carbon or titanium cages, or with an anterior lumbar interbody fusion (ALIF) by means of an autologous bone graft or a Hartshill horseshoe. Pure stenoses of the spinal canal without instability are decompressed by the Roy-Camille technique (11), which does not require arthrodesis.

Since October of 1992 we have been using the SIR device in the treatment of various spinal disorders. All components of this device are made of titanium (Ti6A14V) because of its high mechanical resistance and the magnetic resonance imaging (MRI) compatibility that is, in our opinion, an essential requisite of any modern spinal fixator.

The spine gripping elements in this system are hooks and screws (Fig. 1) with a

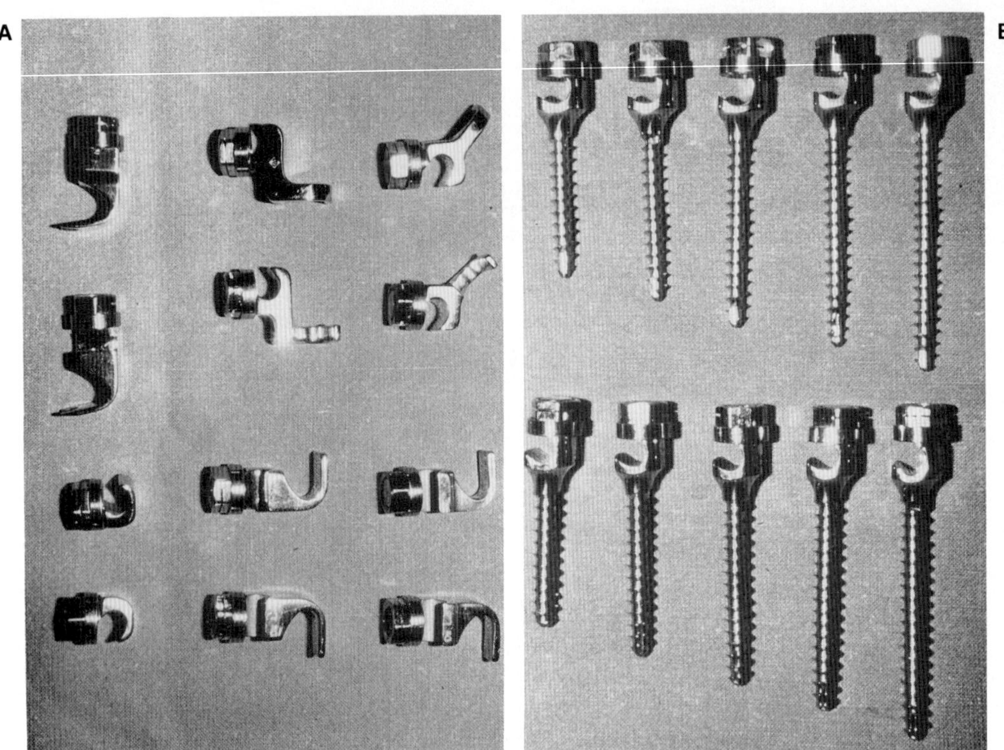

**FIG. 1.** SIR instrumentation. **A:** The four types of hooks. **B:** The pedicular screws.

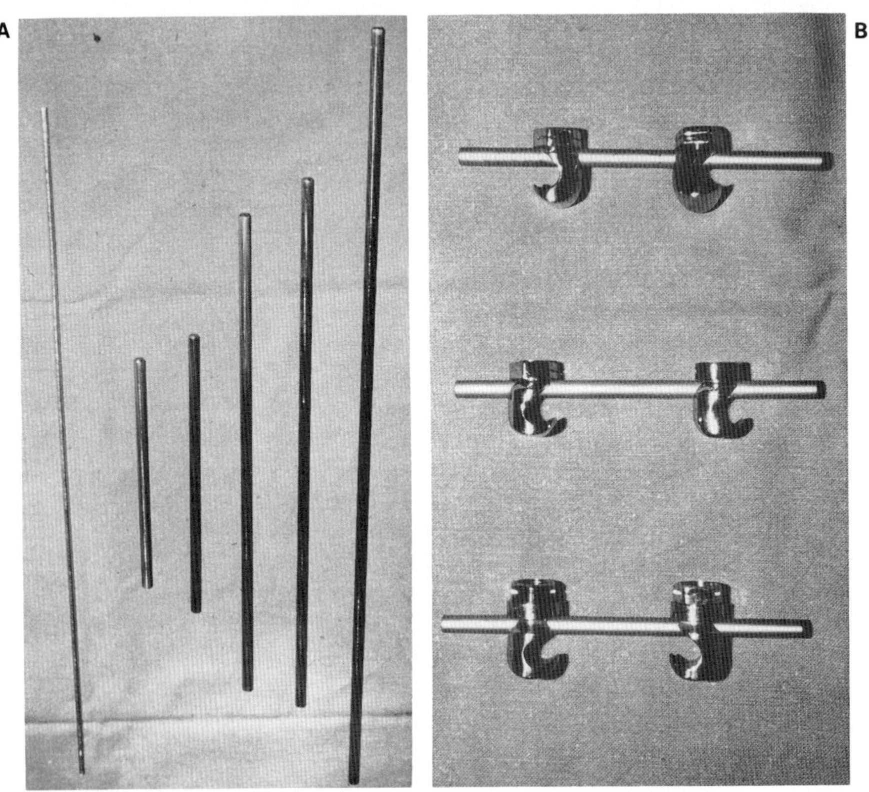

**FIG. 2.** SIR instrumentation. **A:** The titanium rods. **B:** Transversal traction device.

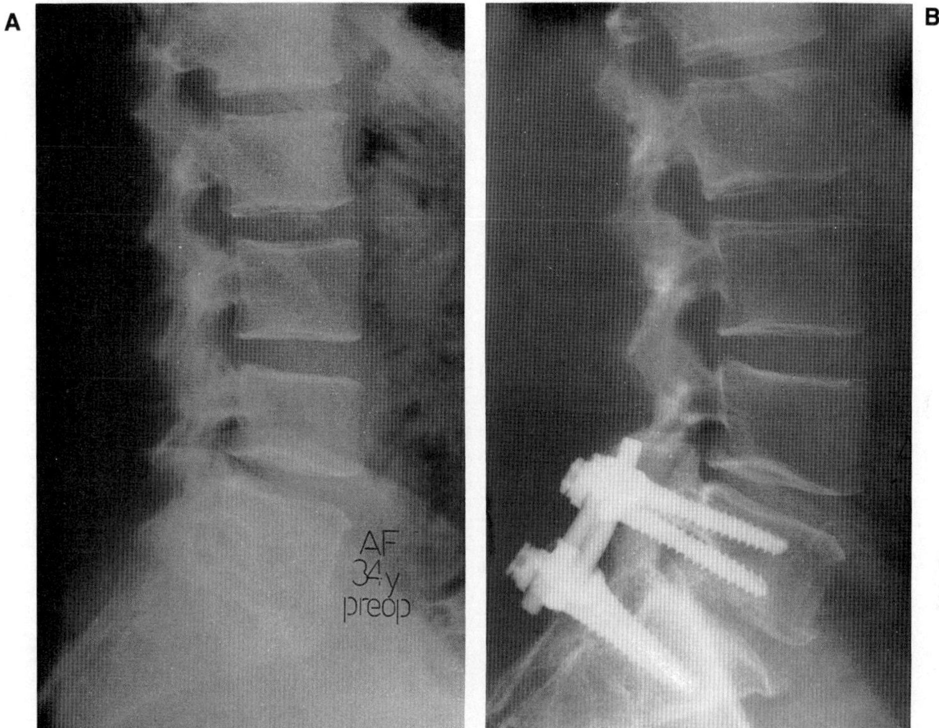


**FIG. 3.** Male patient, 34 years old, with unilevel instability, treated by posterior arthrodesis and PLIF (carbon cages). **A:** Preoperative radiograph. **B:** One-year follow-up.

right- or left-sided opening, the connecting element consisting of a moldable knurled rod (Fig. 2A) measuring 6 mm in diameter. Four types of hooks are available: laminar, with 6- or 9-mm-wide blades; pedicular, with a forked blade measuring 9 mm in width; offset body; and oblique, characterized by the position of the blade. Pedicular screws in diameters of 4, 5, 6 and 7 mm and in lengths ranging from 30 to 55 mm are also available. The core of the screw thread, which was initially cylindrical, has been changed to conical to double its resistance. The screws are self-threading, with rounded tips. The rod is available in lengths of 11, 14, 17, 21, 32, and 45 mm and can be cut with nippers to obtain the desired length. The knurling is of the "parallel-line" type, as this has proved optimal in various tests for preventing the hooks from slipping on the rod. The rod is fixed to the spine gripping elements by direct tightening of a hexagonal nut applied to the upper part of the hook or screw. Before the nut is tightened, it allows the rod to slide, although preventing it from slipping out during distraction or compression maneuvers. A transverse traction device (TTD) (Fig. 2B), consisting of two small hooks and a rod, can connect the implant rods for a greater resistance to torsional stresses.

Preoperative clinical investigations include conventional standard and dynamic radiographs and MRI, because of its indispensable information about neural components and the disc structures. Computed tomography (CT) is used in cases of marked stenosis because of its greater definition of bony structures.

From October 1992 to October 1994, we applied the SIR device in 19 patients with instability of the lumbar spine, 12 women and seven men with a mean age of 49 years

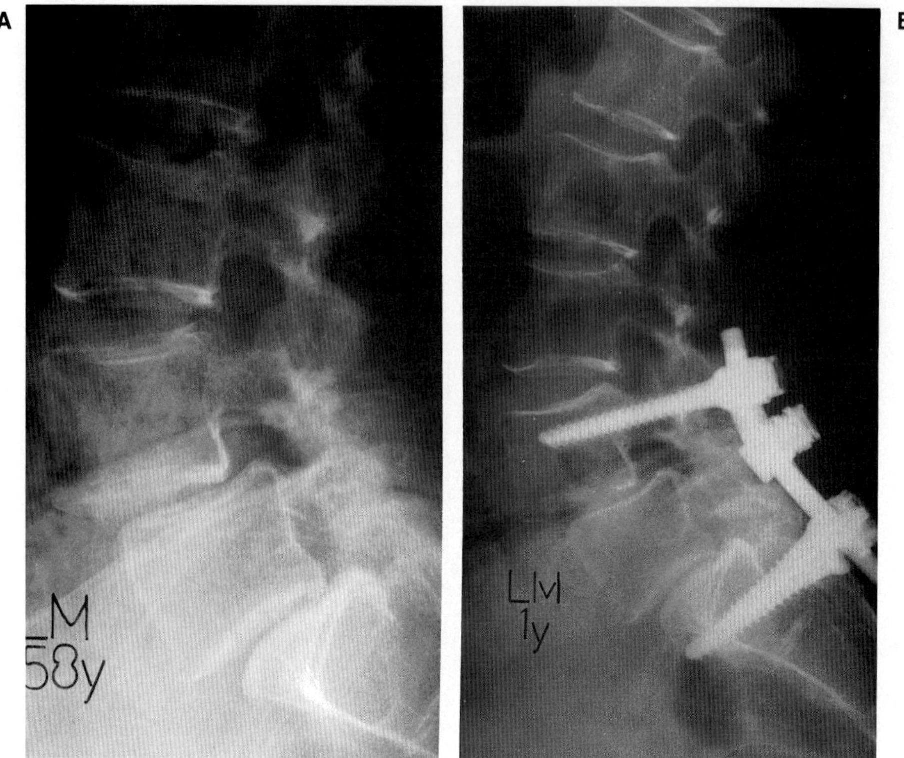

**FIG. 4.** Female, 58 years old, with multilevel instability, treated by posterior arthrodesis. **A:** Preoperative radiograph. **B:** One-year follow-up.

(range 30–69 years). Six patients were suffering from unilevel instability (including two postsurgical cases), eight from multilevel instability (three postsurgical), three from adult degenerative scoliosis, and two from flat back. In four patients with severe instability, SIR was combined with interbody fusion (PLIF in three cases, ALIF in one case). The mean follow-up period was 27 months (range 11–35 months).

The cases can be subdivided into the following four groups.

### Unilevel Instability

We treated six patients (four men, two women; mean age 41 years, range 33–47 years) for unilevel instability, two of whom had undergone previous surgery. The levels involved were L5–S1 in five cases (Fig. 3) and L4–L5 in one case.

Four patients presented with sensory deficits in the preoperative period and two with sensorimotor deficits. All patients complained of low back pain, sometimes associated with sciatica, which was resistant to treatment.

Disappearance of the symptoms and neurologic disorders was observed postoperatively. Only one case exhibited mild symptoms of sciatica, which disappeared by 1 year postoperatively. There is no evidence to date of device failure or pseudoarthroses.

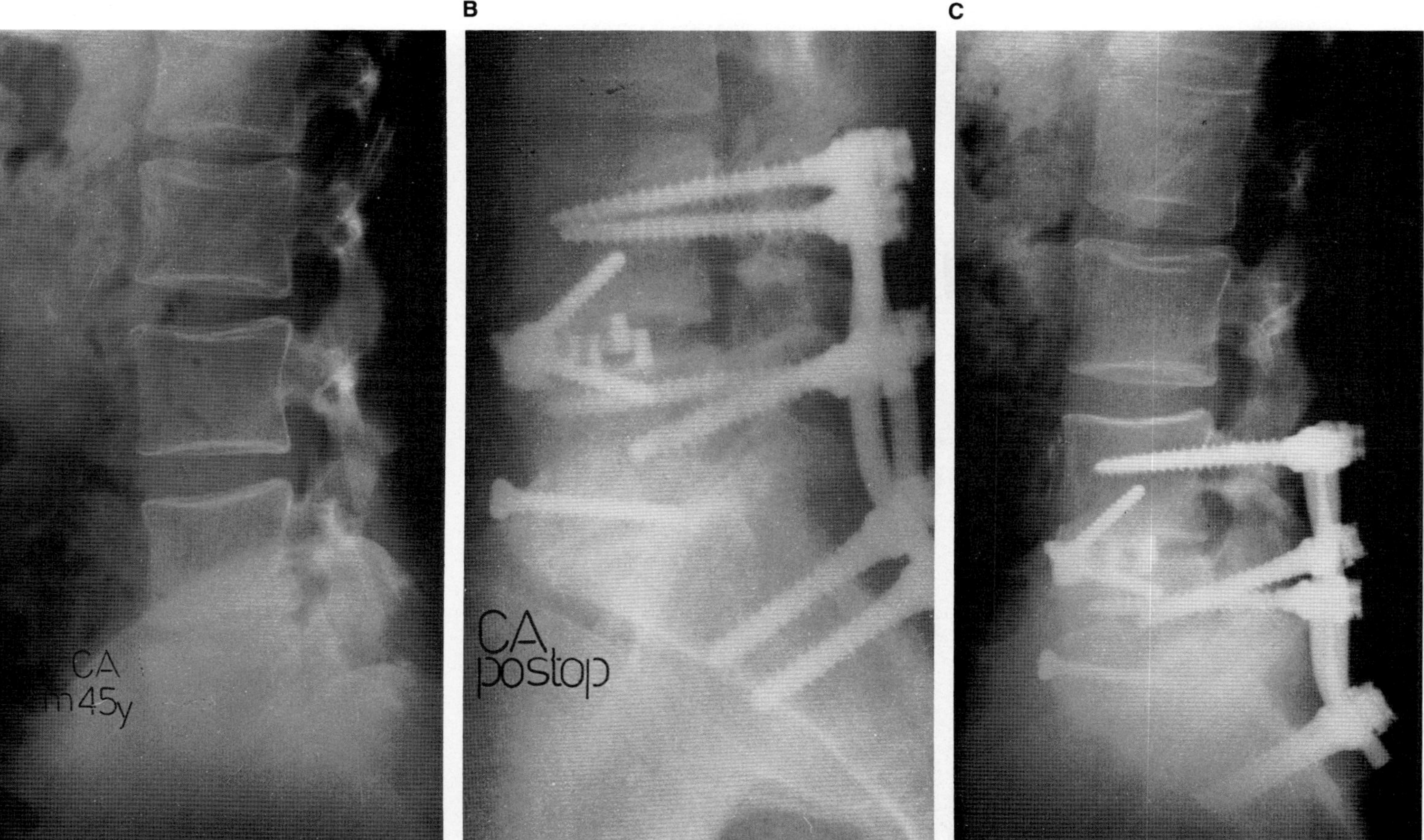



**FIG. 5.** Male, 45 years old, with multilevel instability, treated by posterior arthrodesis, anterior fusion at L5–S1 by autologous bone graft and at L4–L5 by Hartshill horseshoe. **A:** Preoperative radiograph. **B:** Postoperative radiograph. **C:** One-year follow-up.

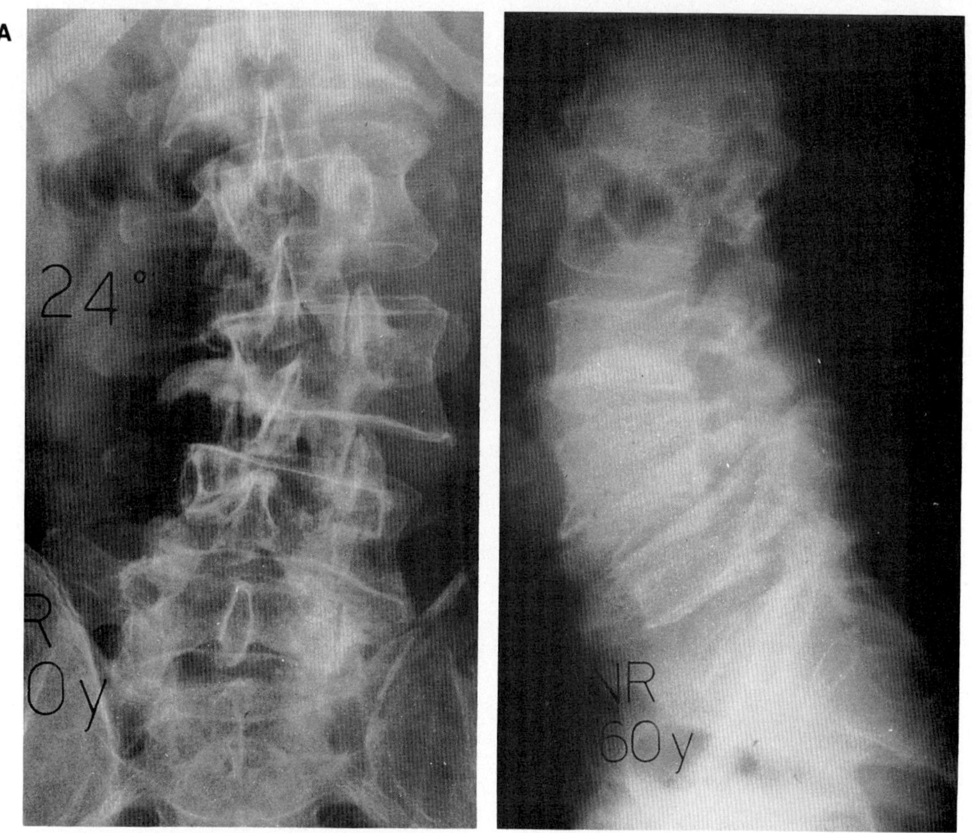

**FIG. 6.** Male patient, 60 years old, with lumbar degenerative scoliosis, treated by posterior arthrodesis and decompression L3–L4. **A, B:** Preoperative radiographs. The curve entity (Cobb's method) is 24°.

## Multilevel Instability

Eight patients (four women, four men; mean age 53 years, range 39–69 years) have been treated for multilevel instability, three of whom had undergone previous surgery. The levels involved were L4–L5 and L5–S1 (Figs. 4 and 5) in six cases and L3–L4, L4–L5, and L5–S1 in the other two cases.

Three patients presented with sensory deficits, two with motor deficits, and three with sensorimotor deficits preoperatively. All patients complained of low back and leg pain, which disappeared during the postoperative period.

One patient experienced intolerance of the hardware 1 year postoperatively, due to subcutaneous protrusion of the device. Consolidation of the arthrodesis enabled us to remove the device, with resolution of the symptoms. No device failures or pseudoarthroses have been noted up to now.

## Degenerative Scoliosis

Three patients with degenerative lumbar scoliosis (Figs. 6 and 7) (two women, one man; mean age 59 years, range 57–61 years) have been treated with correction–

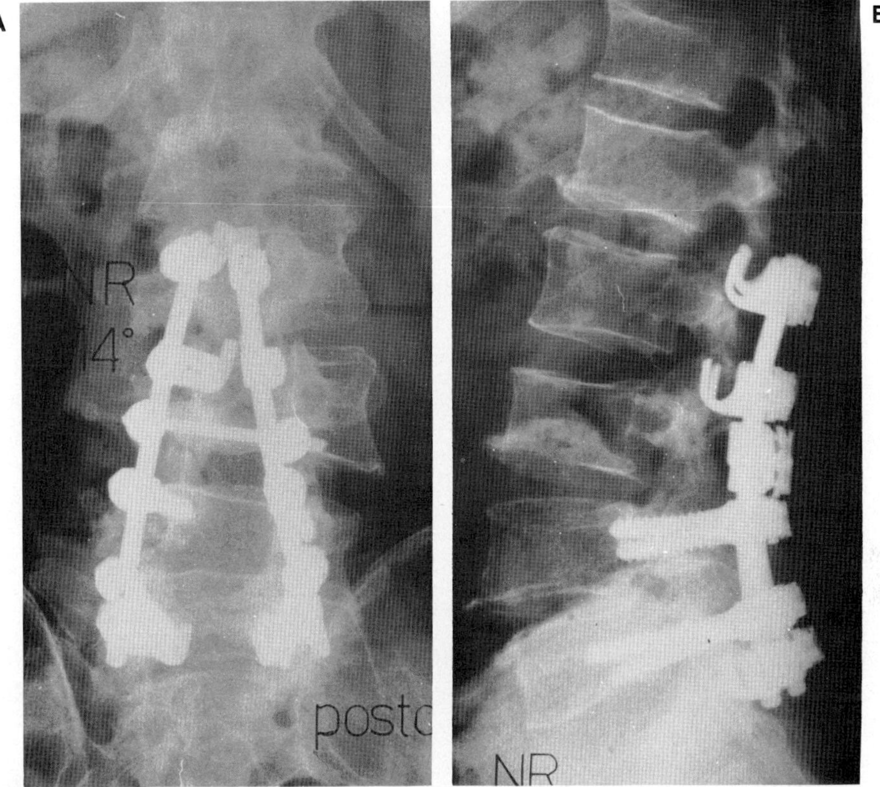

**FIG. 7.** Same case as in Fig. 6. **A, B:** Postoperative radiographs: The amount of the curve is decreased to 14°.

stabilization and posterior fusion. All patients complained of intractable chronic low back pain. The mean extent of the scoliotic curvature was 44°.

In one patient the condition was associated with an 86° dorsolumbar kyphosis with an altered load axis. Correction of the curve in the frontal plane therefore had to be combined with restoration of normal load axis in the sagittal plane by means of a lumbar osteotomy. The mean curvature correction was 38%.

The only complication observed has been a partial muscle deficit affecting the quadriceps in a patient treated by corrective osteotomy, although this deficit subsequently regressed. Disappearance of symptoms was achieved in all patients.

### Flat Back

The flat back in patients treated with correction and fusion for scoliosis can be regarded as a particular form of chronic instability, since a severely altered load axis is produced in the sagittal plane.

Two female patients aged 39 and 40 years were submitted to a posterior closing-wedge lumbar osteotomy at L3–L4 level for flat back as a late complication of surgical correction of double primary curve scoliosis (Fig. 8). Restoration of normal load axis in the sagittal plane was obtained in both cases.

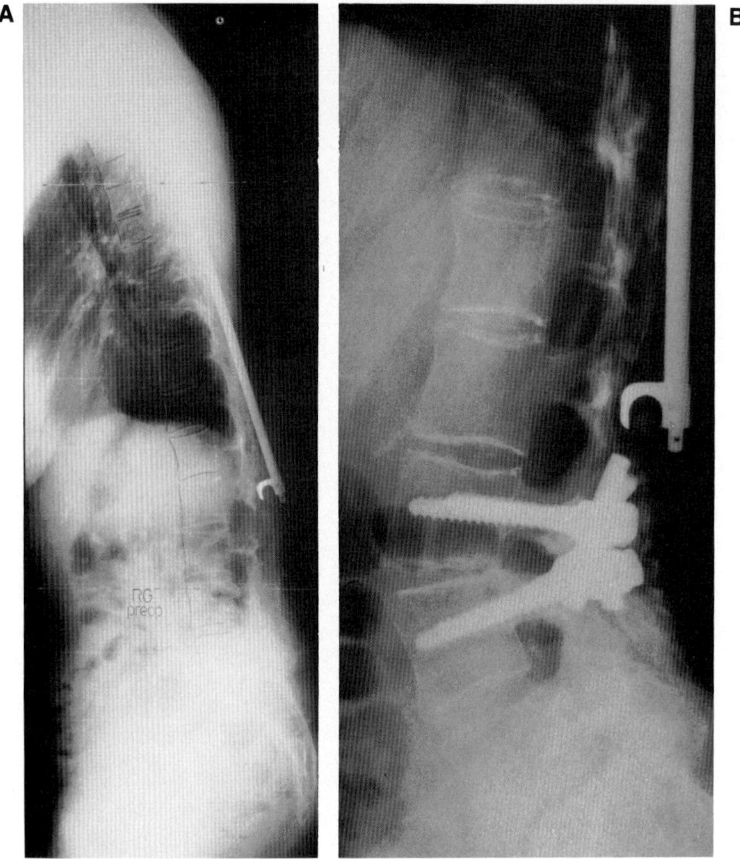

**FIG. 8.** Female, 40 years old, with postsurgery flat back. **A:** Preoperative radiograph. The spinal load axis is altered. **B:** The osteotomy L3–L4. Normal load axis and physiologic lordosis are restored.

## CONCLUSIONS

Surgical spinal fusion for degenerative instability of the lumbar spine is necessary when all other therapeutic measures have failed. A high percentage of pseudoarthrosis has been demonstrated if posterior fusion is performed (7–59%) without instrumentation (2,4–7,10,12,14,16–19).

Most of the risks of neurologic lesions can be avoided by correct surgical technique (1,3,8), because such complications are less attributable to the hardware (particularly the pedicular screws) than to the experience needed for correct application of the devices.

Another possible complication related to the use of the hardware is device failure or breakage, which largely involves the sacral screws. It is well known that at the level of the lumbosacral hinge the greatest stresses are concentrated, because of the contrast between the high degree of mobility of the lumbosacral hinge and the rigidity of the devices. We have overcome this problem by using screws with a conical rather than a cylindrical thread core and with a diameter of 7 mm at sacral level (3), combined with a posterior (PLIF) or anterior (ALIF) interbody fusion (9), whenever the high degree of instability or an altered load axis, calculated according to the Vidal method (15), indicates a high risk for device failure. In addition, the patients are fitted postoperatively with a plastic jacket combined with an extension-locked thigh brace to reduce the movement of the lumbosacral hinge when the segment to be fused includes the lumbosacral passage (13). Thanks to these protocols, to date we have had no device failures in any of our patients.

In view of the good results obtained, we can safely claim that when surgery is indicated for degenerative instability of the lumbar spine, instrumented posterior fusion is the best option available. In particular, the SIR device has proved to be safe, complete, and simple for this surgery.

## REFERENCES


1. Bartolozzi P, Cassini M, Pasquetto D, Sandri A, Girardi P. Il trattamento delle spondilolistesi mediante stabilizzazione posteriore. *Progressi Patologia Vertebrale* 1994;17:129–38.
2. Dawson EG, Lotysch M, Urist MR. Intertransverse process lumbar arthrodesis with autogenous bone graft. *Clin Orthop* 1981;154:90–6.
3. Dickman CA, Fessler RG, MacMillian M, Haid RW. Transpedicular screw-rod fixation of the lumbar spine: operative technique and outcome in 104 cases. *J Neurosurg* 1992;77:860–70.
4. Grubb SA, Lipscomb HJ. Results of lumbosacral fusion for degenerative disc disease with and without instrumentation: two to five-year follow-up. *Spine* 1992;17:349–55.
5. Heggeness MH, Esses SI. Translaminar facet joint screw fixation for lumbar and lumbosacral fusion. A clinical and biomechanical study. *Spine* 1991;16:266–9.
6. Hellstadius A. Experiences gained from spondylo-synthesis operations with H-shaped bone transplantations in the case of degeneration of discs in the lumbar back. *Acta Orthop Scand* 1955;24:207–15.
7. Kimberley AG. Low back pain and sciatica. *Surg Gynecol Obstet* 1937;65:195–216.
8. Krag MH, Fredrickson BE, Yuan HA. Biomechanics of transpedicle spinal fusion. In: Weinstein JN, Wiesel SW, eds. *The lumbar spine*. Philadelphia: WB Saunders, 1990:916–40.
9. Kumano K, Miyashita H, Hirabayashi S, Takahashi S, Ishii J. Cotrel-Dubousset pedicle screw fixation for unstable lumbar spine due to spondylolisthesis. *Proc 6th Int Congr Cotrel-Dubousset Instrumentation*. Montpellier: Sauramps Medical, 1989:141–6.
10. Lorenz M, Zindrick M, Schwaegler P, et al. A comparison on single-level fusions with and without hardware. *Spine* 1991;16:S455–8.
11. Roy-Camille R, Saillant G, Doursounian L, Rolland E. Traitement chirurgical des stenoses du canal lombaire. In: *Encyclopedie Medico-Chirurgicale; Techniques Chirurgicales; Orthopedie et Traumatologie*. Paris: Techniques Chirurgicales, Orthopedie-Traumatologie, 1992:44–181.
12. Shaw EG, Taylor JG. The results of lumbo-sacral fusion for low back pain. *J Bone Joint Surg* 1956;38-B:485–97.
13. Sunny SK, Denis F, Lonstein JE, Winter RB. Factors affecting fusion rate in adult spondylolisthesis. *Spine* 1990;15:979–84.
14. Unander-Scharin L. On low back pain with special reference to the value of preoperative treatment with fusion. *Acta Orthop Scand* 1950;5(suppl 18):12–21.
15. Vidal J, Marnay T. La morphologie et l'équilibre corporel antéro-postérieur dans le spondylolisthésis $L_5$–$S_1$. *Rev Chir Orthop* 1983;69:17–28.
16. Wood GW, Boyd RJ, Carothers TA, et al. The effect of pedicle screw-plate fixation on lumbar/lumbosacral autogenous bone graft fusions in patients with degenerative disc disease. *Spine* 1995;20:819–30.
17. Zagra A, Lamartina F, Giudici F, Zagra L. L'artrodesi vertebrale nella patologia degenerativa del rachide lombare. *Progressi Patologia Vertebrale* 1994;17:69–81.
18. Zdeblick TA. A prospective randomized study of lumbar fusion. *Spine* 1993;18:983–91.
19. Zucherman J, Hsu K, Picetti G, White A, Wynnie G, Taylor L. Clinical efficacy of spinal instrumentation in lumbar degenerative disc disease. *Spine* 1992;17:834–7.

# 19

# The BWM Spinal Fixator System

## Hein J. A. Kruls and Ad F. A. van Beurden

*Ignatius Ziekenhuis, NL-4800 RK Breda, The Netherlands*

The BWM spine system was developed at the Werner Wicker Klinik, Bad Wildungen, Germany, as a single system for use in the treatment of spinal instability of all etiologies occurring in the spine from the T4 to the S1 level. It is a pedicle screw-based device which can be inserted posteriorly and/or anteriorly. The system has two interconnecting possibilities: a fixator module and a distractor module. The spinal fixator module is mainly suited for use in cases of instability such as fractures, spondylolisthesis, and postlaminectomy syndromes, whereas the spinal distractor module has rods and is used in the degenerative spine and for curvature deformities, such as scoliosis, for which distraction is necessary. To facilitate the treatment of conditions such as scoliosis, a range of hooks is also available.

The key element of the BWM system is the design of the pedicle screw, which has a tapered inner diameter and a cylindrical outer diameter. The design produces a thread profile that is deepest at the tip of the screw providing maximal purchase in the anterior body of the vertebrae (Fig. 1).

The standard pedicle screw used has a diameter of 6.5 mm; a 7.5-mm screw is sometimes used for the sacrum and a smaller 5.5-mm screw is also available for patients with smaller pedicles. Pedicle screws of seven different lengths are available (25 to 55 mm). The radially serrated head of the screw provides a secure connection with the radially serated heads of the spacer element and the caudal end of the rod system. These are firmly connected by an articular screw.

The pedicle screws articulate with the spacer elements and can be rotated to achieve the desired degree of sagittal realignment required. Rotation with the axis of the spacer element is also possible, so that a three-dimensional correction can be achieved. The spacer element acts as a mechanical bridge between the pedicle screws and allows distraction or compression of the instrumented vertebrae.

By rotating the spacer element sleeves, shortening or lengthening can be obtained for precise matching of interpedicular distances. The spacer elements are available in seven different lengths. The separation distance with this system ranges from 24 to 86 mm; each element has a range of extension of up to 10 mm. Once the desired alignment has been achieved, the articular screw is tightened to form a solid connection between the pedicle screw and the spacer head. The spacer element sleeve

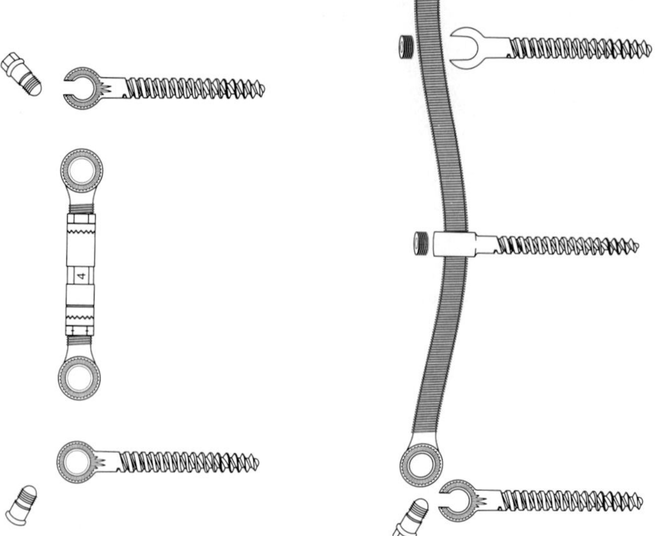

**FIG. 1.** BWM fixator. **Left:** Spacer element module. **Right:** Short fusion rod module.

can then be rotated to compress or distract the vertebrae. Finally, tightening of the end nuts on the spacer element sleeve immobilizes the entire system.

It is also possible to use the distractor rod as a mechanical bridge between two pedicle screws. Instead of the original or top-loading pedicle screw, a tulip pedicle screw is used at the cranial end of the rod, which is then fixed and secured with a flat closure screw. Placement and configuration of the top open and tulip pedicle screws with the short fusion rod module are quick and easy to perform (see Fig. 1). Because the pedicle screw and the interconnecting device, either spacer element or rod, can be connected in every physiologic angle, especially in the lumbosacral area, this system can achieve good physiologic realignment. The modular nature of the system also allows interconnection of multiple spacer elements. Therefore, multiple segments can be instrumented, either by insertion of pedicle screws into each segment or by bridging of segments as required.

The primary function of a spinal fixator system is to provide immediate stability in a corrected alignment that can be maintained and that will not interfere with the bone grafting process. Maximization or optimization of fusion and less morbidity to the patient constitute the main goals.

The success of posterior lumbar instrumentation fusion is dependent on more than merely the hardware insertion. To obtain a stable lumbosacral fixation, the sacral anchoring is important. The placement of the sacral screws must be convergent, and they may pass the anterior cortex or end in the sacral endplate. The extent of the fusion, either posterior/posterolateral and/or anterior, is often a subject of debate. Cases of spondylolisthesis, fractures, and extensive postdecompressions show the mechanical limitations of a rigid posterior segmental system. Anterior column instability needs to be treated at the same time by anterior grafting to prevent hardware failure.

## CASE HISTORY 1

The patient was a 41-year-old man who was treated for degenerative discopathy with prolapse, stenosis, and instability at the L4–L5 level. Surgery involved decompression, discectomy, and posterolateral fusion of one level with autograft bone harvested from the iliac crest (Fig. 2).

## CASE HISTORY 2

This patient was a 61-year-old woman who was admitted for treatment of a degenerative spondylolisthesis at the L4–L5 level, together with spinal stenosis as revealed by myelo–CT scan (Fig. 3A,B). She underwent a follow-up assessment 1 year postoperatively after decompression and posterolateral fusion with the BWM fixator implants at L4–S1 (Fig. 3C,D).

## CASE HISTORY 3

This patient was a 42-year-old woman who was admitted with a burst fracture of L1 (Fig. 4A,B). She underwent posterior decompression, distraction, and stabilization with the BWM rod fixation module at T12–L2, and a corresponding anterior strut graft was also inserted at T12–L2 (Fig. 4C,D).

## CASE HISTORY 4

The patient was a 38-year-old woman treated for failed back syndrome due to a pseudarthrosis after instrumentation for a spondylolysis at the L5 level. Her revision surgery involved a decompression and posterolateral fusion from L4–S1, with posterior BWM instrumentation. An anterior fusion was also performed, with an autograft over these two levels (Fig. 5).

## CASE HISTORY 5

Figure 6 shows a patient who underwent a massive posterolateral fusion at L4–S1 after implantation of the BWM pedicle screw fixator. Note the alternative divergent placement of the pedicle screws at S1.

## CLINICAL STUDY

During the past 4 years we have participated in an international multicenter clinical study to assess the use of the fixator module of the BWM spine system. This study has recently been completed and work is under way to prepare a publication of the full study results.

The following data, from the first 200 patients to complete the 2-year study, are based on a preliminary report of the data that is scheduled to be published in *Spine* during 1996. The study, known as the BWM Spinal Fixator International Multicentre Clinical Study, was conducted at the following Canadian, British, Dutch, German, Swedish, Swiss, and Italian Clinics: Victoria Hospital, University of Western Ontario, London, Ontario, Canada. (S. I. Bailey and K. R. Gurr); Clinica Ortopedica di Verona, Policlinico Borgo Roma, Verona, Italy. (P. Bartolozzi); Orthopädische Abteilung, Chirurgie Kliniken der Universität Göttingen, Germany (R. Bertagnoli); Department of Orthopaedics, Sunderland District General Hospital, Sunderland, UK (A. T. Cross); Ignatius Ziekenhuis, Breda, The Netherlands.

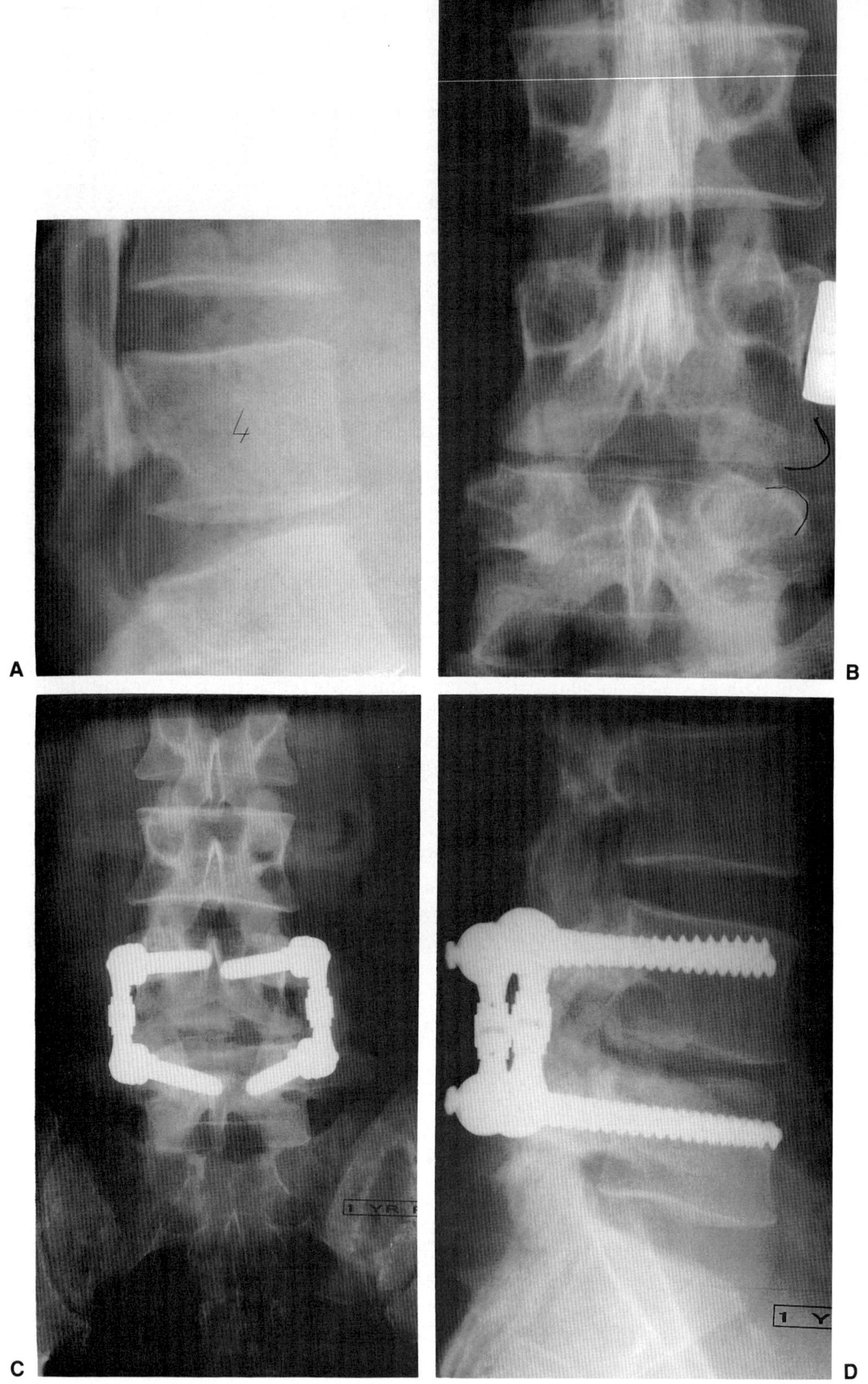

**FIG. 2.** Case history 1. **A,B:** Preoperative views; **C,D:** postoperative views.

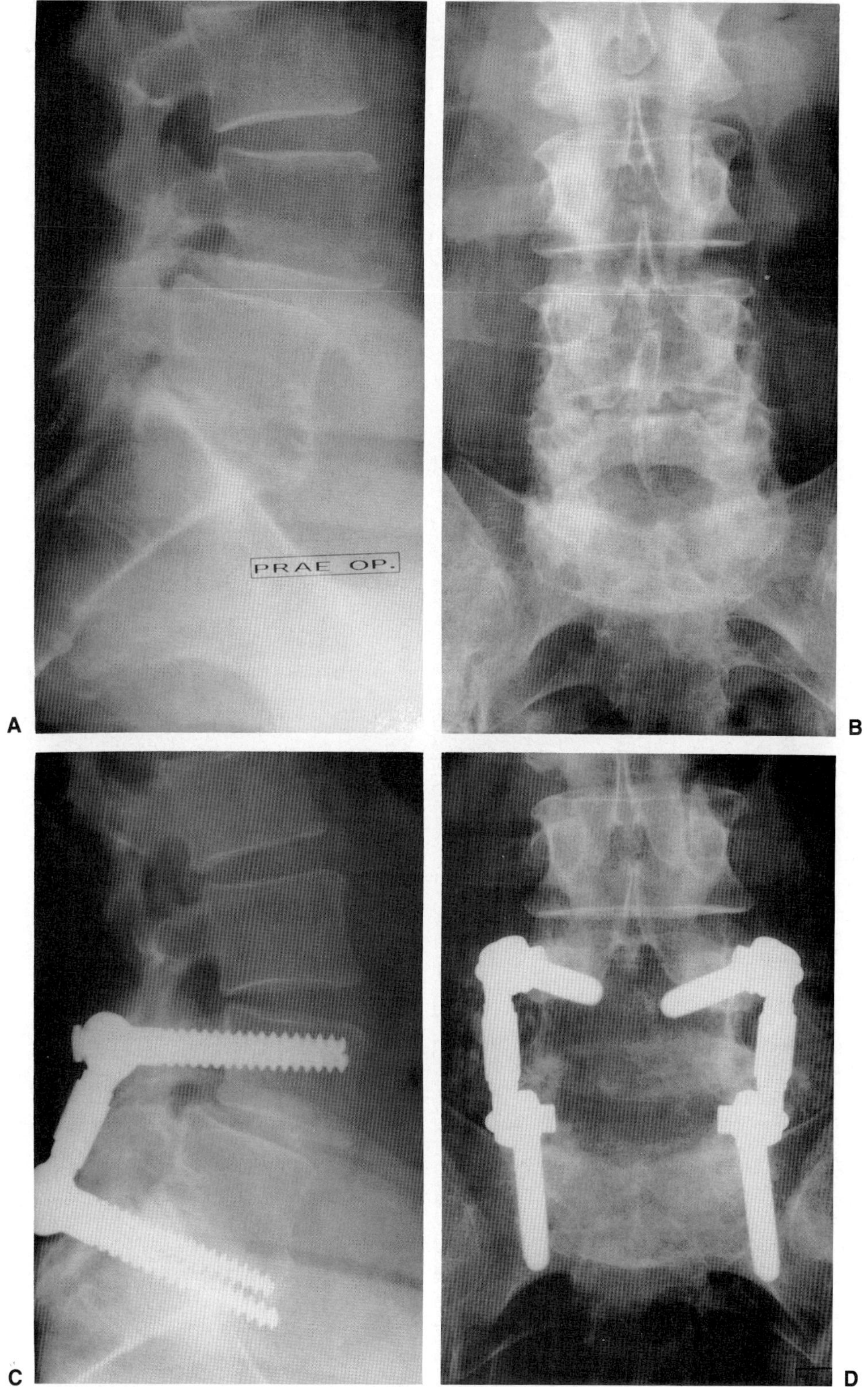

**FIG. 3.** Case history 2. **A,B:** Preoperative views; **C,D:** postoperative views.

225

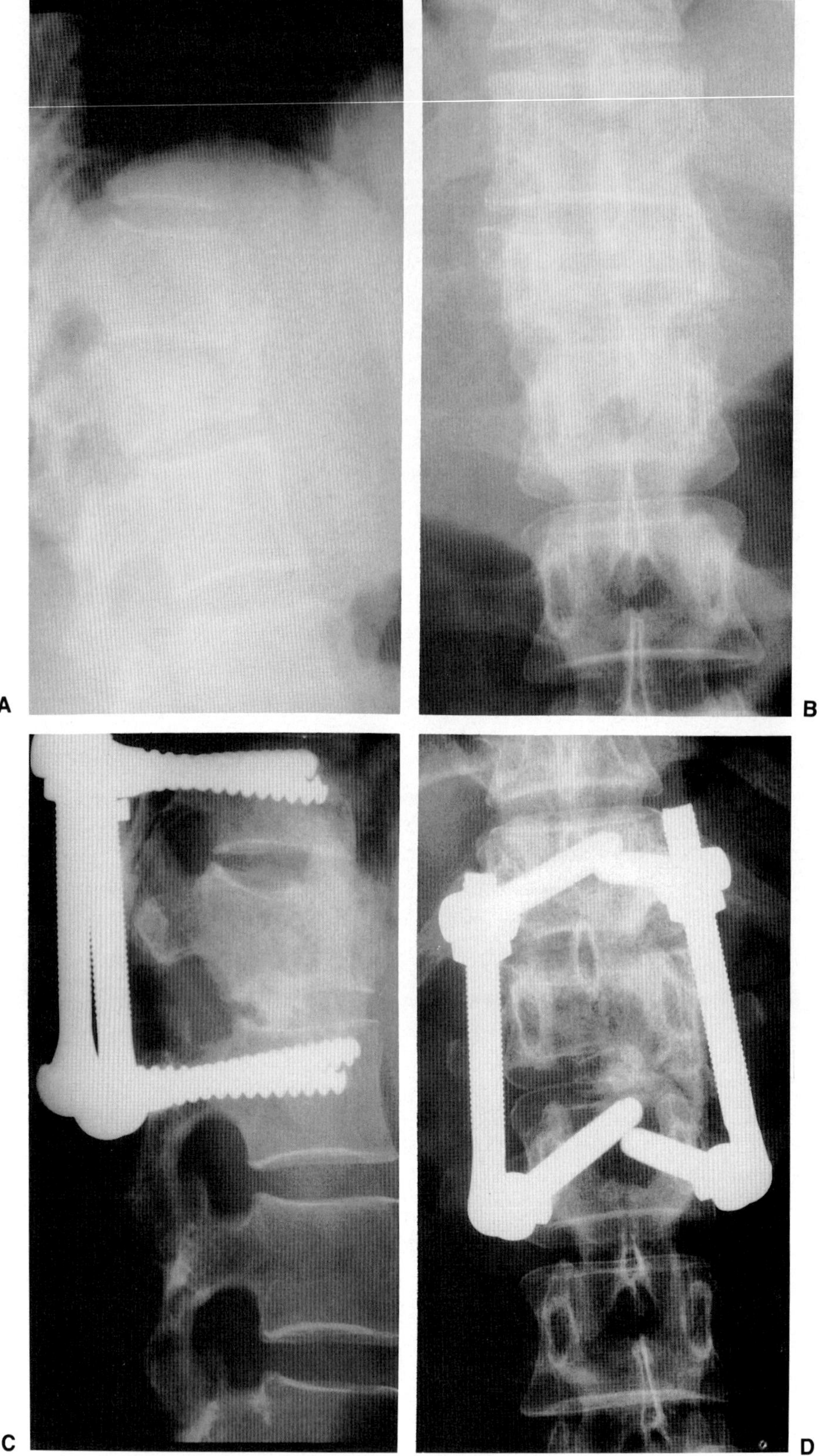

**FIG. 4.** Case history 3. **A,B:** Preoperative views; **C,D:** postoperative views.

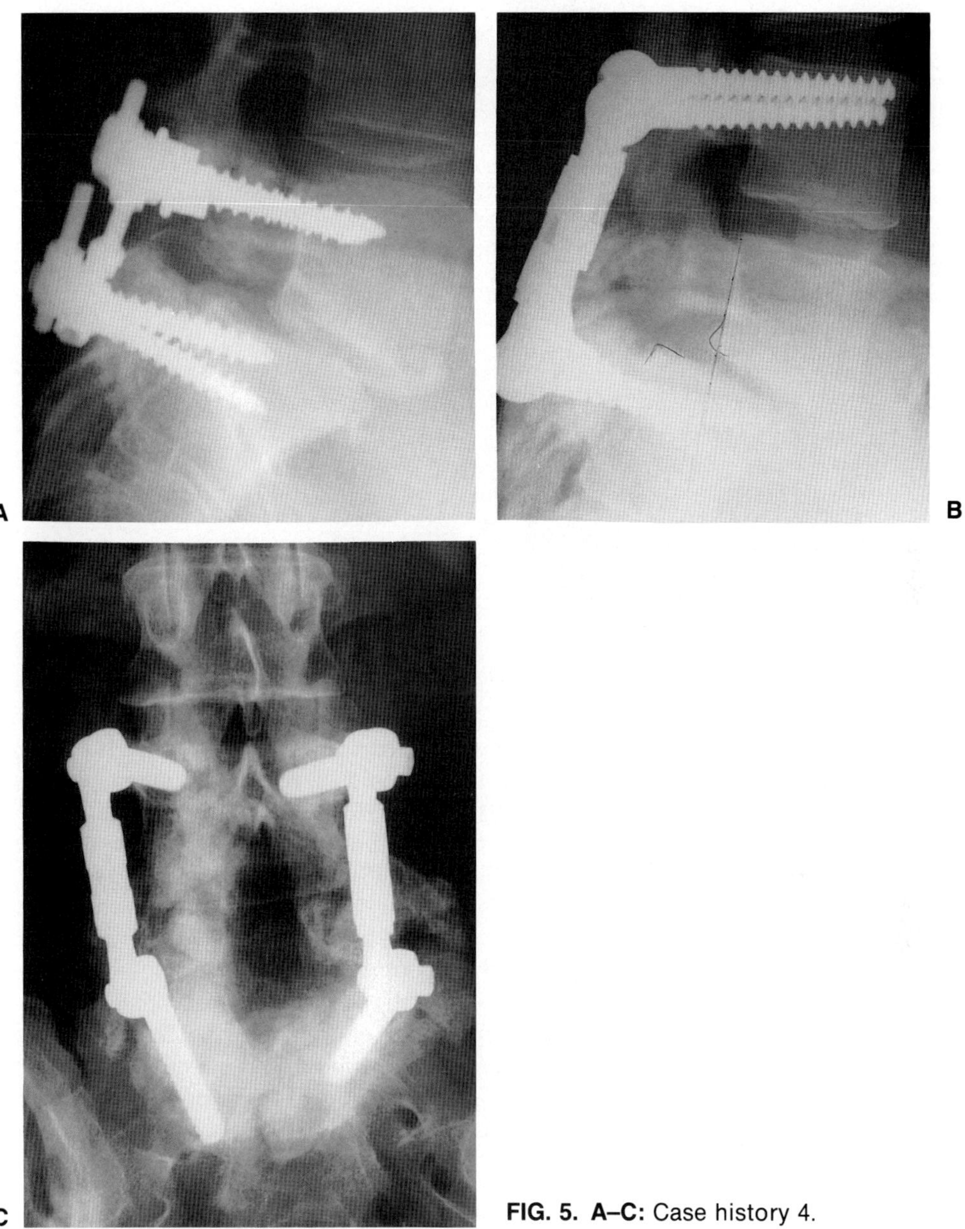

**FIG. 5. A–C:** Case history 4.

(H. J. A. Kruls and A. F. A. van Beurden); Skoliose Department II, Werner Wicker Klinik, Bad Wildungen, Germany (P. Metz-Stavenhagen); Istituti Ortopedici Rizzoli, Bologna, Italy (S. Boriani); Orthopädische Klinik, Medizinische Akademie "Carl Gustav Carus," Dresden, Germany (K-J Schulze); Klinik und Poliklinik für Allgemeine Orthopädie, Wilhelms Universität, Münster, Germany (H. Halm); Klinik für Unfallchirurgie, Universitätsspital Zürich, Switzerland (H. P. Friedl and K. Kaech); and Department of Orthopaedics, Malmo Allmanna Sjukhus, Malmo, Sweden (A. Ohlin).

The main study objective was to assess the efficacy of the system. (More detailed

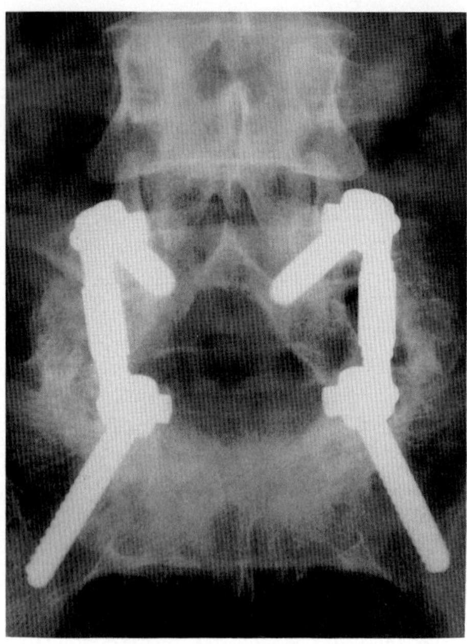

**FIG. 6.** Case history 5.

features, together with an interim statistical analyses, will be published in *Spine* during 1996).

The patients in this study group included 105 men and 95 women with a mean age of 46.1 years. Preoperatively, the patients were diagnosed with following conditions: degenerative spine (including degenerative spondylolisthesis), 75 patients; failed back syndrome, 46 patients; fracture, 33 patients; nondegenerative spondylolisthesis, 30 patients; spondylitis, 13 patients; and spinal tumor, three patients (Fig. 7).

The surgical technique used to insert the BWM system followed the routine operative procedures at each of the participating centers, provided that these conformed to the guidelines provided with the system. In this group, all 200 patients received posterior instrumentation with posterior and/or anterior bone grafting. When an anterior approach was also performed, either strut grafts or tricortical stabilization was undertaken. Postoperative spinal support, either a cast or orthosis, was recommended for 8–12 weeks after surgery, and deep sitting posture was to be avoided for at least 12 weeks after lumbosacral operation.

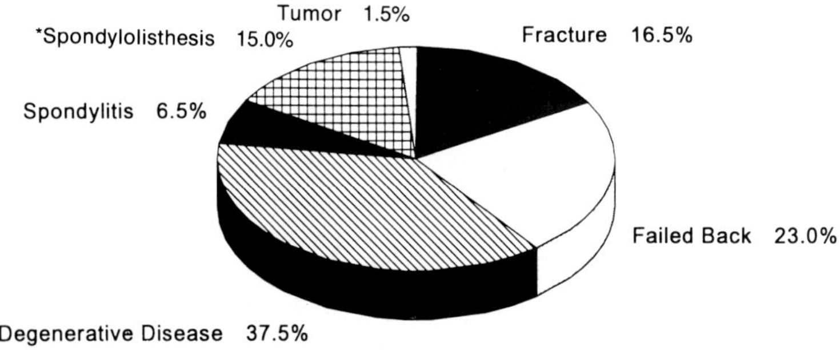


**FIG. 7.** Diagnosis (*n* = 200 patients). *Refers to nondegenerative spondylolisthesis patients.

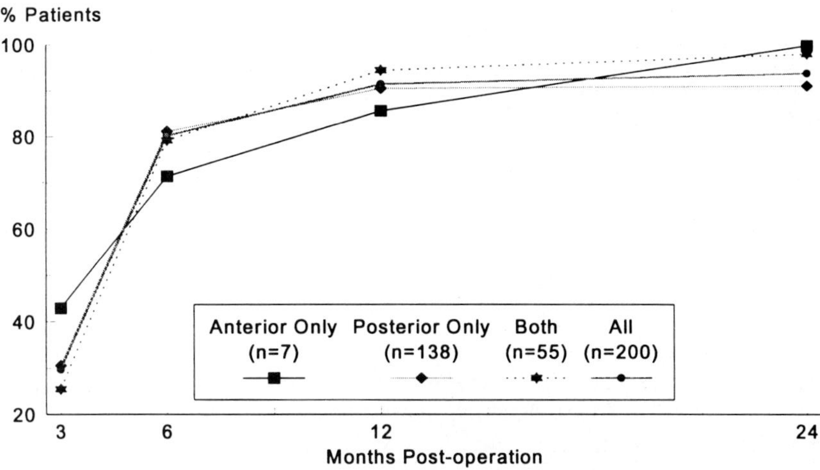



**FIG. 8.** Overall rate of graft consolidation.

Seven patients died during the 2-year follow-up period, but none of the deaths was related to the fusion or the implant.

The patients were assessed according to the schedule identified in the study protocol, i.e., preoperatively, perioperatively, before discharge from hospital, and at 3, 6, 12, and 24 months postoperatively. The primary effectiveness variable was bone graft consolidation.

Graft consolidation (Fig. 8) was observed in 188 (94%) patients at 24 months. When the location of bone graft was considered, 100% of the seven patients with anterior grafting, 126 (91.3%) of the 138 patients with posterior grafting, and 54 (98.2%) of the patients with both were observed to have graft consolidation at the end of the study.

A total of 61 device problems were seen in 52 patients. Twenty-one of the 856 implanted pedicle screws failed (2.5%), and 10 of 446 spacer elements broke (2.2%). Thirteen of the 21 broken pedicle screws were implanted in the sacrum, and it was this finding that prompted the introduction of the 7.5-mm-diameter pedicle screws, which provided greater strength, for use in the lumbosacral region. There have been no reported failures of these new 7.5-mm pedicle screws. The implant failures are

**TABLE 1.** *Device failures[a]*

| Type of failure | Number of items failed | Number of items implanted | Percentage of items implanted | Percentage of patients ($n$ = 200) |
|---|---|---|---|---|
| Articular screw loosening | 21 | 856 | 2.5 | 10.5 |
| Pedicle screw loosening | 2 | 856 | 0.2 | 1.0 |
| Pedicle screw failure | 21 | 856 | 2.5 | 10.5 |
| Spacer element failure | 10 | 446 | 2.2 | 5.0 |
| Spacer element loosening | 3 | 446 | 0.7 | 1.5 |
| 4-mm rod failure | 1 | 12 | — | — |
| Other | 3 | — | — | — |

[a] Some patients had a combination of device failures.

**TABLE 2.** *Activity level, function–walking, and pain score assessment scales*

| Activity level | Function–walking score | Pain score |
|---|---|---|
| 1  Needs assistance for all activities | 1  Unable to walk | 1  Totally disabling |
| 2  Independent in self care | 2  Indoors or <200 m | 2  Severe |
| 3  Indoor activities of daily living | 3  15 min or 500 m | 3  Moderate |
| 4  Outdoor activities of daily living | 4  30 min or 1,000 m | 4  Mild |
| 5  Low-stress sports | 5  60 min or 2,000 m | 5  None |
| 6  High-stress sports | 6  Unlimited | |

summarized in Table 1. Improvements in pain score and quality of life were assessed using the graded score systems as shown in Table 2.

Preoperative pain score was assessed on admission to the hospital using a 5-point scale, from grade 1 for totally disabled to grade 5 for no pain; mean preoperative pain score for the entire group was grade 3, moderate pain.

As detailed in Fig. 9, the pain score at the 24-month assessment was unchanged in 36 (18%) of the patients, whereas it has improved by one grade in 63 (31.5%) of the patients and by a minimum of two grades in 82 (49.1%). Of the entire series of 200 patients, 145 (72.5%) patients had improvement in their pain score (Fig. 9).

The 33 patients who underwent surgery for the treatment of a spinal fracture are not included in the assessments of activity level and function–walking score because these patients were immobilized post trauma before surgery.

As described in Table 2, the daily activity level was assessed using a 6-point scale, ranging from grade 1, where patients "required assistance with all activities," to grade 6, where patients were "able to do high-stress sports." The mean preoperative activity score in the nonfracture group (167 patients) was between grades 3 and 4. Of this patient group, 64 (38%) improved by one grade and 39 (23.4%) improved by at least two grades (see Fig. 10). At 24 months, 80% of patients were capable of a minimum of normal outdoor activities (grade 4).

Walking ability was also scored on a 6-point scale (Fig. 11). The mean preoperative function–walking score in the nonfracture patient group was between score 3 (15 min or 500 m) and score 4 (30 min or 1,000 m). In the nonfracture group, 35 (21%) had

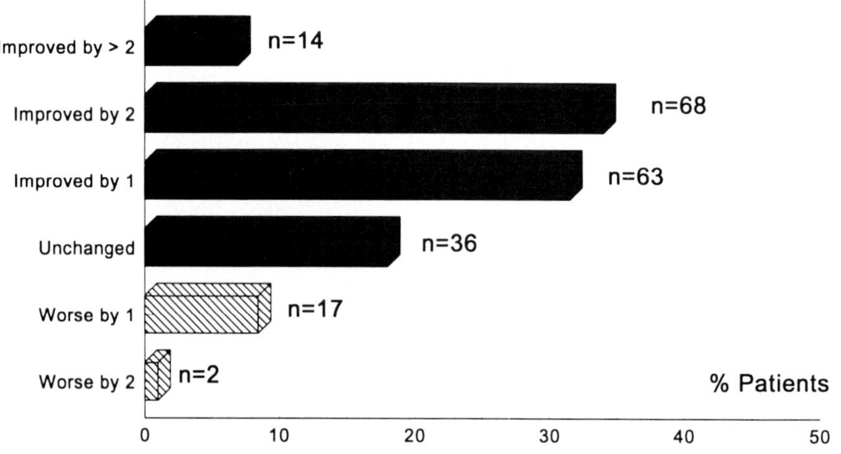


**FIG. 9.** Changes in pain score at 24 months from preoperative level (all patients); *n* = 200.

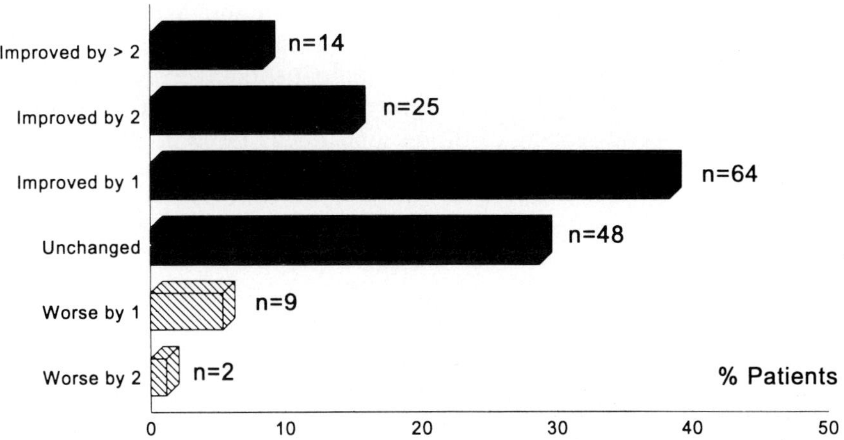


**FIG. 10.** Changes in activity level at 24 months from preoperative level (nonfracture patients); *n* = 167.

improved by one grade and 81 (48.5%) had improved by at least two grades (Fig. 11).

The clinical results of these first 200 patients at the 2-year postoperative assessment are promising and are comparable with the results of other spinal pedicle screw-based devices. The procedure enables patients to improve their quality of life, especially in terms of being able to enjoy outdoor activities, usually accompanied by a reduction in pain.

We are aware of the ongoing arguments related to the topic of spinal fusion:

When is it indicated?
Should it be performed with or without instrumentation?
Should pedicle fixation always be used?

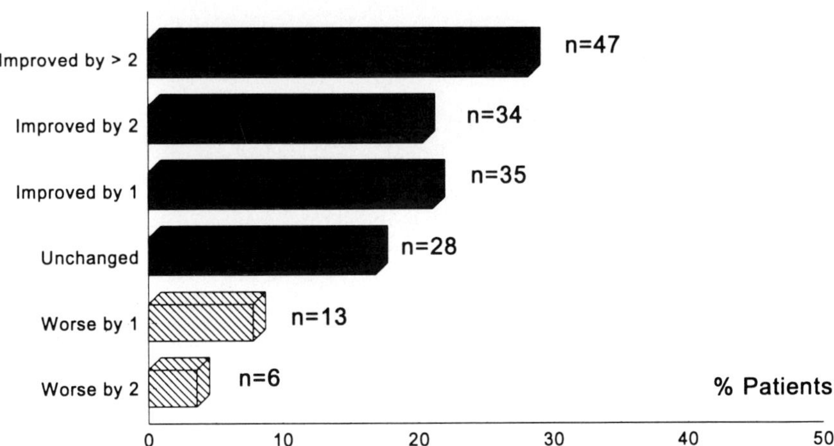


**FIG. 11.** Changes in function–walking score at 24 months from preoperative level (nonfracture patients); *n* = 167.

Evaluating the efficacy of a fusion is a complex matter and involves consideration of many more items than those given above. The results from this multicenter trial appear to indicate a reasonable outcome for the patients involved, but further experience of the system will enable us to have a better overview of its performance. We therefore recommend reading of the Second Focus Issue of Spine, devoted to lumbar spine fusion (*Spine,* volume 20, supplement 24S, December 15, 1995).

*Instrumented Fusion of the Degenerative
Lumbar Spine: State of the Art, Questions,
and Controversies,* edited by M. Szpalski,
R. Gunzburg, D. M. Spengler, and
A. Nachemson. Lippincott–Raven
Publishers, Philadelphia © 1996.

# 20

# The Treatment of Chronic Discogenic Low Back Pain by the Bagby and Kuslich Method of Interbody Fusion

Stephen D. Kuslich

*Department of Orthopaedic Surgery, University of Minnesota; and St. Croix
Orthopaedics, Stillwater, Minnesota 55082*

The diagnosis and treatment of chronic low back pain remain among the most challenging and rewarding activities in the arena of orthopedics and neurosurgery. Significant progress has been made in understanding the origin of back pain (11,20,24, 27,33,39,45). Magnetic resonance imaging (MRI) and discography can provide us with clear insight into the status of specific spinal tissues and the disease processes involved.

Most cases of acute low back pain resolve spontaneously, with or without treatment. However, perhaps as many as 10% become chronic. Spinal fusion is one option in such cases. Of the several techniques available, many surgeons prefer to use internal fixation in addition to bone grafting. However, this can produce new and sometimes serious complications (48).

A smaller number of surgeons advocate circumferential fusion with interbody graft, posterolateral graft, and pedicle fixation (28), but these techniques subject the patient to an even higher rate of complications (47). Interbody fusion techniques abound (7,8,14–18,21,23,25,26,29–32,35,37,38,40–43,46).

Bagby (1) invented the "Bagby Basket" to treat wobbler syndrome in the horse (Fig. 1). This porous, hollow stainless steel cylinder encloses the bone graft and protects it from excessive compression and migration. In a manner similar to the Cloward anterior cervical fusion, Bagby successfully fused the cervical spine of horses by distracting the intervertebral space using a slightly oversized basket, and filled the basket with local autogenous bone graft (1,9,44). Bagby called the procedure a "distraction–compression stabilization."

With the assistance of Butts and Bechtold, I studied the Bagby principle of distraction–compression stabilization by performing biomechanical experiments on bovine and porcine spines. Two parallel implants, interposed between lumbar vertebral bodies in a manner similar to Wiltberger's bone graft (46) and distracting the annulus about 2–3 mm, resulted in marked stabilization of the motion segment during flexion–extension and side bending (4). I collaborated with Bagby and a group of bioengi-

*233*

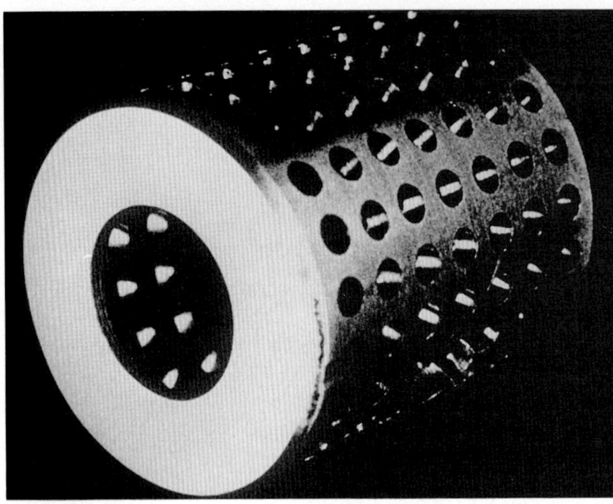

**FIG. 1.** The Bagby Basket—the stainless steel hollow cylinder used to perform cervical anterior interbody fusions in horses with "wobbler syndrome." (Reprinted from ref. 1, with permission.)

neers to develop the Bagby and Kuslich implant (BAK) for use in the human spine (34). The current BAK System (Spine-Tech, Inc., Minneapolis, MN) includes many sizes of the device and the special tools required for its safe implantation.

The BAK device is a hollow, porous, square-threaded, slightly tapered cylinder, made of a titanium alloy. The implant provides the stability necessary for arthrodesis to occur (Fig. 2). The device is sufficiently rigid to withstand the spinal forces without deformation or fracture, yet porous enough to allow through-growth of cancellous bone, thereby inducing interbody arthrodesis (34). Zdeblick and associates (3) at the University of Wisconsin at Madison performed a biomechanical study demonstrating that the BAK system stabilized the lumbar motion segment in a manner superior to PLIF bone graft alone and equivalent to the use of PLIF bone graft and a pedicle screw–rod construct (Fig. 3).

Grobler and others (19) performed a controlled study of the anteriorly implanted

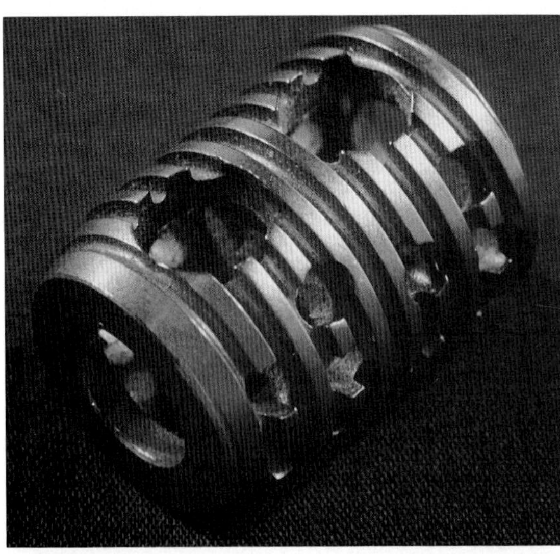

**FIG. 2.** The BAK implant—the hollow titanium alloy cylinder we use to perform lumbar interbody fusions in humans.

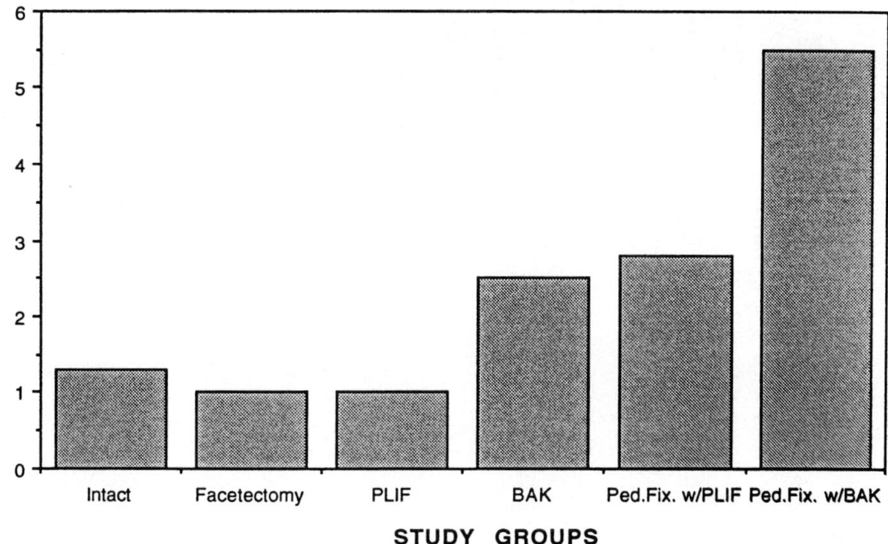


**FIG. 3.** Biomechanical study showing comparison of BAK device with other methods of spinal stabilization. (Reprinted from ref. 3, with permission.)

BAK versus anterior interbody allograft in the baboon. That study concluded that the BAK was vastly superior to allograft in terms of radiographic and histologic rates of fusion. Human clinical trials of the BAK have been completed in the United States. Since 1992, over 2,000 patients have been implanted with the devices during surgical procedures performed by over 50 surgeons at more than 30 United States, Canadian, European, Asian, and Australian medical centers. Most patients have been treated for painful degenerative disc disease of the lower lumbar spine, but similar devices are available for and have been used in the thoracic and cervical

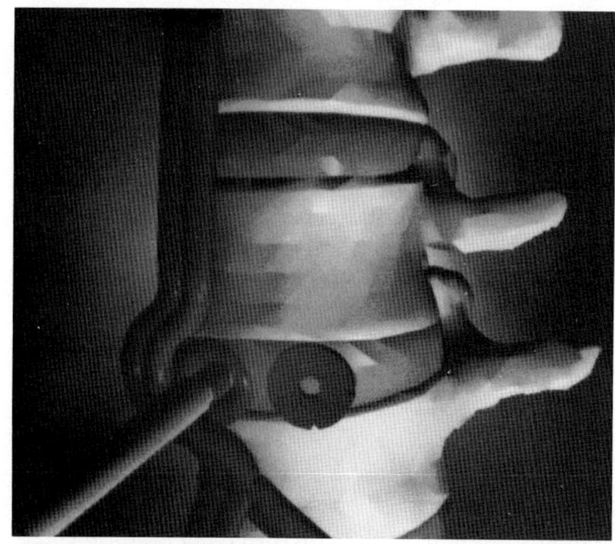

**FIG. 4.** The great vessels are retracted laterally in the anterior approach to allow preparation and implantation of the BAK devices.

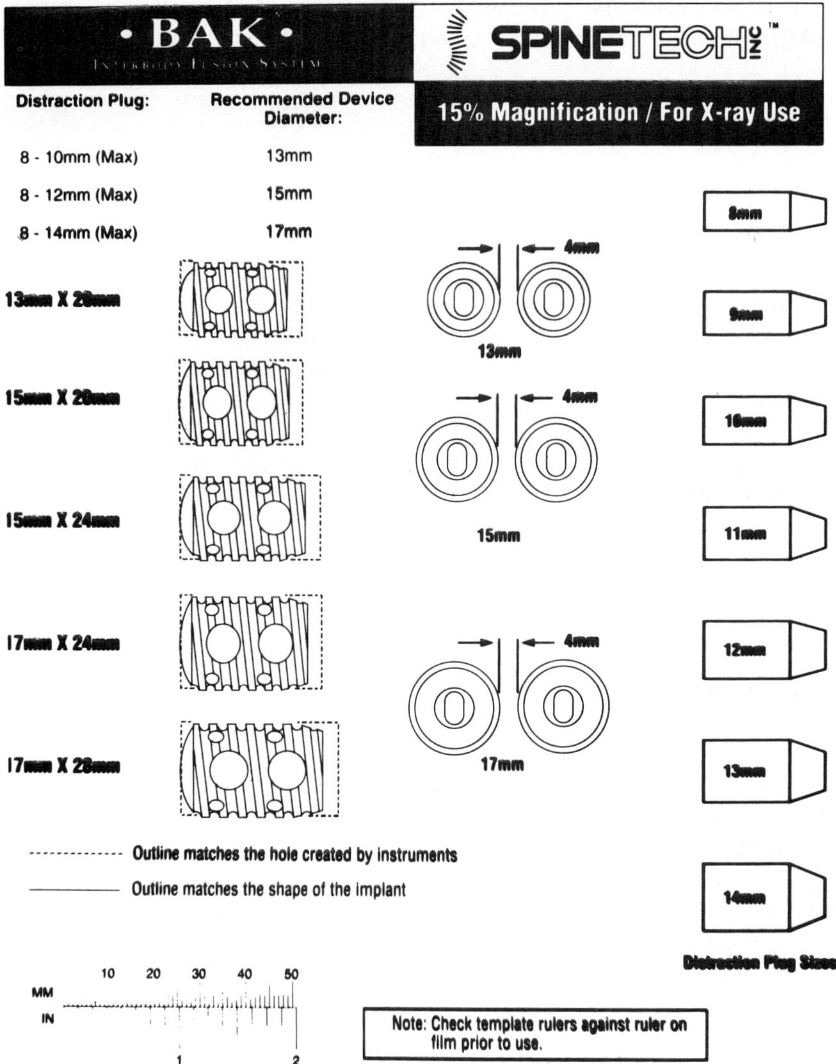



**FIG. 5.** Sizing template used to predict appropriate size of BAK implant.

spine. A majority of the patients were implanted by the open posterior laminotomy or open anterior retroperitoneal route, but some surgeons insert the devices by means of thoracoscopic and laparoscopic techniques. Results of the prospective, multicenter United States trial of lumbar open anterior and open posterior implantations are included in this chapter.

The indications for the procedure include painful degenerative disc disease at one or two contiguous levels of the lumbar spine in patients between the ages of 21 and 65 years, and chronic, disabling low back pain of at least 6 months' duration in patients who are unresponsive to an adequate trial of conservative treatment. The contraindications include active infection, osteopenia, symptomatic vascular disease, active malignancy, gross obesity, greater than grade 1 spondylolisthesis, and pregnancy. The diagnosis of chronic, disabling discogenic low back pain is established by generally accepted methods, including history and physical examinations, x-rays, MRI, and discography when necessary.

## SURGICAL METHOD

### Anterior Retroperitoneal Approach

The patient is placed in the supine position and a general anesthetic is administered. A pad is placed under the lumbar spine to maintain lordosis. The lumbar spine is exposed through a paramedian or low transverse incision, and a retroperitoneal plane is developed, exposing the large vessels (Fig. 4), the ureter, and the sympathetic trunk on the left side. A vascular surgeon usually provides the exposure while the spine surgeon assists and performs the implantation. Normally, the L5–S1 disc level can be exposed below the bifurcation of the great vessels, whereas L4–L5 and above requires that the left iliac vein and/or the vena cava be mobilized to the right side. Segmental vessels may need to be identified, ligated, and sectioned to provide adequate exposure. Great care, skill, and experience are necessary to safely expose

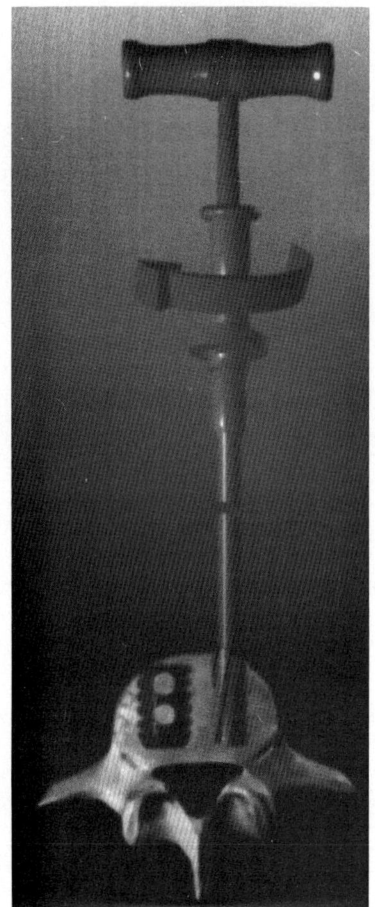

**FIG. 6.** Distraction plug on the left provides equalized annular distraction of the interspace. Drill guides with safety stops ensure proper position and depth of the implant cavity.

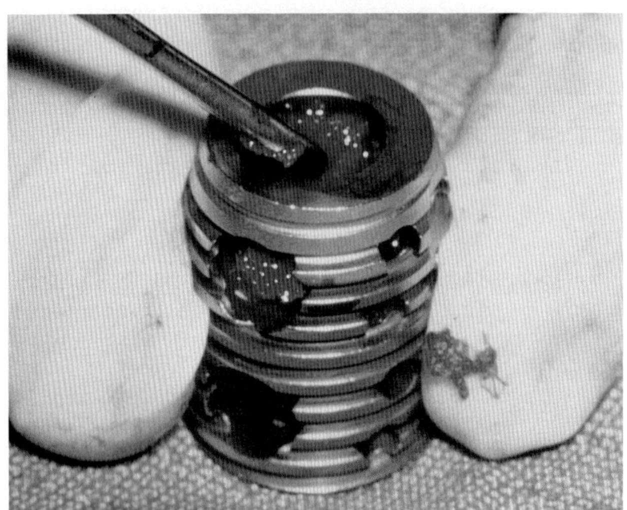

**FIG. 7.** The distal chamber of the BAK device is filled with morselized bone graft before insertion into the prepared space. The proximal chamber is filled after insertion.

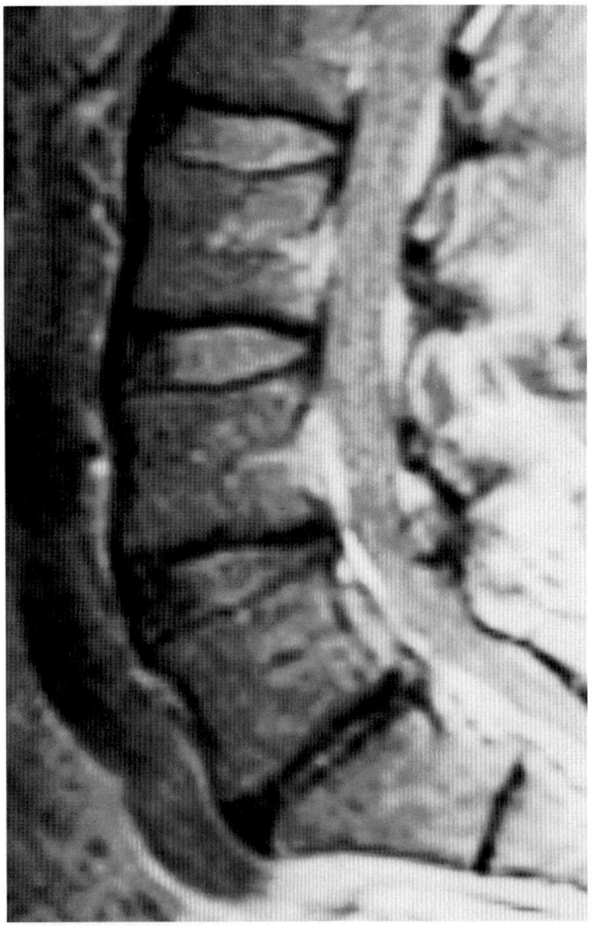

**FIG. 8.** Preoperative sagittal MRI of the lumbar spine. The diagnosis is degenerative disc disease at the L5–S1 disc with anterior and posterior disc bulging.

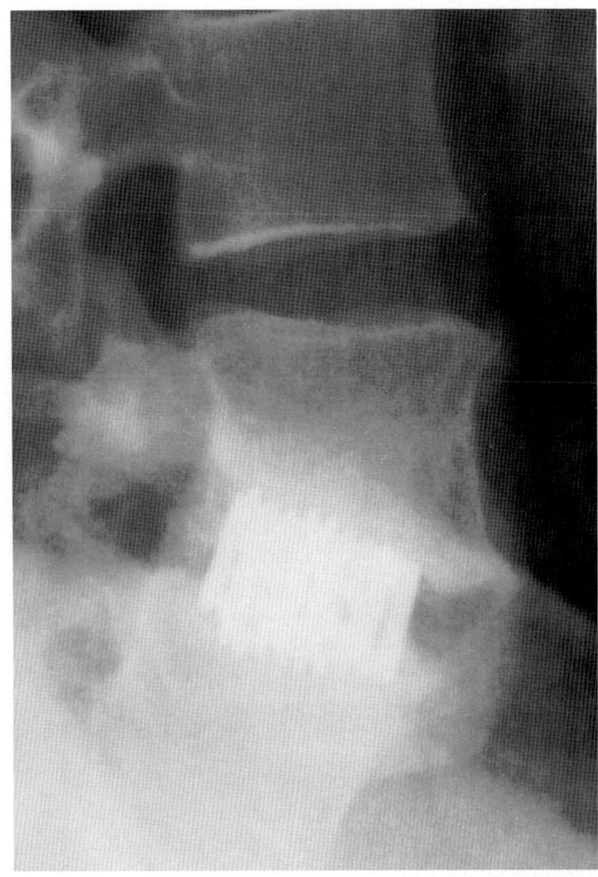

**FIG. 9.** Lateral radiograph of a patient at 2 years postoperatively. Note the anterior bridging osteophytes. This patient has resumed normal activities and reports no back pain.

the spine from the anterior approach, and therefore only surgeons who are properly trained and skilled should attempt this operation.

Sufficient bone graft is harvested from the anterior iliac crest in cases of one-level fusion, but a preliminary posterior iliac graft harvest may be necessary for two-level fusions. About 5–7 cc of compacted cancellous graft is necessary for each of two implants per level.

### Posterior Laminotomy Approach

The patient is placed in the kneeling–sitting position on an Andrews or similar frame. Spinal, general, or "progressive local anesthesia" (24) may be used. The paravertebral muscles are retracted laterally to the outer edge of the facet joint. A laminotomy of sufficient size is developed to accommodate the bilateral drill tubes.

### *Maneuvers Common to Both Anterior and Posterior Approaches*

Special proprietary instruments are necessary to safely and effectively implant the devices. After the spinal midline is established by anterioposterior x-ray, the proper entrance holes are drilled on each side of the spinal midline using a guide. A distraction plug is then inserted into one side of the disc space. When the appropriate distraction plug is in place, the disc space is distracted in a manner that stabilizes the motion segment by circumferential tension on the annulus and allows equal bone drilling on both sides of the interspace.

X-rays or fluoroscopic images are taken in both AP and lateral planes. Special templates for x-ray and for computed tomography (CT) and MRI scans are used to determine the proper implant size (Fig. 5).

All preparation and implantation from this point forward is carried out through specially designed proprietary tubes that protect the dura in the case of posterior approaches or the great vessels in the case of anterior approaches. On the side of the disc opposite the distraction plug, a hole is drilled (Fig. 6), removing most of the nuclear material and cartilaginous endplate, cutting into the edges of the vertebral bodies above and below. The surgeon than taps the resulting hole and securely screws the device filled with compressed cancellous bone graft into place (Fig. 7). After removing the distraction plug, curretting the remaining disc material, and performing a similar implantation procedure on the opposite side, the surgeon takes

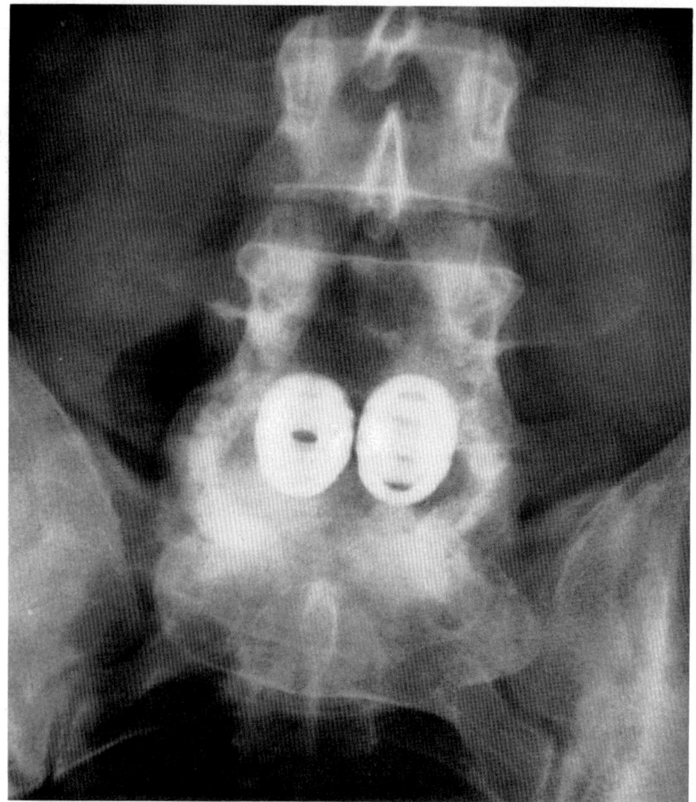

**FIG. 10.** Anteroposterior x-ray at 2 years postoperatively. The patient reports no pain and has resumed all preoperative activities. Note the trabecular bone lateral to the implants.

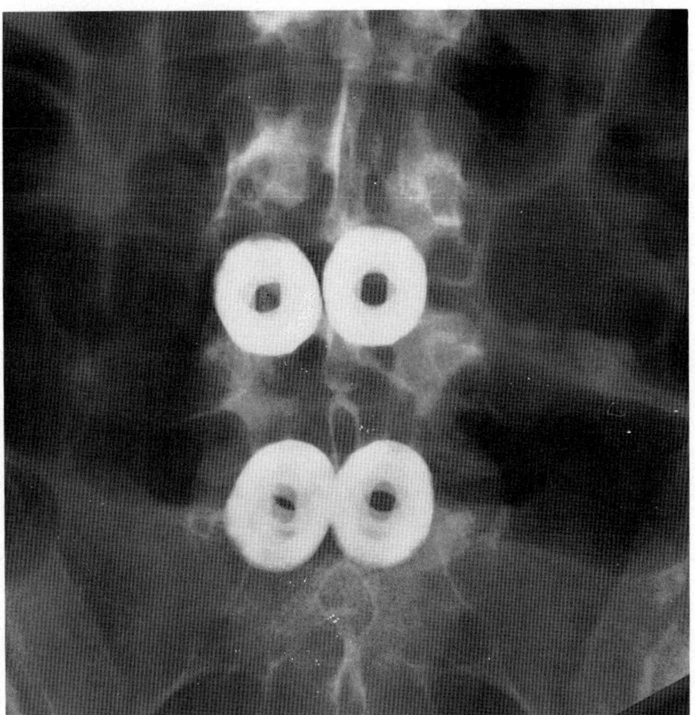

**FIG. 11.** A postoperative AP showing a two-level (L4–L5, L5–S1) anterior interbody fusion using BAK.

final x-rays and makes appropriate final adjustments. In the posterior surgery cases, a polyethylene end cap is applied to the posterior surface of the implant, thereby preventing adherence of the dura to the internal bone graft. During the anterior approach, no such end cap is needed because the posterior annulus is maintained as a barrier to dural adherence.

Additional bone graft can be inserted between and around the implants if desired. In most cases the implants occupy most of the interbody space except for the outer annulus, and therefore no additional graft is necessary. We do not utilize additional means of fixation such as facet screws or pedicle fixation systems. The incision is closed in the usual manner. External braces may be worn for comfort, but they are not required for the clinical study. Walking with or without assistance is encouraged as soon as possible after the procedure.

We obtain x-rays, including flexion–extension lateral views, at 1- and 2-year follow-up visits to assess the degree of stability and to determine whether or not fusion has occurred.

### Case Examples

Figure 8 shows the lumbar MRI of a patient with painful degenerative disc disease at L5–S1. He is a 54-year-old man whose prior treatments consisted of two decompressions at L5–S1, chiropractic treatments for 2 years, physical therapy in the form

**TABLE 1.** *Surgical data*

|  | Surgery time (min) | Blood loss (ml) | Length of hospital stay (days) |
|---|---|---|---|
| All | 194 | 446 | 4.8 |
| Anterior level | 146 | 249 | 4.4 |
| Anterior 2 levels | 212 | 515 | 5.2 |
| Posterior 1 level | 228 | 592 | 4.5 |
| Posterior 2 levels | 279 | 785 | 6.2 |

of traction and bracing, and steroid injections. None of his previous treatments provided significant relief of the low back pain. Before the onset of back problems he worked in heavy labor and participated in light recreational activities such as roller skating, walking, and dancing. At the time of surgery he was unable to participate in any of these activities. This patient had virtually complete relief of his preoperative leg and back pain at 3 months postoperatively and was participating in all his preoperative activities by 1 year postoperatively. The 2-year lateral film (Fig. 9) shows a bridging osteophyte anteriorly. The AP film at 2 years demonstrates no radiolucency around the implant (Fig. 10).

The second case is a 35-year-old woman who experienced repeated low back pain episodes for more than 20 years. Laminectomy had been performed for a herniated disc in 1992. Leg pain was improved but low back pain continued in spite of extensive conservative treatment. MRI demonstrated isolated severe degenerative disc disease at L4–L5 and L5–S1. A two-level anterior interbody fusion using BAK was performed in May of 1993 (Fig. 11). CT scanning with three-dimensional rendering at 1 year postoperatively (Figs. 12 and 13) revealed solid fusion at both levels. She was back to normal activities, with a majority of her original low back pain relieved.

## RESULTS

This chapter describes 187 patients with 2-year follow-up. A total of 121 patients underwent anterior implantations and 66 underwent posterior implantation. The following surgeons provided patients for the multicenter, prospective United States clinical trial: John Sherman, William Taylor, David Arnold, Guy Danielson, Edgar Dawson, Randall Dryer, Donald Erickson, Bruce Frederickson, Thomas Highland, Eric Widell, Hansen Yuan, Thomas Zdeblich, and James Zuckerman.

### SUMMARY OF THE UNITED STATES PROSPECTIVE, MULTICENTER CLINICAL TRIAL OF BAK LUMBAR INTERBODY FUSION

A total of 187 patients underwent surgery at 247 levels (Tables 1 and 2). At the anterior level were 121 patients (166 levels total): one level, 76 patients (76 levels);

**TABLE 2.** *Efficacy of surgery*

|  | Levels fused/ levels operated | Fusion (%) | Pain reduced (%) | Function improved (%) |
|---|---|---|---|---|
| All groups | 226/247 | 91.5% | 86.5 | 93.6 |
| 1 level anterior | 74/76 | 97.4 | 88.1 | 94.9 |
| 2 level anterior | 81/90 | 90.0 | 86.1 | 97.2 |
| 1 level posterior | 47/51 | 92.2 | 88.9 | 94.4 |
| 2 level posterior | 24/30 | 80.0 | 80.0 | 80.0 |

**TABLE 3.** *Comparison of patient population and overall fusion rates for BAK anterior procedures and ALIF studies*

| Reference | n | Mean age (yr) | % female | % failed fusion | % fusion success |
|---|---|---|---|---|---|
| Greenough 1994 (18) | 151 | 41 | 49 | — | 76 |
| Knox 1993 (23) | 22 | 40 | 77 | 0 | 45 |
| Neuman 1992 (32) | 36 | 38 | 58 | 0 | 89 |
| Gill 1992 (16) | 53 | 34 | 32 | — | 80 |
| Kim 1993 (22) | 24 | 41 | 52 | — | 78 |
| Kim 1991 (21) | 75 | 41 | 71 | — | 77 |
| Linson 1991 (28) | 35 | 36 | 51 | — | 80 |
| Cheng 1989 (5) | 20 | 41 | 65 | — | 65 |
| Dennis 1989 (10) | 29 | 43 | 66 | — | 68 |
| Loguidice 1988 (29) | 85 | 41 | 48 | 19 | 75 |
| Blumenthal 1988 (2) | 34 | 36 | 38 | 0 | 73 |
| Thomasen 1985 (42) | 312 | 39 | 51 | — | 84 |
| Raustad 1982 (36) | 45 | 38 | 58 | — | 81 |
| Fujimaki 1982 (15) | 150 | 42 | 50 | 19 | 96 |
| Chow 1980 (6) | 97 | 43 | 29 | 0 | 63 |
| Flynn 1979 (12) | 50 | 40 | 36 | 14 | 56 |
| Sorenson 1978 (40) | 98 | 40 | 62 | — | 91 |
| Stauffer 1972 (41) | 68 | 42 | 55 | 60 | 56 |
| Goldner 1971 (17) | 100 | — | — | 30 | 81 |
| Freebody 1971 (14) | 243 | 45 | 66 | 5 | 85 |
| Total | 1,726 | | | | |
| Mean ± SD | — | 40.1 ± 2.6 | 53 ± 12 | 14 ± 18 | 75 ± 12.5 |
| (range) | | (34–45) | (29–77) | (0–60) | (45–96) |
| All BAK | 166 levels | 41.7 | 66% | 6.6% | 93.4% |
| Anterior levels | 155 fused | | | Not fused | Fused |

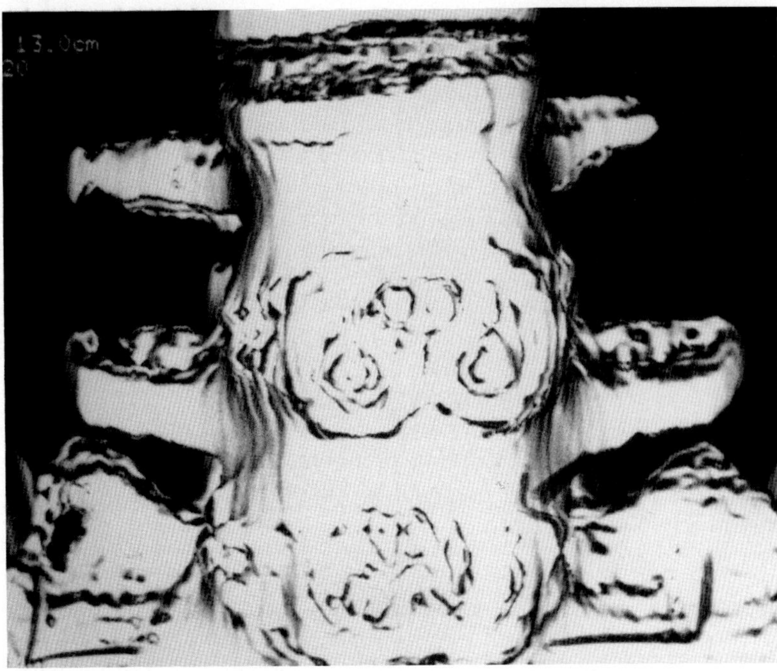

**FIG. 12.** Anteroposterior view of a three-dimensional CT scan showing bone growth in the annulus at both instrumented levels.

**TABLE 4.** *Comparison of patient population and overall fusion rates for BAK posterior procedures and PLIF studies*

| Reference | $n$ | Mean age (yr) | % female | % failed fusion | % fusion success |
|---|---|---|---|---|---|
| Schechler 1991 (38) | 24 | 37 | 26 | 0 | 96 |
| Mitsunaga 1991 (31) | 27 | — | — | 0 | 81 |
| Rish 1989 (37) | 250 | — | — | 0 | 86 |
| Prolo 1986 (35) | 34 | 45 | 35 | — | 94 |
| Ma 1985 (30) | 100 | 41 | 24 | 9 | 74 |
| Lin 1983 (25,26) | 465 | 40 | 44 | 24 | 88 |
| Cloward 1982 (7,8) | 100 | — | 35 | — | 82 |
| Verlooy 1993 (43) | 20 | 42 | 65 | — | 80 |
| Total | 1,019 | | | | |
| Mean ± SD | — | 41 ± 2.6 | 38 ± 14 | 7 ± 9 | 85.1 ± 6.9 |
| (range) | | (37–45) | (24–65) | (0–24) | (74–96) |
| All BAK | 81 levels | 40.6 | 44 | 12.3% | 87.7% |
| Posterior procedures | 71 fused | | | Not fused | Fused |

two levels, 45 patients, (90 levels). At the posterior level were 66 patients, (81 levels total): one level, 51 patients (51 levels); two levels, 15 patients (30 levels).

# A COMPARISON OF BAK FUSION RESULTS WITH PUBLISHED SERIES OF ALIF AND PLIF PROCEDURES USING BONE GRAFT WITHOUT INTERNAL FIXATION

## Fusion Results

Table 3 compares the results of BAK fusion to other reported series of anterior lumbar interbody fusions. The fusion rate for anterior BAK patients was over 93.4%, exceeding the mean fusion rate of these 20 reported series by more than 18%.

Table 4 compares the BAK posterior fusions to a literature survey of eight posterior lumbar interbody fusion series using bone graft. Posterior BAK results exceed the mean fusion rates for this type of operation.

The mean pain score improved by an average of 2 out of 5 points at 2 years. This change is significant, ($p < 0.0001$). The mean neurofunctional impairment score improved by 7.2 points. Mean preoperative score was 20.7 and postoperative was 13.5. This change is also significant ($p < 0.0001$).

## Return to Work Data

Of the patients, 41.8% were working preoperatively and 66.7% were working postoperatively. A total of 64.6% received Workers' Compensation preoperatively, but postoperatively 69.5% did not.

## Complications

There were no deaths related to the procedure. Two postoperative deaths (1.4%) were unrelated to the procedure: one thoracic aortic aneurysm 24 months after fusion and one bowel infarction after gynecologic surgery 28 months post fusion.

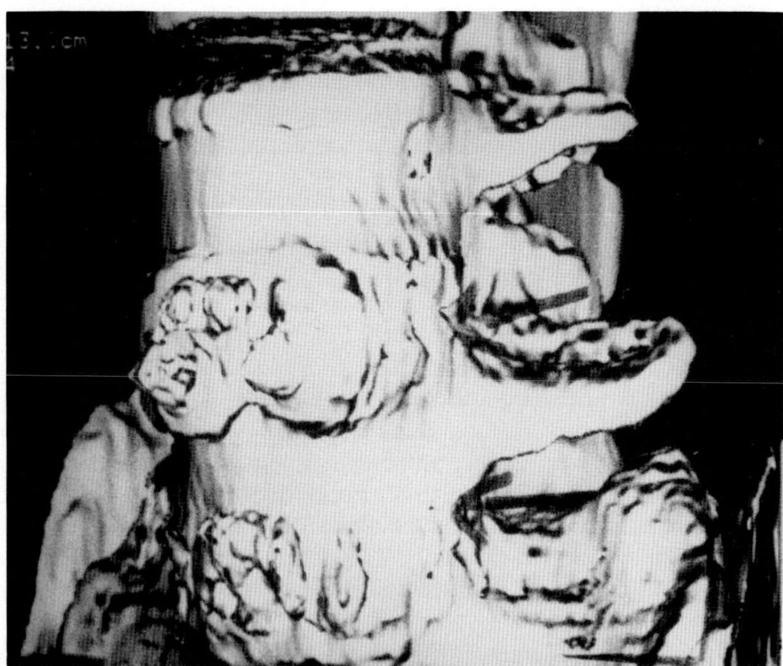

**FIG. 13.** Oblique view of a three-dimensional CT scan showing fusion at both instrumented levels.

Reoperation was required in 19 patients (10.2%). Five of these (2.7%) were device-related (device migration). No implant fractures or deformities occurred. Fourteen (7.5%) were not device-related: 10 cases of fusion augmentation (5.3%), two cases of nerve root decompression (1.1%), and two cases in which an additional level underwent fusion (1.1%). Other non–device-related complications are shown in Table 5.

## SUMMARY

Can bone grow through a rigid or semi-rigid device when the device itself may "stress shield" the internal bone graft? Does this violate Wolff's Law?

**TABLE 5.** *Other non–device-related complications*

| Complication | n | % |
|---|---|---|
| Major paralysis (i.e., cauda equina syndrome) | 0 | 0 |
| Deep infection | 0 | 0 |
| Superficial infection | 5 | 2.7 |
| Retrograde ejaculation | 3 | 1.6 overall, 2.5% of anterior cases |
| Thromboembolism | 2 | 1.1 |
| Nerve palsy (persistent) | 4 | 2.1 |
| Pneumonia | 3 | 1.6 |
| Iliac vein laceration | 3 | 1.6 overall, 2.5% of anterior cases |
| Dural tear | 7 | 3.7 overall, 10.6% of posterior cases |
| Paresthesia (other than transient) | 2 | 1.1 |
| Incisional hernia | 1 | 0.5 overall, 0.8% of anterior cases |

We do not at present understand all of the laws that govern the behavior of bone. Perhaps hydrostatic forces continue to stress the graft inside and around the rigid implant. We do know that bone did grow into and through a very rigid stainless steel "Bagby Basket" in the cervical spine of the horse (1,9). We do know that bone did grow into and through a very rigid BAK device in the lumbar spine of the baboon (19). And, although we do not at this time have confirmatory autopsy material to demonstrate the same in humans, we do have dynamic x-ray and CT evidence that strongly suggests that interbody fusion is being achieved by means of the BAK device in humans. We also know that union rates in excess of 90% are possible with this technology. And finally, we believe that the method can provide results that are superior to noninstrumented fusions and are comparable to circumferential fusions using pedicle fixation.

Chronic low back pain can be a serious, disabling disease. It produces difficulty and frustration for the surgeon and large expenses for employers and insurers. Whether or not surgery has a place in the treatment of this condition remains a subject of great controversy. For example, Franklin et al. (13) have concluded that fusion has little or no place in the management of low back pain in Workers' Compensation cases. They reported that only 32% of lumbar fusion patients returned to work. Furthermore, they found that less than 50% of fusion patients were improved by surgery. The re-operation rate at 2 years was 24%.

The results of our multicenter, prospective BAK study contrast sharply with Franklin's conclusions. We had 65% of patients returning to employment, over 80% reporting pain relief and improved function, and our re-operation rate was only 10%.

The primary goal of BAK stabilization is pain relief by interbody fusion. We assume that many spine surgeons are capable of properly selecting patients that are good candidates. No procedure can produce good results when the wrong patient is operated on, or when the wrong diagnosis is considered, or when a poorly skilled or inadequately trained surgeon performs the procedure. It is our hope and expectation that only fulled qualified spine surgeons will perform BAK procedures on only qualified patients.

A secondary goal of the BAK system is to decrease intraoperative and postoperative morbidity. The results to date indicate that this goal is also being met, with decreased blood loss, shorter hospital stays, and lower re-operation rates compared to the alternative procedures. Finally, a relatively low incidence of complications implies an improved margin of safety when this procedure is performed according to protocol by appropriately trained surgeons.

In summary, BAK technique of intervertebral stabilization can provide several advantages over alternative procedures for the treatment of chronic low back in selected patients with degenerative disc disease.

## REFERENCES

1. Bagby GW. Arthrodesis by the distraction-compression using a stainless steel implant. *Orthopaedics* 1988;11:931–4.
2. Blumenthal S, Baker J. The role of anterior lumbar fusion for internal disc disruption. *Spine* 1988; 13:566–9.
3. Brodke DS, Dick JC, Zdeblick TA, et al. Biomechanical comparison of posterior lumbar interbody fusion including a new threaded titanium cage [Abstract]. *Proc Soc for the Study of the Lumbar Spine,* 1993;108.
4. Butts MK, Kuslich SD, Bechtold JE. Biomechanical analysis of a new method for spinal interbody

fusion. Presented at the annual winter meeting of the American Society of Mechanical Engineers, Boston, MA, December, 1987.

5. Cheng CL, Fang D, Lee PC. Anterior spinal fusion for spondylolisthesis and isthmic spondylolisthesis. *J Bone Joint Surg* 1989;71B:264–7.

6. Chow SP. Anterior spinal fusion for deranged lumbar intervertebral disc: a review of 97 cases. *Spine* 1980;5:452–8.

7. Cloward RB. The treatment of ruptured intervertebral discs by vertebral body fusion. *Ann Surg* 1952;136:987.

8. Cloward RB. Long-term result of PLIF. In: Lin PM, ed. *Posterior lumbar interbody fusion*. Springfield, IL: Charles C Thomas, 1982.

9. DeBowes RM, Grant BD, Bagby GW, et al. Cervical vertebral interbody fusion in the horse: a comparative study of bovine xenografts and autografts supported by stainless steel baskets. *Am J Vet Res* 1984;45:191–9.

10. Dennis S. Comparison of disc space heights after anterior lumbar interbody fusion. *Spine* 1989;14: 876–8.

11. Falconer MA, McGeorge M, Begg AC. Observations on the cause and mechanism of symptom production in sciatica and low back pain. *J Neurol Neurosurg Psychiatry* 1948;11:13–26.

12. Flynn JC, Hogue MA. Anterior fusion of the lumbar spine. *J Bone Joint Surg* 1979;61A:1143–50.

13. Franklin GM, Haug J, Heyer NJ, et al. Outcome of lumbar fusion in Washington State workers' compensation. *Spine* 1994;19:1897–903.

14. Freebody D. Anterior transperitoneal lumbar fusion. *J Bone Joint Surg* 1971;53B:617–27.

15. Fujimaki A, Crock HV, Bedbrook GM. The results of 150 anterior lumbar interbody fusion operations performed by two surgeons in Australia. *Clin Orthop Relat Res* 1982;165:164–7.

16. Gill K, Blumenthal SL. Functional results after anterior lumbar fusion at L5–S1 in patients with normal and abnormal MRI scans. *Spine* 1992;17:940–2.

17. Goldner LJ, Urbaniak JR, McCollum DE. Anterior disc excision and interbody spinal fusions for chronic low back pain. *Orthop Clin North Am* 1971;2:543–68.

18. Greenough CG. Anterior lumbar fusion: a comparison of non-compensation patients with compensation patients. *Clin Orthop Relat Res* 1994;300:30–7.

19. Grobler LJ, Wilder DG, Ahern JW, Reinsel TR, Hardin NJ, Pope MH. BAK vertebral stabilization system: an experimental comparative investigation to evaluate this implant in a primate model. Presented at the eighth annual meeting of the North American Spine Society, San Diego, CA, 1993.

20. Hirsch C. An attempt to diagnose the level of disc lesion clinically by disc puncture. *Acta Orthop Scand* 1948;18:132–40.

21. Kim NH, Kim DJ. Anterior interbody fusion for spondylolisthesis. *Orthopaedics* 1991;14:1069–76.

22. Kim NH, Kim HK, Suh JS. A computed tomographic analysis of changes in the spinal canal after anterior lumbar interbody fusion. *Clin Orthop Relat Res* 1993;286:180–91.

23. Knox BD, Chapman TM. Anterior lumbar interbody fusion for discogram concordant pain. *J Spinal Dis* 1993;6:242–4.

24. Kuslich SD, Ulstrom CL. The tissue origin of low back pain and sciatica: a report of pain response to tissue stimulation during operations on the lumbar spine using local anesthesia. *Orthop Clin North Am* 1991;22:181–7.

25. Lin PM. Posterior lumbar interbody fusion technique: complications and pitfalls. *Clin Orthop* 1985; 193:16–9.

26. Lin PM, Cutilli RA, Joyce MF. Posterior lumbar interbody fusion. *Clin Orthop Relat Res* 1983;180: 154–68.

27. Lindblom K. Diagnostic puncture of intervertebral discs in sciatica. *Acta Orthop Scand* 1948;17: 231–9.

28. Linson MA, William H. Anterior and combined anteroposterior fusion for lumbar disc pain: a preliminary study. *Spine* 1991;16:143–5.

29. Loguidice VA, Johnson RG, Guyen RD, Stith WJ. Anterior lumbar interbody fusion. *Spine* 1988;13: 366–9.

30. Ma GC. Posterior lumbar interbody fusion with specialized instruments. *Clin Orthop Relat Res* 1985;193:57–63.

31. Mitsunaga MM, Chong G, Maes KE. Microscopically assisted posterior lumbar interbody fusion. *Clin Orthop Relat Res* 1991;263:121–7.

32. Newman MH, Grinstead GL. Anterior lumbar interbody fusion for internal disc disruption. *Spine* 1992;17:831–3.

33. Nystrom B. Open mechanical provocation under local anesthesia—a definitive method for locating the focus in painful mechanical disorder of the motion segment [Abstract]. *Proc Swedish Orthop Soc* 1992;73.

34. Oxland TR. Biomechanics of lumbar interbody fusion presentation. Presented at International Meeting of Self-contained Instrumented Interbody Fusion. Minneapolis, MN, October, 1994.

35. Prolo DJ, Okund SA, Butcher M. Toward uniformity in evaluating results of lumbar spine operations: a paradigm applied to posterior lumbar interbody fusions. *Spine* 1986;11:601–6.

36. Raugstad TS, Harbo K, Oogberg A. Anterior interbody fusion of the lumbar spine. *Acta Orthop Scand* 1982;53:561–5.
37. Rish BL. A critique of posterior lumbar interbody fusion—a 12 years' experience with 250 patients. *Surg Neurol* 1989;31:281–9.
38. Schechler NA, France MP, Lee CK. Disc disease update—painful internal disc derangements of the lumbosacral spine: discogenic diagnosis and treatment by posterior lumbar interbody fusion. *Orthopaedics* 1991;14:00–00.
39. Smyth MJ, Wright V. Sciatica and the intervertebral disc. An experimental study. *J Bone Joint Surg* 1958;40:1401–18.
40. Sorenson KH. Anterior interbody lumbar spine fusion for incapacitating disc degeneration and spondylolisthesis. *Acta Orthop Scand* 1978;49:267–77.
41. Stauffer RN, Coventry MB. Anterior interbody lumbar spine fusion. *J Bone Joint Surg* 1972;54A:756–68.
42. Thomasen E. Intercorporal lumbar spondylosis. *Acta Orthop Scand* 1985;56:287–93.
43. Verlooy J, Smedt KD, Selosse P. Failure of a modified posterior lumbar interbody fusion technique to produce adequate pain relief in isthmic spondylolytic grade 1 spondylolisthesis patients: a prospective study of 20 patients. *Spine* 1993;18:1491–5.
44. Wagner PC, Grant BD, Bagby GW, et al. Evaluation of spine fusion as treatment in the equine wobbler syndrome. *J Vet Surg* 1979;8:84–8.
45. Wiberg G. Back pain in relation to the nerve supply of the intervertebral disc. *Acta Orthop Scand* 1950;19:211–21.
46. Wiltberger BR. Intervertebral body fusion by the use of posterior bone dowel. *Clin Orthop* 1964;35:69–79.
47. Wood GW, Boyd RJ, Carothers TA, et al. The effect of pedicle screw/plate fixation on lumbar/lumbosacral autogenous bone graft fusions in patients with degenerative disc disease. *Spine* 1995;20:819–30.
48. Zucherman J, Hsu K, Picetti G III, et al. Clinical efficacy of spinal instrumentation in lumbar degenerative disc disease. *Spine* 1988;13:570–9.

*Instrumented Fusion of the Degenerative Lumbar Spine: State of the Art, Questions, and Controversies*, edited by M. Szpalski, R. Gunzburg, D. M. Spengler, and A. Nachemson. Lippincott–Raven Publishers, Philadelphia © 1996.

# 21

# PLIF with the Ray Fusion Cage: Indications and Results

Robert Schönmayr, *Charles D. Ray, Christiane Melzer, Michael Melzer, and Selcuk Babacan

*Department of Neurosurgery, Dr. Horst Schmidt Clinic, 65119 Wiesbaden, Germany; and *Institute for Low Back and Neck Care, Minneapolis, Minnesota 55407, and Spinal Research and Education Foundation, Norfolk, Virginia*

## WHY FUSE THE SPINE?

Fusion of a vertebral segment is used primarily to arrest disabling back pain that arises from degeneration of that segment. Philosophically, the concept appears on the surface to be contradictory, in that the fusion benefits the patients by permanently destroying the mobility of a vertebral segment. However, the early observation that patients with long-lasting, severe, painful degenerative spinal disease often experienced marked relief after spontaneous fusion had for a long time stimulated biomechanical interest and study by physicians and scientists. They postulated that if fusion or full immobilization of a vertebral segment could reduce or eliminate the persistent back pain, then the apparent pathologic mobility must be the major cause of that pain.

During the natural course of degenerative spinal disease, pathologic segmental mobility results from degenerative changes of the intervertebral disc (8). As the disc loses height, the facet joints are increasingly exposed to more sagitally directed forces, commonly resulting in rapid and severe arthrotic changes. In addition, loosening of the segment usually produces inappropriate or unbalanced wear of the endplates and the involved ligaments. The abnormal mechanical stress on all these structures can create pain. Moreover, the circumferentially positioned annular free nerve endings (pain fibers) are exposed to increased concentrations of toxic anerobic metabolites released by the disintegrated disc nucleus through radial tears in the annular fibers. The pain increases as heavy, long-lasting axial or torsional strain is exerted on the damaged segment. When accompanied by secondary reflex muscle tension, the pain may persist even during phases of rest.

Many patients with low back pain experience relief from spinal immobilization. Therefore, external stabilizing devices, such as braces and corsets, have been employed throughout history. However, when the use of such external aids is prolonged, muscular atrophy may occur, inducing still greater segmental destabilization. Therefore, a wide variety of permanent internal (i.e., surgical) solutions for segmental instability (SI) have been developed. The basic principle of all such methods is the bony fusion of one or more painful vertebral segments. The fusion creates full immobilization of the segment and stops the movement-induced destruction of segmental structures such as facet joints, capsules, and ligaments, as well as the pain arising from the mechanical or chemical irritation of nerve endings in these structures. After successful fusion, the patients' sufferings are usually significantly reduced.

Mechanical back pain related to pathologic problems other than those caused by instability will not be influenced by the attainment of a solid fusion. Pain can be generated by the compression of nerve roots or their vascular supply, or by the involvement of other adjacent or remote segments. Even distant structures, such as the sacroiliac joints, may add to the clinical problem. Commonly, involvement of both segmental and the long back muscles plays an important role in the origin of pain. Most potential fusion candidates suffer a variety of pathologic mechanisms in their long history of complaints and trials employing several different treatments. It should be stressed that any recognized pathologic entity may or may not contribute to the pain, and it is incumbent on the surgical team to identify the true pain generators as clearly as possible. For patients in whom severe disabling pain inhibits both work and a normal active lifestyle, psychological and drug-related difficulties commonly add to the physical disease. Depression may overlie the initial somatic pain and finally dominate the clinical picture. Increasing drug, alcohol or nicotine consumption may lead to habituation or addiction and a decline in general health. As the patients' occupational, recreational, social, and family activities decline, they suffer further isolation and reduction in quality of life. We find that most patients with chronic back pain have additional physical ailments as well as psychological and social problems. This is especially true of patients with previous (sometimes multiple) surgery of the spine (15). In many such cases, it is quite difficult to clearly ascertain if the instability of a given segment plays the leading role in the patient's pain generation. Although it would be naive to believe that all of these complex problems can be solved by any surgical approach, it is also clear that under certain circumstances, when the source of the accumulated difficulties can be traced to spinal instability, fusion may well be indicated. Clearly, the principal and often highly difficult task of the physician in charge is to select the patients who have the best opportunity to benefit from surgical fusion.

## WHO WILL BENEFIT FROM A FUSION? PATIENT SELECTION

Our list of possible indications for fusion is shown in Tables 1–3. One major point of discussion is the assessment of SI. In some patients the instability is quite evident, so that the typical clinical picture is well matched with the radiologic findings. The latter principally consist of segmental hypermobility shown in dynamic x-ray images. More difficult to assess is the clinical correlation with radiologic evidence in advanced changes in multilevel segmental degeneration. Forward displacement, retrolisthesis, or laterolisthesis (usually combined with torsion) of the upper vertebra of a segment, in combination with narrowing of the intervertebral space, suggests at least microinstability at a given level (Fig. 1). Typically, deformity and sclerotic

**TABLE 1.** *Indications for fusion: primary segmental instability*

In congenital spondylolisthesis (<grade 1)
As a result of discopathy
In combination with a disc prolapse
In combination with spinal stenosis
   Hypertrophic facet joints
   Spondylotic osteophytes
   Hypertrophic ligaments
In combination with a disc prolapse and spinal stenosis

appearance of the vertebral endplate are usually accompanied by calcification or ossification of the surrounding ligaments. Prominent osteophytic spurs mark the natural attempt to reinforce the tissue structures against abnormal forces. If the intervertebral space collapses asymmetrically, the radiologic findings are unilaterally pronounced, resulting in scoliosis with compensatory curvature of the neighboring spine sectors (Fig. 2).

As a result of chronically increased abnormal loads, facet joints undergo hypertrophic degeneration, and these deformities may reach monstrous dimensions (Fig. 3). If consequent narrowing of the spinal canal is substantial, the significant clinical findings of central stenotic spinal claudication are present. If foraminal impingement is marked, lateral stenotic nerve root compression causes radicular pain and/or neurologic deficits of radicular distribution. Disc protrusion or prolapse contributes to such compressions and may acutely increase the respective symptomatology. Spinal SI is also highly influenced by and dependent on the paraspinal muscle situation and vice versa. Reflex increase in muscle tension blocks movements of the spine to avoid pain (antalgic posturing), but constantly increased muscle tone will provoke intrinsic muscle pain, adding to the problems.

Many potential candidates for lumbar fusion surgery have a long history of pain and a variety of treatment methods and many have undergone prior spine surgery (4). To identify those who are the best candidates for fusion can be exceedingly difficult. We have found that patient selection is enhanced by the response to 10 key questions.

1. Patient history: is it typical for lumbar SI?
2. Orthopedic and neurologic examination: are signs of SI present?
3. Radiology: do we see direct or indirect signs of SI?
4. Provocative discography: does it reproduce the ''typical'' pain pattern and character?
5. Local anesthesia of the facet joints (with or without steroids) at the suspected level: does it eliminate the pain? If so, for how long after injection?
6. Periradicular anesthesia: to what extent is the segmental nerve root involved?
7. External immobilization: how does it influence the patient's complaints?

**TABLE 2.** *Indications for fusion: secondary segmental instability*

As a result of disc surgery
As a result of decompressive surgery such as
   Laminectomy and/or
   Facetectomy
As a result of decompressive and/or disc surgery
If other fusion techniques have failed

**TABLE 3.** *Indications for fusion: if secondary segmental instability is expected*

If extensive decompressive surgery must be done
  Laminectomy
  Facetectomy
  Discectomy
  Combinations thereof
If decompressive surgery must be done and signs of instability are already present
If disc surgery must be done in patients professionally required to lift or carry heavy loads

8. Adjacent segments: is SI already present there or is there a likelihood of developing SI?
9. Patient's psychological and social situation: can we expect improvement at all?
10. Drug consumption: can we expect the patient to refrain from abuse?

The Wiesbaden study included 63 patients who received 187 threaded fusion cage (TFC) implants at 94 lumbar spinal segments. The diagnostic program (Table 4) included plain x-ray images in anterior–posterior and oblique projections and in flexion/extension with weights. They often performed lumbar myelography, again with flexion/extension. Immediately after myelography, a computed tomography (CT) scan (still with intrathecal contrast) was obtained. In some patients a magnetic imaging resonance (MRI) study was performed, and in patients with previous surgery prescanning intravenous gadolinium contrast was used to visualize the extent of scar formation.

If disc protrusion and nerve root compression were present, provocative discography was accomplished at each suspected target level using an injection of a non-irritating, non-ionizable contrast medium with subsequent CT scan. This demonstrated ruptures or tears of the annulus and the posterior longitudinal ligament and provoked pain if the pain was discogenic in origin (normal disc spaces rarely hurt).

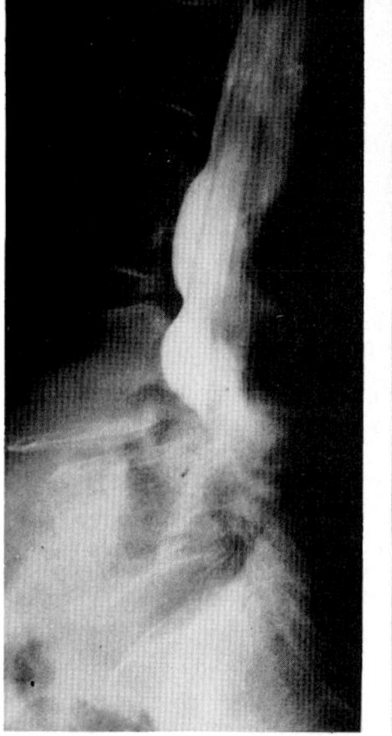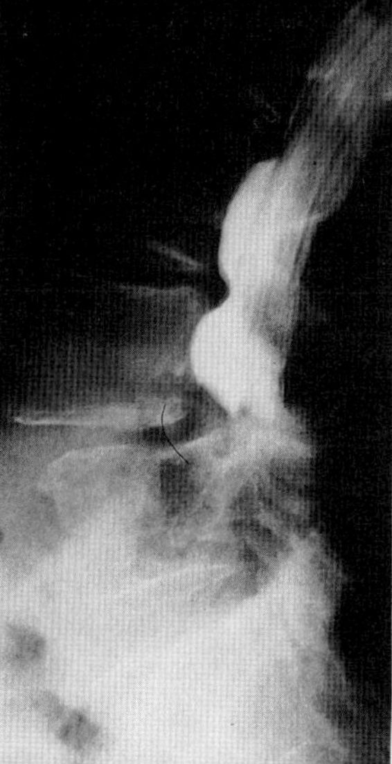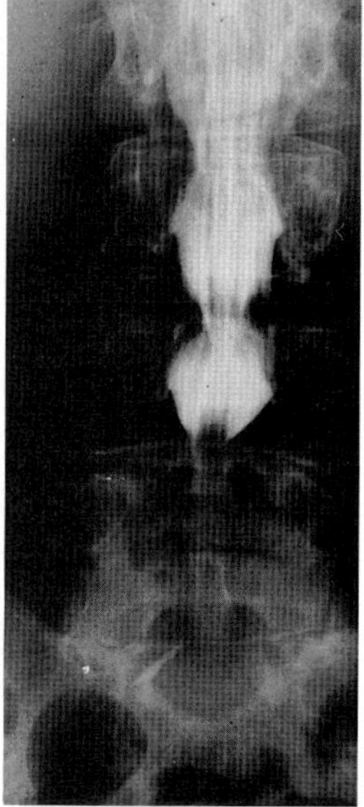

**FIG. 1.** Dynamic myelogram, showing degenerative instability and reactive changes.

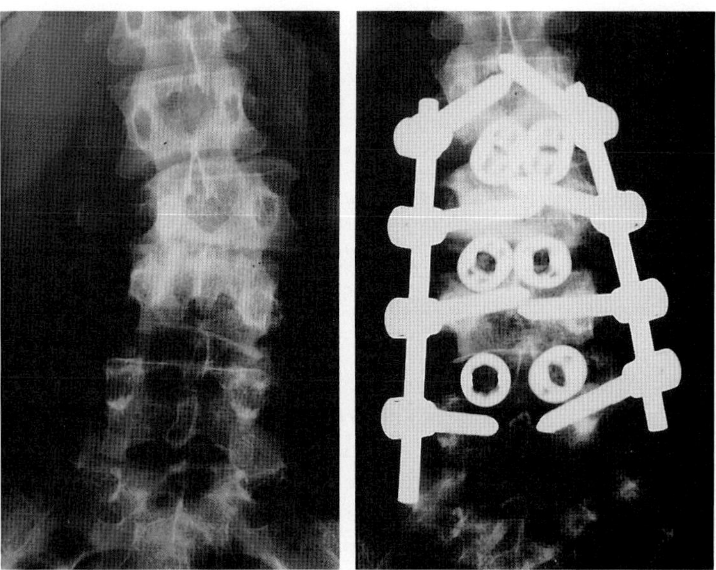

**FIG. 2.** Instability with scoliotic deformity, showing realignment by transpedicular fixation and PLIF with TFC in three levels.

If the patient experienced "typical" pain during discographic injection, it was important to ascertain that this pain was actually related to the disc pathology. Similarly, test injections of local anesthetics were used in nerve roots and/or facet joints. These tests are valuable in localizing the sources of pain and in clarifying the evidence, if SI is to be regarded as the main pathophysiologic cause of the pain syndrome.

The United States program was a Federal Drug Administration Investigational

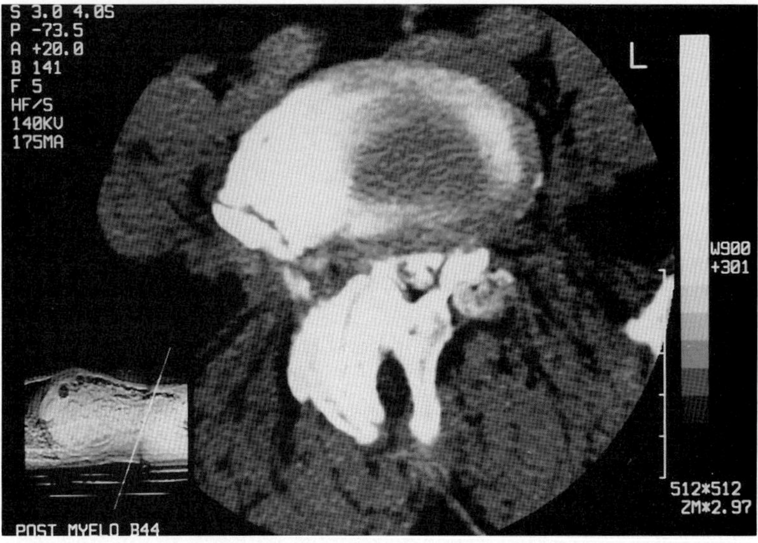


**FIG. 3.** CT scan after myelography, revealing hypertrophic facet joint and stenosis of the spinal canal at L4–L5.

**TABLE 4.** *Diagnostic program*

X-ray in 2 or 4 planes
Functional x-ray
CT scan
MRI scan
Myelography (with CT)
Discography (with CT)
Scintigraphy
Mineralometry
Periradicular infiltration
Facet infiltration
Iliosacral infiltration

Device Exemption (FDA/IDE) sanctioned study of 236 patients with 588 TFC implants at 298 levels. This study was performed at nine different medical centers and utilized similar diagnostic tests and selection criteria as the Wiesbaden study. Routinely obtained were plain anterior–posterior and lateral x-ray films, flexion/extension x-ray views. Many MRI scans, facet injections, and discography (frequently accompanied by postdiscographic CT scanning) (14) were also performed. Myelography was seldom utilized.

When a patient in the Wiesbaden group was found to be qualified for a fusion, the candidate was provided with a corset to wear at home for 3–6 weeks. If significant improvement was seen, the evidence was included, together with the results of the other diagnostic information, in arriving at a final decision regarding surgery. In the United States group, wearing of a brace preoperatively was not included in the selection criteria, although patients wore a rigid shell thoraco–lumbar–sacral orthosis (TLSO) brace postoperatively for 3 months to limit spinal mobility and to remind the patient to be cautious.

In 98% of the United States group of 236 patients, the chief complaint was severe disabling low back pain, and included cases having prior surgery (principally failed back surgery syndrome) in 106 of 236 (46%) of patients, and spondylolisthesis (grade 1 or less) in 11 of 236 (5%).

In the 63-patient Wiesbaden cohort, the principal indication for fusion also was disabling low back pain associated with failed back surgery syndrome (FBSS) in 29 (46%) of cases, spinal stenosis combined with instability in 20 (32%), primary instability in 9 (14%), and spondylolisthesis (grade 1 or less) in 5 (8%).

From the outset of this clinical investigation, the patient selection criteria between our two studies were closely correlated.

## METHODS FOR FUSION OF A LUMBAR VERTEBRAL SEGMENT

A large number of techniques for lumbar fusion surgery are available (1–3,7,9–11,13,16–19). If a physiologic contour in the sagittal and frontal planes is reestablished when complete bony fusion is achieved by any method, it is our opinion that an optimal distribution of spinal forces can be expected. If the spinal canal and its contents are not involved and if there is no reason to access those structures, we would prefer an anterior approach for interbody fusion, except at the L5–S1 level in male patients (particularly young males). In most patients, nerve root compression, stenosis of the spinal canal, or scar formation already plays an important role, which often makes a dorsal approach necessary. In patients with previous surgery, a dorsal access enables one to assess nerve structures, remove scar tissue, and decompress nerves by resection of hypertrophic bone or disc fragments. Moreover, when the dorsal approach is limited to a bilateral laminotomy with preservation of the interspinous ligament and at least a significant portion of each facet joint, no additional instability will be created. Similarly, resection of osteophytic spurs of the medial part of the facets will be well tolerated. If the dorsal structures have already been damaged either by a degenerative process or by prior surgery, additional stabilization, such as by transpedicular fixation, may be necessary.

From a biomechanical point of view, the interbody fusion approach is preferred. In the past, many different materials and methods for interbody fusion have been developed. Autologous bone grafts have many advantages over allografts or xenografts as far as fusion rate and ultimate solidity are concerned, but the initial strength of the harvested grafts is usually poor, especially in patients with osteopenia. To avoid these problems, most fusion studies have shown that the best results are obtained when an autologous bone graft (or substitute) is combined with an implanted mechanical support device (5). At present, the most commonly employed fusion devices are pedicle screws and plates or rods, methods known to involve inherent technical problems and a long learning curve for the surgeons.

## THE RAY TFC AND METHOD

The Ray TFCs (Fig. 4) have been found to be an improvement over pedicle screw methods of fusion because of their simplicity, safety, rapidity of implantation, and relative overall economy. The TFCs are strong medical-grade titanium alloy cylinders with 70% of their strong but thin superior and inferior walls having up to 25 1.5 × 3.5-mm elliptic perforations, while the lateral walls are blocked. TFCs are made with external diameters of 12, 14, 16 or 18 mm and lengths of 21 or 26 mm, to accommodate virtually all disc spaces in large and small patients. The bone graft material needed to fill each cage varies with the internal volume but ranges from 2 to 8 cc each.

The implantation requires bilateral hemilaminotomy with limited resection of the spinous process and preservation of the interspinous ligament. Partial removal of the

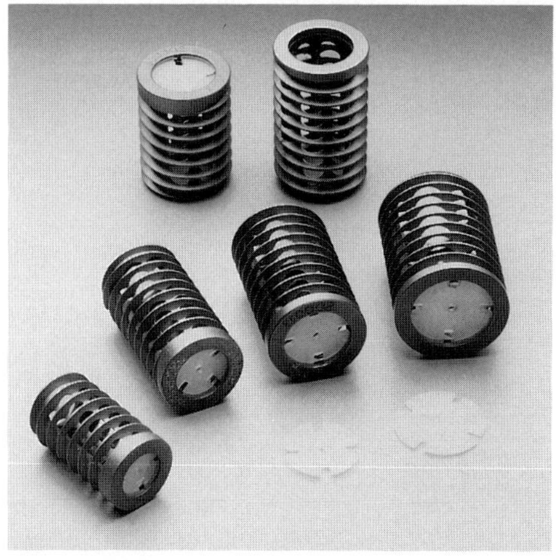

**FIG. 4.** Ray threaded fusion cage of different sizes.

medial facets is necessary to gain room for the implants. While protecting the dura and nerve roots with a special retractor device, each of the two parallel interbody holes is drilled. The holes are deeply tapped into the adjacent endplates, penetrating into each vertebra about 3 mm, and the TFCs are screwed into place. It is important and unique that the recipient bed bone threads actually project well inside the TFC cavity to provide intimate and immediate contact between the recipient bed and the small volume of autologous cancellous bone (or other graft material) as it is packed inside the cage. It appears that the graft grows rapidly through the TFC perforations and into the vertebral bodies. The blocked walls are oriented to face the open disc space (Fig. 5A) and to guard against remnant disc tissue invading the graft, a source of PLIF failure in the past. The lateral walls also provide strength to the cages, giving them the necessary solidity to sustain even extraordinary loading. The matched threads between the TFC and the recipient bone bed prevent dislocation. The multiple openings are wide enough to allow sufficient bony growth and transmission of spinal loading into the graft through the TFC (Fig. 5B). The cages become surrounded by bone and never have to be removed, since they create no discomfort to neighboring tissues.

The newly designed cylindrical retractor device is highly functional, safe, and easy to use. As the side tangs or tapered lateral guides of this device are driven into the disc space, they distract the disc appropriately and correctly orient the subsequent drilling, tapping, and cage insertion. The retractor also serves to protect the dura, nerve root, and ganglion. The procedure can be performed with greater rapidity than

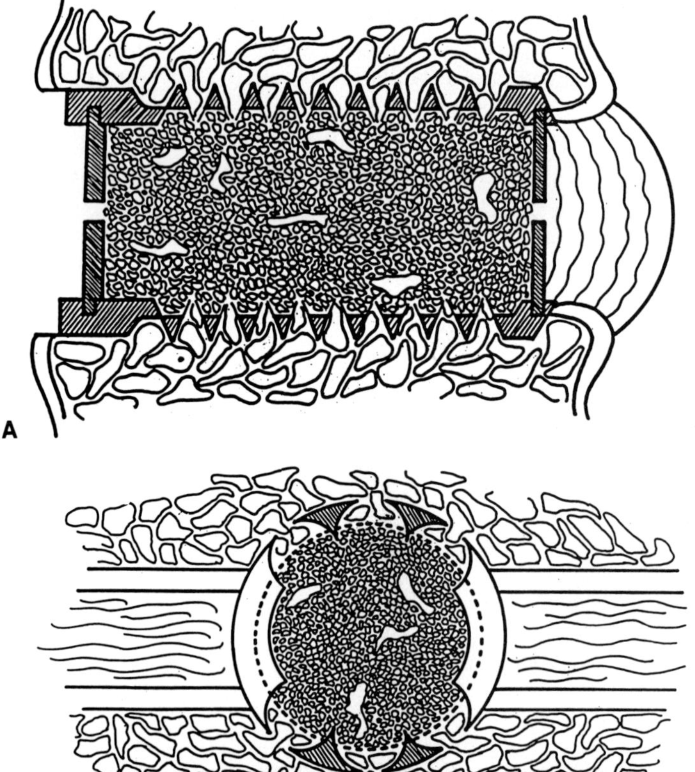

FIG. 5. A: TFC in situ, lateral view. B: TFC in situ, anteroposterior view.

almost any other fusion method. Several single-level, uncomplicated cases have been completed in 90–100 min. Additional spinal stabilization or bone grafting is rarely required. Only in patients who manifest severe inadequacy of the annulus, instability of the dorsal segmental structures, or severely scoliotic deformities needing realignment is additional transpedicular fixation required. In a few cases, we have performed PLIFs with TFCs at three or four spinal levels to attain full fusion without additional stabilization (Fig. 6A,B).

## POSTOPERATIVE FUSION CRITERIA

The determination of solidity of fusions is not without controversy. For the TFC, our principal criteria are:

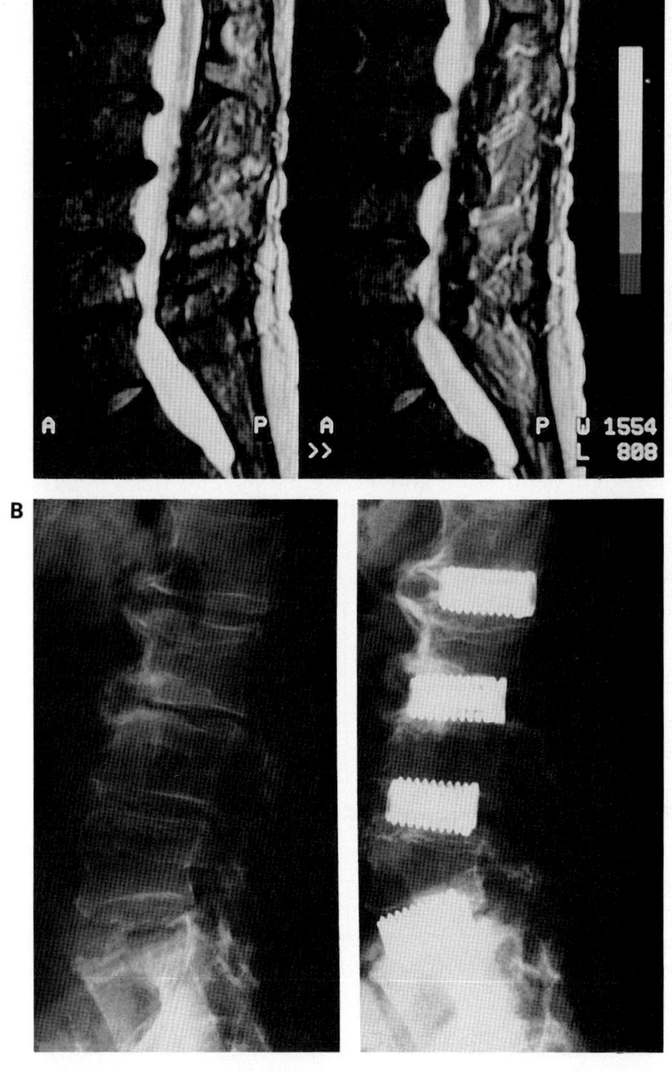

**FIG. 6. A:** MRI, showing discogenic lumbar stenosis at four levels. **B:** PLIF with TFC at four levels.

1. Absence of any discernible movement (roughly more than 2° angular change) at the segment seen on flexion/extension x-ray films.
2. Absence of a halo formation around the cage or marked, new sclerosis of the endplates, as seen in lateral x-ray images.
3. Bone visible inside the cage on Ferguson view x-rays.
4. Normal or reduced enhancement at the fused level on bone scintigraphy.

In the United States study group, criteria 1, 2, and 3 were principally used to assess attainment of fusion at 6 months' follow-up and beyond. In the Wiesbaden group of cases, criteria 3 and 4 provided key assessments.

## RESULTS

Among the 236 patients in the United States cohort, a fusion rate of 82% was seen at the postoperative follow-up interval of 6 months and a 96% fusion rate at 12 and 24 months. The disc height was measured at predetermined intervals during the first 24 months of follow-up. The average posterior disc height was increased by the initial surgery and remained greater than the preoperative measurement by 2.3 mm at 6 months' follow-up and 1.6 mm at 2 years' follow-up (5). There was no apparent collapse of any implanted disc space. The longest follow-up United States cases are now more than 6.5 years post surgery. By use of an outcomes assessment scale (Prolo Scale for symptomatic status and social/occupational function), 84% of the United States group reported fair to excellent clinical results; 14% reported a poor result.

For the Wiesbaden cohort of 63 patients (Figs. 7 and 8), the age distribution is shown in Fig. 9. Fifty-six of these patients have had a follow-up of more than 6 months, 33 of more than 1 year, and five of more than 18 months. In the 33 patients with a follow-up of more than 12 months, there were two patients (3%) in whom fusion according to the above-mentioned criteria was not complete, but no case reported clinical signs of persistent SI. We probably underestimated the negative effects of preoperative psychological depression and weakened psychosocial behavior in at least two patients of the Wiesbaden cohort and a proportionate number in

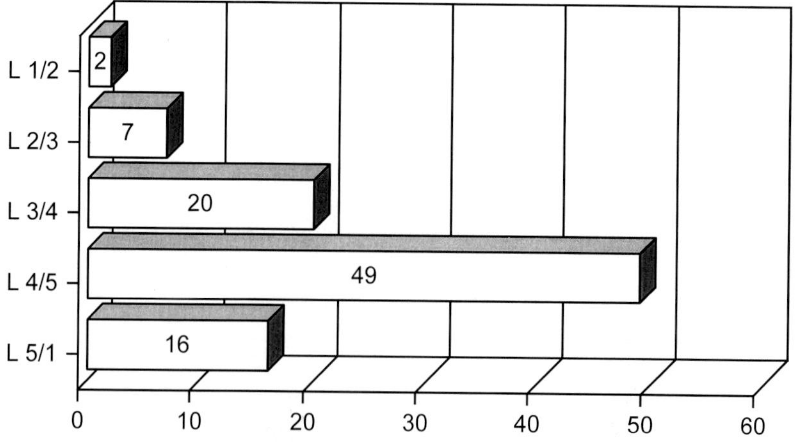


**FIG. 7.** Level of fusion with PLIF and cage (*n* = 94).

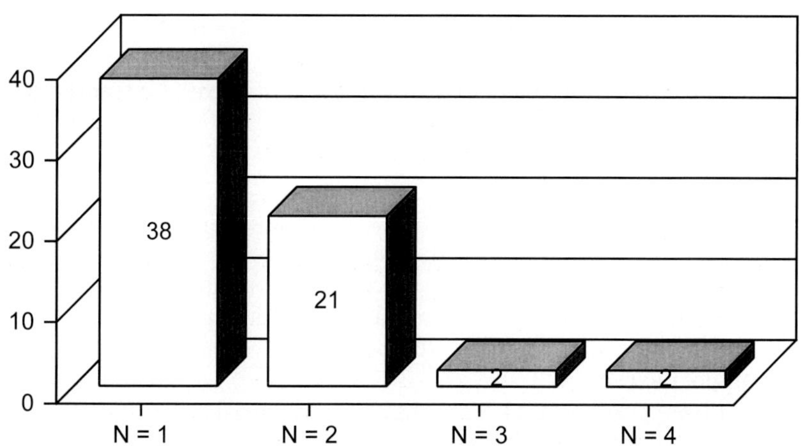



**FIG. 8.** Fused segments with PLIF and fusion cage.

the United States group, as these factors appeared to have contributed to some of the reported unsatisfactory clinical outcomes. In all considerations, these outcome results compare quite favorably with other contemporary, important fusion methods (6,7,12,13).

## COMPLICATIONS

In the United States IDE/FDA study, there was an overall complication rate of less than 1%; none was considered major. The complications included:

Five superficial wound and two deep fascial infections, each of which cleared on antibiotic treatment
Three cages had minor placement revisions (within 1 month)
One cage showed a mild crack but without interference in fusion formation

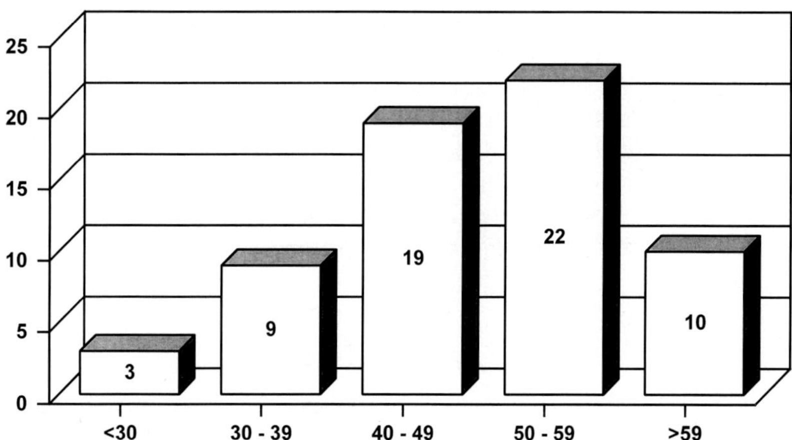



**FIG. 9.** Age distribution of patients in years (37 males, 26 females).

Seventeen patients who had intraoperative dural tears were repaired without consequence

Three patients developed pseudarthrosis, which was resolved by transpedicular fixation.

In the Wiesbaden patients there were:

One case of CSF fistula with postoperative mild meningitis that was successfully treated with antibiotics and lumbar drainage

Two patients who developed mild discitis, cleared on antibiotic treatment

One patient who needed surgical revision because of an epidural hematoma

One patient who had a postoperative temporary motor and sensory deficit of the adjacent (upper) nerve root

Seven minor intraoperative dural tears that were repaired without consequence.

## DISCUSSION

When a lumbar fusion is the goal, we consider PLIF with the Ray TFC a safe, reliable, and effective method. The implantation is only moderately difficult. Dissection of the scar tissue around the nerve roots in patients who have had previous surgery may be time-consuming and requires a microsurgical technique. The complications appear no more often and are no more hazardous than those seen in ordinary discectomy surgery. The surgeon must decide whether to implant the cages from an anterior or a posterior approach, usually depending on whether or not structures within the spinal canal are involved in the patient's clinical problem.

To prove a solid fusion by any means remains controversial. Decisions regarding solidity based on imaging procedures, including CT or MRI scans, are difficult because of artifacts (although much less with the TFC than with stainless steel fusion instrumentation), poorly reproducible density measurements, or inaccuracies in spine positioning during flexion/extension examinations. In the United States study, the first three of our four listed postoperative fusion criteria were used; radioactive uptake scans were not. In the rare case of fusion failure among the United States cases, there was a close correlation between these three criteria and the persistence of low back pain. Among the Wiesbaden patients, all four criteria were utilized but the principal guides were bone density within the cages and bone scintigraphy as an indicator of metabolic activity. Flexion/extension x-rays, even with weights, were felt in Wiesbaden to be inconclusive indicators. In both studies these films nevertheless permitted identification of segmental macroinstability.

Striving toward excellence in clinical outcome for all patients, we are sufficiently assured by this combined study that a solid fusion, or at least a reasonable segmental stabilization, can be reliably created in 96% or more of selected cases. A key element of concern still remains: Is fusion the right solution for the individual patient's back pain?''

## REFERENCES

1. Branch CL, Branch CL Jr. Posterior interbody fusion with the Keystone graft: technique and results. *Surg Neurol* 1987;27:449–54.
2. Cloward R. The treatment of ruptured lumbar intervertebral discs by vertebral body fusion. Indications, operative techniques, after care. *J Neurosurg* 1953;10:154–68.

3. Collis JS. Total disc replacement: a modified posterior lumbar interbody fusion. Report of 750 cases. *Clin Orthop* 1985;193:64–7.
4. Davis RA. A long-term outcome analysis of 984 surgically treated herniated lumbar discs. *J Neurosurg* 1994;80:415–21.
5. Dennis S, Watkins R, Landaker S, Dillin W, Springer D. Comparison of disc space heights after anterior lumbar interbody fusion. *Spine* 1989;14:876–8.
6. Hutter CG. Posterior intervertebral body fusion: a 25-year study. *Clin Orthop* 1983;179:86–96.
7. Inoue S, Watanabe T, Hirose A, et al. Anterior discectomy and interbody fusion for lumbar disc herniation. A review of 350 cases. *Clin Orthop* 1984;183:22–31.
8. Junghanns J, Schmorl G. *The human spine in health and disease.* New York: Grune & Stratton, 1977.
9. Lin PM. *Posterior lumbar interbody fusion.* Springfield, IL: Charles C Thomas, 1981.
10. Lin, et al. Posterior lumbar interbody fusion. *Clin Orthop* 1983;180:154–68.
11. Ma GWC. Posterior interbody fusion with modified instruments. *Clin Orthop* 1985;193:57–63.
12. Prolo DJ, Oklund SA, Butcher M. Toward uniformity in evaluating results of lumbar spine operations: a paradigm applied to posterior lumbar interbody fusions. *Spine* 1986;11:601–6.
13. Rish BL. A comparative evaluation of posterior interbody fusion for disc disease. *Spine* 1985;10:855–7.
14. Schechter NA. Painful internal disc derangements of the lumbosacral spine: discographic diagnosis and treatment by posterior lumbar interbody fusion. *Orthopedics* 1991;14:447–51.
15. Sepulveda R. Chemonucleolysis failures treated by PLIF. *Clin Orthop Relat Res* 1985;193:68–74.
16. Simmons JW. Posterior lumbar interbody fusion with posterior elements as chip grafts. *Clin Orthop Relat Res* 1985;193:85–9.
17. Stonecipher T, Wright S. Posterior lumbar interbody fusion with facet-screw fixation. *Spine* 1989;14:468–71.
18. Takeda M. Experience in posterior lumbar interbody fusion: unicortical versus bicortical autologous grafts. *Clin Orthop* 1985;193:120–6.
19. Tunturi T, Kataja M, Keski-Nisula L, et al. Posterior fusion of the lumbosacral spine. *Acta Orthop Scand* 1979;50:415–25.

*Instrumented Fusion of the Degenerative Lumbar Spine: State of the Art, Questions, and Controversies,* edited by M. Szpalski, R. Gunzburg, D. M. Spengler, and A. Nachemson. Lippincott–Raven Publishers, Philadelphia © 1996.

# 22

# Utilization of the Spine System in Degenerative Lumbar Pathology

Thierry Marnay and Jean Huppert

*Clinique du Parc, 34171 Castelnau le Lez, France*

## LUMBAR INTERVERTEBRAL ARTHRODESES

Vertebral arthrodesis often becomes necessary in degenerative spinal pathology that involves disc failure, destabilization and curvatures (e.g., scoliosis and kyphosis), and fixed displacements (dislocations, spondylolisthesis). Arthrodesis should be used locally to restore patency of the foramina and regionally for correction of lordosis and restoration of sagittal balance. This procedure is used for rigid stabilization of the affected area and for correction of unstable conditions such as kyphotic progression, fixed but progressive displacements, spontaneous horizontal displacements (i.e., spinal instability), and instrumented lumbar stenoses.

## DEVICE

The Spine System device consists of titanium implants, screws and hooks. These can be securely joined together independently of rods because they utilize a self-retaining clamp, either transverse pedical or laminar. The diameter of the junction rods is 5–6 mm.

For short fixations at one or two levels, a three-branched plate can be used to obtain a more rigid stabilization. The transverse junction process is achieved with a plate that can be placed directly on the implants or on the riders. Connection is done with an open screw locked by a conical nut, which ensures complete security of the fixation.

## ONE-SEGMENT POSTERIOR ARTHRODESIS

### Principles and Indications

The affected intervertebral space is stabilized by a rigid bony fusion. Therefore, it can be used in a variety of unstable conditions, assuming that other patient factors are favorable. These conditions include the following: kyphotic progression of the intervertebral space or retrolisthesis in extension (i.e., fixed displacement), in which horizontal displacement may be exacerbated by shear movement; associated posterior joint arthrosis, particularly when this has been confirmed by computed tomography (CT) scan; previous surgery involving multiple discs, including nucleo-orthesis and chemonucleolysis; a positive corset test, especially in patients with a history of multiple surgeries and those in whom imaging reveals direct instability (e.g., pseudoarthrodesis), in which case the external fixation test can be performed to obtain a prognosis for the success of arthrodesis (2); treatment of intracanicular conditions or revision treatments that require extensive posterior widening, including the bony structures of joints; and intraforaminal stenosis due to fibrosis. Perioperative observation of abnormal intervertebral mobility and the necessity for arthrectomy should guide the therapeutic decision.

The presence of degenerative lesions previously observed at adjacent intervertebral spaces should also be taken into consideration, because this increases loads. The risk for decompensation and degeneration (3) of other lumbar segments when discopathy is present may lead to a poor clinical result. Treatment in such cases should be directed at conservation and restoration of disc function.

Arthrodesis and osteosynthesis are clearly necessary in case of kyphotic discopathy, destabilization [e.g., horizontal shear movement, degeneration of the plates as seen on magnetic resonance imaging (MRI)], or recurrent herniation. A four-point osteosynthesis can achieve stable fixation.

Rigid osteosynthesis allows primary consolidation of the posterolateral joint area. This can be performed in patients who have advanced instability and little residual mobility, when no important reduction of the displacement is necessary. Rigid osteosynthesis is particularly indicated in patients with both anterior and posterior arthrosis or these with extensive arthrodesis (i.e., more than two levels).

Connections between the vertebral implants (pedicle screws) can be obtained with the use of either plates or rods. A 5-mm-diameter rod represents a good compromise between rigid and semi-rigid fusion. The stability of the fixation system on rotation must be ensured by a transverse connection system. Titanium implants are compatible with MRI and thus permit easier intracanicular control.

### Technique: Posterior Arthrodesis with Four-Point Osteosynthesis

The patient is placed in the ventral decubitus position without execessive flexion of the hips, to avoid fusion of the spine in a delordotic or a kyphotic position. A posterior midline approach is used to expose the upper arthrodetic vertebrae because of the projection into the space below of the upper pedicle of the fixation system. Exposure continues laterally until the transverse process is reached (5). Insertion of the pedicle screws must be slightly more exterior at the base of the upper joint and in front of the transverse process. Making an entry at the joint avoids limitation of inververtebral extension of the upper space in the fixation system (7).

Alignment of the screws during positioning makes later connection of the rod easier. Screwing is performed in the same way for all lumbar pedicles. For the S1 pedicle, the entry point can be slightly lower to avoid posterior implant contact L5 and S1 in cases of pronounced lordosis and to aim at the anteriosuperior corner of the sacrum, at which bone gripping by the screw will be better.

Intra-joint grafting must be performed before the connecting rods are placed, to allow the best positioning. An iliac grip of the graft must be achieved at the beginning of the procedure rather than after osteosynthesis has been completed. Once osteosynthesis has been performed, the posterolateral graft can be placed (9). Intra-joint grafting is more difficult after laminectomy because of the risk for intraforaminal migration of the graft. Two transverse plates placed directly on the vertebral implants enable the construct to be assembled into a frame.

Ambulation is possible on the second day after surgery. A corset may be required, depending on the condition of the individual patient.

## INTERVERTEBRAL LUMBAR ARTHRODESIS BY THE POSTERIOR APPROACH (PLIF)

This procedure is always combined with osteosynthesis and a graft to the joint column.

### Principles and Indications

Interest of grafting to the anterior column in the posterior approach has been increased by the addition of a posterior osteosynthesis (1). Previously, the operative difficulty, the risk for posterior migration, the potential for neurologic problems, and the frequency of pseudoarthrosis (often occurring some time after surgery) made this a marginal technique. However, the use of this technique has now been increased by progress in methods of anesthesia, the ability to reduce bleeding, and routine combination with osteosynthesis.

Recently, the use of cages that decrease the risk for graft breakdown by maintaining the intervertebral space and ensuring greater rigidity of the fixation system has also increased the applicability of this technique. The cage maintains the patency of the foramen and obviates stenosis of the lateral recess. In addition, it increases the surface area available for fusion and decreases disc debris. It can be used to preserve disc height in cases of early kyphosis, horizontal displacement (spondylolisthesis), or arthrectomy. However, it may be entirely contraindicated in cases of intraductal fibrosis (particularly in patients who have undergone multiple surgeries), when mobilization of the nerve roots or the dural sheath is difficult. This is also true of cases in which previous intervention has used a bilateral interlaminar approach. Otherwise, it is the arthrodesis of choice after recurrence of a disc problem. The procedure uses bone from the iliac crest as the source of graft (bank grafts tend to break down or pseudoarthrose) and is always combined with posterior osteosynthesis. To avoid neurologic complications and risk for hemorrhage, it is rarely performed on more than two levels.

Although the cage technique supports the cancellous bone graft and avoids the difficulty of performing three corticocancellous grafts, with maintenance of the intervertebral space, it should only be used in combination with osteosynthesis.

### Technique

#### *PLIF with Iliac Graft*

Graft harvesting is achieved by detachment of the aponeurotic tissue, after which the pyramid is exposed and the graft is taken (two grafts are used in PLIF with posterior osteosynthesis). A wide intralaminar approach is taken, with resection of the yellow ligament and of the inferior area of the upper lamina of from 5 to 8 mm (slightly less on the superior upper lamina). The freed nerve roots are placed inside of the dural sheath. Outside, a 6–8-mm resection of the joints at the disc level must allow an accessible area of approximately 12 to 14 mm. Special care must be taken with the root that lies on the upper pedicle, which is above and medial during its traject to the foramen. In cases of decreased disc height, this root is close to the inferior disc. This disc must be incised and the end plates rasped with care so as not to damage its contact with the bone below. This is better done with a raspatory than with a chisel.

The use of a Lerat (4) distracting device allows restoration of the intervertebral space while avoiding excessive root tensioning. The grafts are inserted from the cortical aspect (in a vertical position), and the cortical crest is pushed to the rear to facilitate graft filling.

Implantation of such grafts requires posterior interlaminar distraction with a Meary-type retractor, and should be performed under radiographic or fluoroscopic control. Care must be taken to avoid kyphosis during this manipulation. By making the the anterior portion of the graft higher than the posterior, restoration of normal lordosis after release of the distraction and posterior compression by osteosynthesis is made easier. The intra-joint graft is performed as previously described, as is osteosynthesis (four points for a single space and six points for two spaces). Posterior compression allows for loads to be applied on lordosis and definitely stabilizes the graft, thus avoiding any neurotoxic migration. Rigid by definition, this fusion of the three columns can be combined by fixation with 5- or 6-mm rods.

Ambulation is allowed between the second and the fourth day after surgery. A corset will provide support and protect the healing area.

### *PLIF with Screw Cages*

This technique allows the use of cancellous bone for intersomatic grafts. It creates a strong chamber for the graft by maintaining the space and enhancing fusion. The graft bone must be compacted and should protrude through the filter openings of the screw cage before placement to achieve the best connection with the bone. The use of the ancillary instrumentation described above makes the implantation easier. Under radiographic control, approximately the same approach is used. The space is prepared with a drill adapted to the height of the cage and screwing is accomplished with a twist drill, with radiographic verification of the direction (parallel to the plates) and depth. The two cages must superimpose exactly on the fluoroscopic lateral view (8). An obturator will avoid any migration of the spongious grafts. Instrumentation, intra-joint and/or posterolateral arthrodesis, and osteosynthesis are performed as described above.

## EXTENDED ARTHRODESIS

### Principles and Indications

Surgery of lumbar stenosis going beyond canal decompression may include arthrodesis and osteosynthesis. Fusion for lumbar stenosis must be discussed in case destabilization includes cases of displacement, curvature, and dislocation. Displacements include hypermobility, instability (excessive motion), and fixed displacements (e.g., spondylolisthesis, retrolisthesis). Curvatures may represent progressive lumbar kyphosis or scoliosis. Dislocations may be open or closed.

### Technique

The patient is placed in the ventral decubitus position, and the pedicle screws are located under fluorscopic control. The extent of the instrumentation depends on the level of the injured disc and the degree of displacement or curvature.

Antero- or posterolateral joint can be performed (the latter, which is more likely to involve extensive bleeding, is performed after the instrumentation at the end of the procedure). More extended and convergent pedicle screwing is necessary because the pedicle is likely to become more fragile after laminectomy. The direction of the screws must take into consideration the orientation of the screw head to the rods and the final degree of lordosis desired. The implanted rods are bent in such a way that physiologic curvature is achieved. To achieve this, osteotomy of the inferior facets of upper segments is necessary. The use of a frame with transverse plates will increase the rigidity of the instrumentation.

## L4–L5 SPONDYLOLISTHESIS

### Principles and Indications

L4–L5 spondylolisthesis, either degenerative or caused by isthmic fracture, leads to severe vertebral instability and lumbar stenosis, particularly in case of degenerative spondylolisthesis. Freeing the nerve root involves ablation of the posterior arch, liberation of L4 in the foramen, and liberation of L5 in the canal. Stabilization of the space is achieved by discectomy. Failures of isolated posterior instrumentations have been reported in the literature. Reduction is not always useful when root liberation is performed, and should be done only by performing an intersomatic graft by the posterior approach, to avoid recurrence of displacement and/or breakdown of the isolated posterior osteosynthesis.

When arthrodesis of the anterior column is not possible, the alternative is an careful posterolateral graft, followed by immobilization in a corset until fusion occurs. A second alternative is reoperation with performance of a second graft by the posterior approach.

### Technique

The technique is the same as for four-point arthrodesis in which the posterior arch is ablated. Displacement caused by sliding between L4 and L5 can be compensated for by driving the L4 screw of the implanted arthrodesis more shallowly or by reduction of the slippage after screwing of the implants (with a rod-pusher if necessary, which pulls back the screw on the rod). In cases of spondylolisthesis caused by isthmic fracture, an intersomatic graft is easy and restoring disc height greatly reduces the slippage.

In cases of degenerative spondylolisthesis, access to the dural sheath by the posterior route is difficult, with the risk for hemorrhage on ischemia of the roots caused by chronic compression. The use of a triple-rod system will ensure maximal rigidity of the fixation system.

## L5–S1 SPONDYLOLISTHESIS

### Principles and Indications

Slippage of L5–S1 involves slippage of the inferior part. Mechanical loads are important and this causes an anteroposterior lack of balance, and the slippage may recur unless it is corrected by reduction. Reduction should focus on correlation of the pelvic retroversion, and an anterior column graft should be routinely used.

### Technique

After liberation of the roots, screws are implanted in the L5 and S1 pedicles. Progressive extension of the lower limbs will bring about anteversion of the pelvis and ensure reduction. In this case, also, use of the rod-pusher will aid in placement of the rod in the L5 screws in difficult cases.

The fixation system can be made more rigid by implantation of triple rods. Sacral anchoring can also be performed, with the sacral plate inserted into the sacral hole by three screw fixation points, two in the partaes lateral sacraes and one in the pedicle.

Grafting of the anterior column can be achieved by a PLIF, a traditional iliac graft, or by a "hollow screw" used as a cage (see above) when there is only slight displacement and no dysplasia.

In other cases, a trans-sacrolumbar graft allows pegging of L5–S1 by a posterior approach. The sacral canal is opened through a posterior window until the S1 pedicle is visible. While the S1 root under this pedicle is controlled, S2 is driven back beyond the median line. Introduction of a perforator and then of a cylindrical rasp with progressive height from S1 to L5 allows the formation of a tunnel through which the graft will be applied. This can be a fibular graft 55 to 60 mm long. A hollow screw full of iliac cancellous bone is used, and the trajectory of the screw is completed with a special drill under fluoroscopy control. The cover of the sacral window is replaced at the end of the intervention.

## ANTEROPOSTERIOR BALANCE

The quality of a lumbar arthrodesis depends on the intervertebral fusion achieved, the physiologic compatibility of the device used, and on the degree of stabilization obtained. It is also dependent on restoration of vertebral stasis, i.e., restoration of normal lordosis and a balance between the lumbosacral and coxofemoral joints (6). Avoiding the possibility for spinal rotation, as well as flexion–extension and lateral inclinations, the stresses of rotation are transmitted to the first mobile disc and will place greater stress on the sacroiliac joints (which in the adult are rarely capable of a slight adaptation to stress but at the cost of pain). This should always be borne in mind when surgery is contemplated.

The patient is usually placed in the ventral decubitus position with flexed hips and the lumbar spine in delordosis to facilitate root liberation, but this position is not ideal for arthrodesis. Before bone fixation, the hips should be repositioned so that lordosis is once again observed. Resection of the head of the facet joints and compression on the fixation device allow restructuring of the lumbar curvature throughout the extent of the fixation system.

## CONCLUSIONS

Arthrodesis has an important place in treatment of lumbar instabilities. By reducing pain and correcting lesions resulting from repeated discectomies, it permits liberation of the nerve root, correction of abnormal curvature, and immediate stabilization. Systematic instrumentation has increased the quality of arthrodesis, with encouraging results (often spectacular after PLIF, particularly with the use of cages), which encourage us to pursue in this direction.

## REFERENCES


1. Cloward RB. Lesions of the intervertebral discs and their treatment by interbody fusion methods. *Chir Orthop* 1963;57:27.
2. Esses SI, Butsford DJ, Kostiuick JP. The role of external spinal skeletal fixation in the association of low-back disorders. *Spine* 1989;14:594–600.
3. Lehman TR, Spratt KF, Tozzi JE, et al. Long term follow-up of lower lumbar fusion patients. *Spine* 1987;12:97.
4. Lerat JL, Basso M, Trillaud JM, et al. Traitement due spondylolisthésis chez l'adolescent at l'adulte par arthrodèse intersomatique par vole posterieure. A propos de 40 cas. *Rev Chir Orthop* 1984; 70(Suppl 2):127–33.
5. Louis R. *Chirurgie due rachis*. Berlin, Heidelberg, New York: Springer-Verlag, 1982.
6. Marnay Th. L'équilibre du rachis et du bassin. Cahiers d'enseignement de la SOFCOT. *L'Expansion Scientifigue* 1988:281–313.
7. Marnay Th. Rachis lombaire dégénératif. Manuel d'ostéosynthèse vertébrale. *Sauramps Med,* 1991.
8. Marnay Th. Arthrodèse vertébrale du segment lombaire inférieur. Instabilitiés vertébrales lombaires. *Exp Sci Française* 1995;155:165.
9. Watkins MB. Posterolateral fusion in pseudoarthrosis and posterior element defect of the lumbosacral spine. *Chir Orthop* 1964;35:80–5.

*Instrumented Fusion of the Degenerative Lumbar Spine: State of the Art, Questions, and Controversies,* edited by M. Szpalski, R. Gunzburg, D. M. Spengler, and A. Nachemson. Lippincott–Raven Publishers, Philadelphia © 1996.

# 23

# Usefulness of Intervertebral Titanium CH Cages for PLIF and Posterior Fixation with Semi-Rigid Isolock Plates

Gilles Perrin

*Department of Neurosurgery, Hôpital Neurologique, F-69003 Lyon, France*

The traditional treatment for lumbar stenosis is a wide laminectomy. This procedure has a high success rate (1,6,17) and a low but not insignificant incidence of complications secondary to the removal of several levels of laminae, supraspinous ligaments, and articular facets (7). According to many reports in the literature, painful recurrence of back pain due to postoperative instability occurred in 15% of patients (16).

Because laminectomy without arthrodesis results in satisfactory outcomes for most patients with uncomplicated medial spinal stenosis, spinal fusions in patients with more important degenerative lesions that threaten spinal stability, such as degenerative spondylolisthesis, degenerative disc disease with severe collapsed disc, or failed back surgery syndrome still remain controversial (5,6,18). As new imaging with computed tomography (CT) scanning and magnetic resonance imaging (MRI) often demonstrates lateral and foraminal stenosis, such extensive lateral nerve root compressions lead the surgeon to be more aggressive, with the risk for iatrogenic instability.

To avoid fusion procedures and internal fixation methods, surgical techniques such as decompressive laminotomy with conservation of the facets were proposed with the aim of decreasing perioperative morbidity and potential long-term destabilizing effects (2,11,14). However, such conservative procedures may not be effective for correcting nerve root entrapment. The difficult portion of this procedure is foraminal decompression through a limited interlaminar approach. Spondylotic lumbar stenosis is often associated with hypertrophy of the superior facet. It is important that the superior tip of the superior facet be amputated to achieve adequate bony decompression in the foraminotomy (13).

If the patient requires foraminotomy and medial facetectomy, stability may be threatened by overzealous or unavoidable sacrifice of a supporting procedure. In such cases, intervertebral fusion is indicated to prevent further subluxation and recurrence of the root compression. Good results have been reported after short-range posterior stabilization with pedicle screw fixation, such as the rigid Cotrel-Dubousset instrumentation (15). The danger of painful postoperative displacement is less troublesome than failure resulting from too limited decompression. Stenosis in the foramen may be caused not only by hypertrophy of the pedicle or enlargement of the superior facet but also by a collapsed disc and loss of intervertebral height. In lateral and foraminal stenosis, a wide decompressive procedure with unroofing of the lateral recess and foraminotomy sometimes requires intervertebral distraction to restore the intervertebral height, to widen the foraminal opening, and to maintain nerve root decompression. This more extensive procedure is justified because of the failures that have previously occurred in patients in whom inadequate decompression had been performed.

Whereas the usefulness of posterior interpedicular fixation combined with intervertebral grafting is well known for achieving definitive stabilization, new interest is centered on posterior interbody fusion (PLIF) to obtain nerve root decompression by its "spacer" effect (8). By restoring the intervertebral height and providing immediate, postoperative stabilization, the foraminal opening is maintained. The purpose of this study was to determine the efficiency of titanium CH cages for interbody fusion and the use of semi-rigid Isolock plates for posterior interpedicular fixation (Fig. 1A,B).

## PATIENTS AND METHODS

In the total group of patients who were operated on for spinal stenosis, only 12% required PLIF and posterior fixation. The others underwent classical surgery with laminectomy or laminotomy with conservation of the articular facets.

From 1978 to 1994, 630 consecutive cases underwent surgery for root decompression and intervertebral stabilization with interbody grafting. A total of 440 patients were operated on for isthmic spondylolisthesis, 72 for discoligamentar unstability and 118 for degenerative disc or spinal disease with lateral and foraminal stenosis. The age distribution was 43–81 years (mean 54 years). The involved sites were mainly L4–L5. All patients suffered from radicular sciatic pain, and intermittent claudication was noted in 83% of the cases.

Radicular decompression was obtained by total foraminotomy by means of resection of the facets and laminectomy. Restoration of the intervertebral height was achieved by using a distracting probe from the smallest size to the largest to spread the intervertebral space until the appropriate space was reached. The CH titanium cage-like implants filled with spongy bone from the laminectomy were deeply inserted. The interbody implants maintained the nerve root decompression and ensured immediate restoration of the spinal column vertical and horizontal stabilization after bone healing.

Anterior arthrodesis was completed by interpedicular posterior fixation to restore the biomechanical tripod well described by Louis, ensuring immediate horizontal and vertical stability and enabling early mobilization without an immobilizing corset or brace. The fixation was performed with little compression, both to restore physiologic lordosis and to protect the anterior implants from possible posterior displacement.

To protect the function and the physiologic dynamic equilibrium of the upper

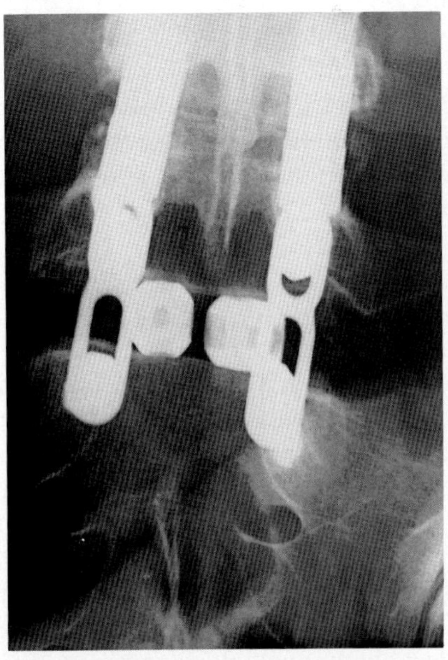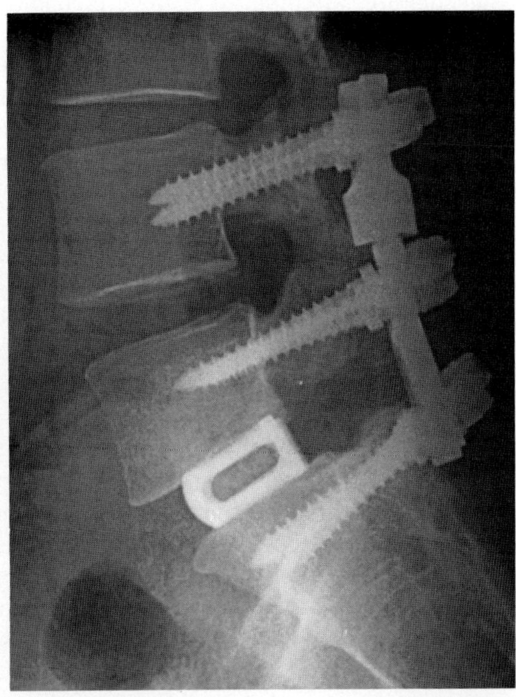

**FIG. 1. A:** Interbody fusion with CH cages: note the wide opening of the foramen through the "spacer effect" of the cages. **B:** Surgical stabilization of L5–S1 isthmic spondylolisthesis with CH cages, PLIF, and bisegmental posterior fixation with Isolock semi-rigid plates. Note the transitional semi-rigid functional zone between the L5–S1 rigid segment and the L3–L4 level with reactional hypermobility.

lumbar spine, the shortest possible fixation was performed. Monosegmental fixation only at the level of degenerative compression or unstable lesions is advisable. However, in the case of pathology adjacent to the arthrodesis disc, it is very important to protect this overlying level by a longer fixation. In our experience, preoperative assessment through MRI examinations of the overlying disc led the surgeon to perform bisegmental fixation in 60% of all the operated cases.

Such lumbar postoperative segmental rigidity is responsible for superjacent compensatory hypermobility. This functional hypersolicitation may induce further clinical deterioration or secondary superjacent destabilization (3,10). Although such risk is low for monosegmental fixation, it must be kept in mind in cases of bisegmental arthrodesis with fixation of three vertebrae. In such cases, we use Isolock semi-rigid plates for interpedicular fixation to create an intermediate transitional functional zone between the rigid arthrodesis and superjacent compensatory hypermobility. This semi-rigid system enables early rehabilitation with no damage to the fixation or screw fracture. It stimulates acceleration of the osteogenic process by maintaining constraints on the cages or the compressed intervertebral grafts. To improve the long-term anatomic and clinical result by preventing the "neo-hinge" or "false joint" phenomenon, we proposed a series of surgical and rehabilitation measures: intervertebral body arthrodesis, semi-rigid posterior fixation, the shortest assembly possible sparing the upper lumbar spine, early rehabilitation to achieve posterior remusculature, attempts to achieve physiologic lordosis, and systematic radiologic assessment of the superjacent spine.

According to these principles, the patient was allowed to walk without bracing the day after the operation. The rehabilitation program began very early, at the fifth postoperative day, with the main purpose of restoration of posterior muscles and normal lordosis. X-ray controls were performed at 3 months and 1 year after the surgical procedure. No breakage or failure of the posterior fixation was radiologically observed. For the PLIF, x-ray controls determined absence of secondary collapse of the intervertebral space, increasing bone density in the cage, and presence of osteogenetic thickening of the vertebral endplates.


## RESULTS

In this series of patients who underwent surgical vertebral fusion with interbody cages and posterior fixation, we observed no postoperative neurologic complication. No patients required further destabilization procedures or removal of the implants.

A total of 32 patients with degenerative diseases treated by intervertebral cages and semi-rigid fixation were reviewed after a follow-up of more than 1 year. The anatomic lesions were degenerative spondylolisthesis in 13 cases, secondary post-laminectomy slipping in three cases, severe degenerative collapsed disc disease with foraminal stenosis in 11 cases, primitive (Fig. 2) or after disc surgery (Fig. 3), and extreme intervertebral disc collapse after lumbar chemonucleolysis in three cases (Fig. 4), or after disc injection of triamcinolone in two cases.

The clinical outcome was excellent in 18 cases (56.2%), fair in 11 cases (34.3%), and poor in three cases (9.5%). According to Beaujon's French clinical scale, the assessment of mean functional benefit was 76%. The mean postoperative working disability was 4.1 months for the nonretired patients.

Radiologic controls after 1 year of postoperative evaluation demonstrated bony fusion in all the cases. Evaluation of osteogenesis was allowed through the large lateral openings by determining the density of the bone filling the implant. In 26 cases (80%), increasing bone density in the cage was observed as early as 3 months after the operation in comparison with early postoperative x-ray controls. After 1 year, hyperdensity of the vertebral endplates facing the cages was noted in all the cases. We observed no early or delayed breakage or failure of the fixation system. No secondary posterior displacement of the cages was noted on the late x-ray controls. These data may indicate that intervertebral fusion and definitive vertebral stabilization were obtained in all the patients.


## DISCUSSION

Once the diagnosis of lumbar spinal stenosis has been established (19), surgery is performed in patients who present with persistent severe low back pain and sciatica, numbness or weakness of the leg, and neurogenic functional claudication. Laminectomy is the procedure of choice, with more or less radical resection of the intervertebral articular facets at one or several levels. Good results with improvement of radicular symptoms and claudication were reported in about 70% of the patients. However, low back pain could not be sufficiently eliminated in many patients. Clin-

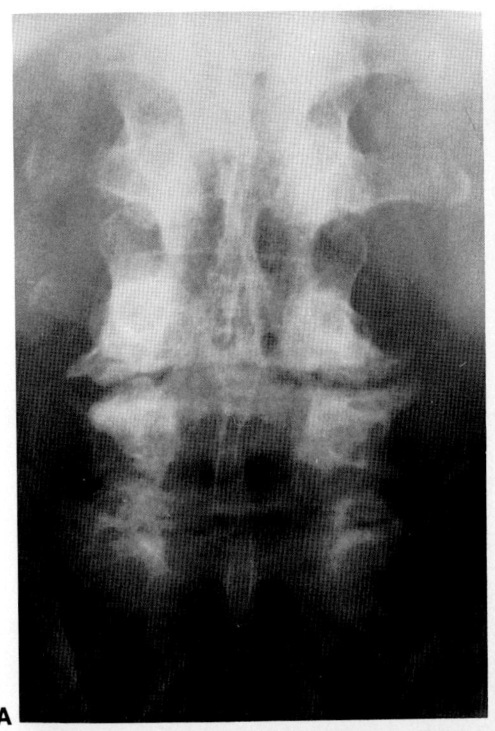

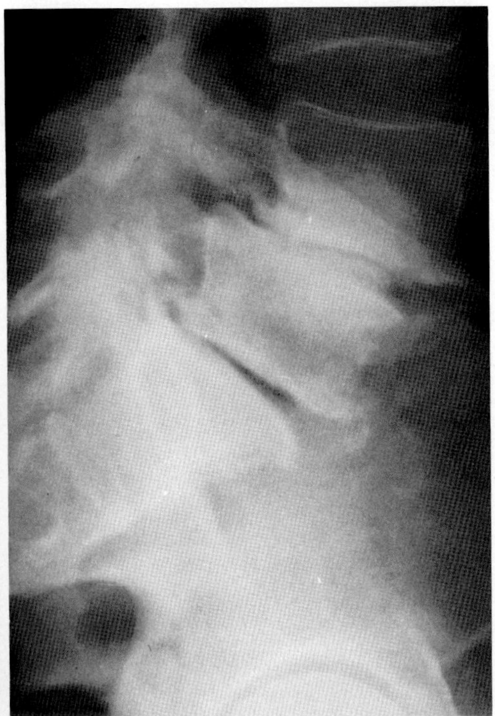

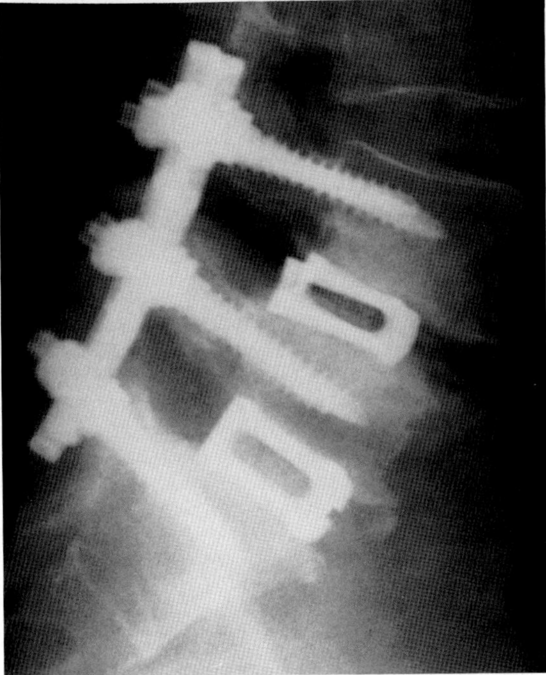

**FIG. 2. A:** Severe lateral and foraminal L4–L5 and L5–S1 stenosis. **B:** Lateral view of the same patient shows severe collapsed discs and important slipping. **C:** Postoperative control: note the restoration of the intervertebral space and the enlarged foramens. Both interbody cages and posterior fixation ensure total horizontal and vertical stabilization through the restoration of the three columns of the biomechanical tripod stand system.

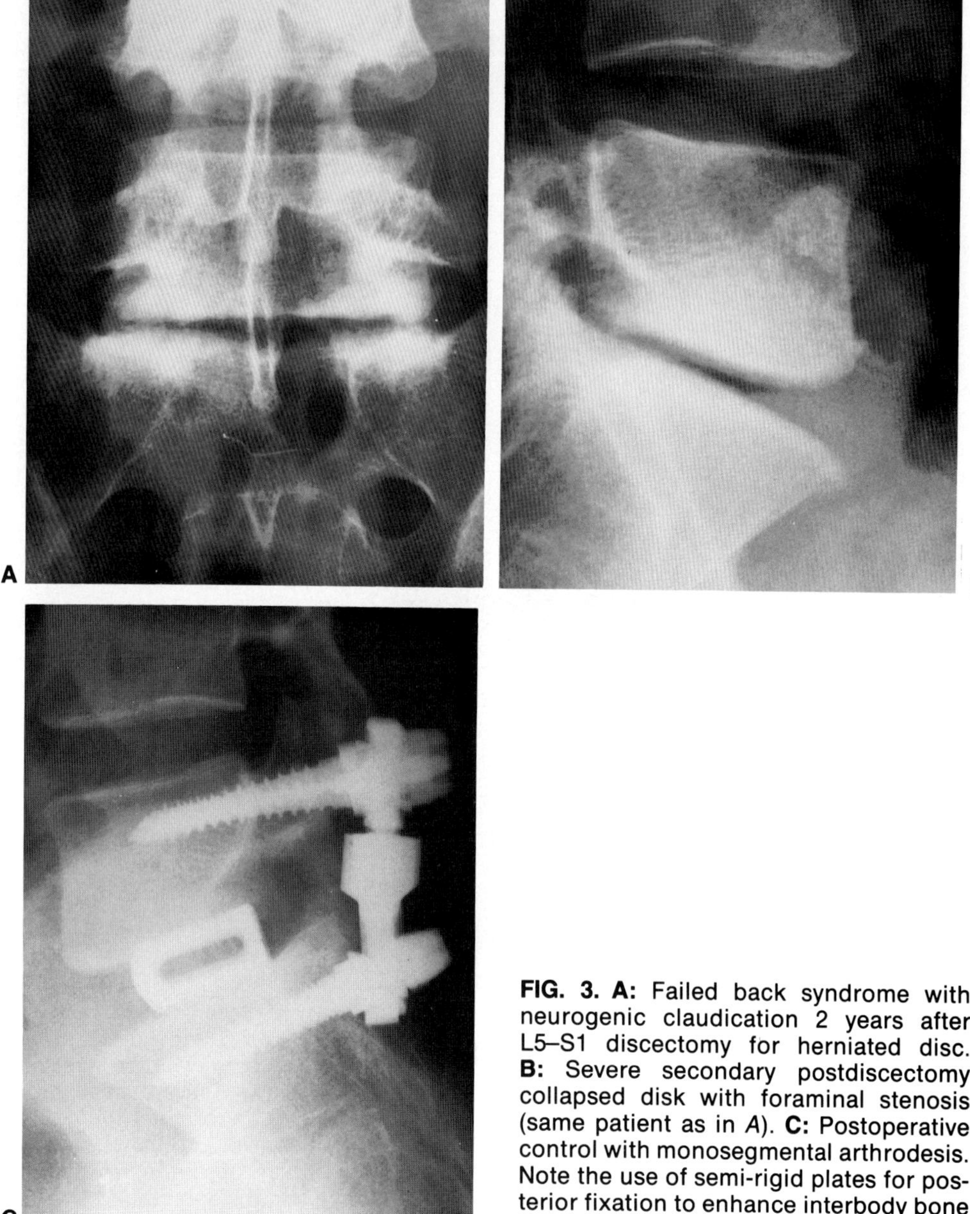

**FIG. 3. A:** Failed back syndrome with neurogenic claudication 2 years after L5–S1 discectomy for herniated disc. **B:** Severe secondary postdiscectomy collapsed disk with foraminal stenosis (same patient as in *A*). **C:** Postoperative control with monosegmental arthrodesis. Note the use of semi-rigid plates for posterior fixation to enhance interbody bone healing.

ical failures were related to inadequate decompression or to further horizontal dislocation due to the removal of intervertebral connecting elements. Intervertebral fusion with posterior instrumentation was proposed in patients either with obvious preoperative instability or in whom the surgeon feared postoperative slipping due to the amount of resection of the facet joints. Another argument in favor of intervertebral fusion and fixation is the pursuit of complete and definitive nerve root de-

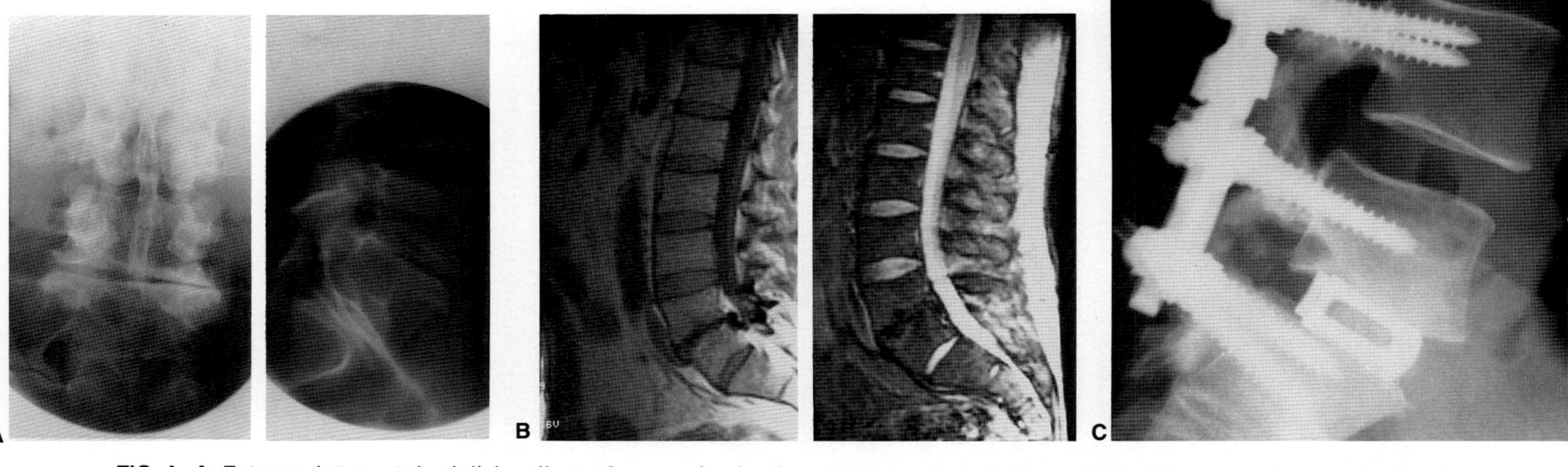

**FIG. 4.** **A:** Extreme intervertebral disk collapse 3 years after lumbar chemonucleolysis in a patient with recurrent severe low back pain and neurogenic claudication. **B:** Severe disc deterioration after chemonucleolysis, well-demonstrated by MRI. **C:** Postoperative control 1 year after surgery. Note the maintained spacer effect, the absence of secondary collapse, and the bone density in the cage.

compression. Intervertebral distraction is an efficient and reliable method for opening the foramen and decompressing the roots.

PLIF is a biomechanically, optimal fusion because the graft maintains the disc height (i.e., the lateral foraminal opening), protects the nerve roots, restores weight-bearing to anterior structures, and immobilizes both horizontal and vertical instability. In our total series of PLIF, the postoperative results were excellent, with an 87% clinical success rate and a 92% fusion success rate. Although autologous bone is undoubtedly the best bone for grafting, most PLIF surgeons prefer processed allograft to avoid donor site mobidity. Fresh allograft is usually avoided because of the risk for transmission of viral diseases. Lyophilized bone is often preferred but may induce altered fusion.

The cage-like implant (CH cages) meets the mechanical requirements for PLIF by serving both a mechanical function and a biologic bone growth function. The cages stretch the intervertebral space to its normal anatomic height and prevent the postoperative collapse of the graft. The implant is hollow to accept packing of autologous bone graft with local cancellous bone obtained from the laminectomy. The lateral windows improve the bony fusion and allow easy assessment of fusion by normal radiographic methods.

The theorical risk for secondary posterior displacement of the cages is well controlled by the optimal position of the implants. They are deeply inserted into the intervertebral space such that two-thirds of the implant is situated in front of the theorical center of intervertebral rotation. The implants are tightly held in place under extreme compression because the cages are inserted after intervertebral distraction and are completely integrated under compression after the slackening of the interbody distractor. The scraped surfaces of the implants ensure anchorage in the bone of the vertebral endplates. It is possible to insert prelordosing implants with front heights greater than rear heights. When used with posterior fixation, the cages cannot be mobilized by micromovements. In our total series, retropulsion of the PLIF grafts was never observed.

Since 1990, anterior stabilization has been completed by a metallic bilateral pedicular posterior fixation to restore a biomechanical tripod stand system. With this technique, earlier fusion without the need for a postoperative brace was observed. The patients were referred very early to a rehabilitation program.

Since 1993, the semi-rigid osteosynthetic plate Isolock System with pedicular screws was used with the aim of ensuring enhanced graft integration by the filtered micromovements and, above all, to ensure that the zones adjacent to the arthrodesis are preserved as long as possible by avoiding stress at those levels. This surgical fixation may prevent the neo-hinge phenomenon through the functional load transitional area between the rigid zone at the level of the arthrodesis and the superjacent compensatory hypermobility. This system may prevent screw loosening or fixation breakage by absorbing most of the mechanical loads induced by early rehabilitation within the semi-rigid connecting element itself rather than letting them affect the bone–screw interface. With the use of both interbody cages and semi-rigid plates, we observed no failure due to continued instability of the surgical construction.

Interbody fusion with cages, semi-rigid posterior fixation, the shortest possible assembly sparing the upper lumbar spine, and early rehabilitation to achieve posterior remusculature and physiologic lordosis are measures that meet all the requirements not only for immediate pain relief but also for definitive stabilization without further and delayed iatrogenic spinal complications.

## REFERENCES


1. Alexander E, Kelly DL, Davis CH, et al. Intact arch spondylolisthesis. A review of 50 cases and description of surgical treatment. *J Neurosurg* 1985;63:840–4.
2. Aryanpur J, Ducker Th. Multilevel lumbar laminotomies: an alternative to laminectomy in the treatment of lumbar stenosis. *Neurosurgery* 1990;26:429–33.
3. Cauchoix J, Benoist M, Chassaing V. Degenerative spondylolisthesis. *Clin Orthop Relat Res* 1976; 115:122–9.
4. Dall BE, Rowe DE. Degenerative spondylolisthesis. Its surgical management. *Spine* 1985;10:668–72.
5. Feffer HL, Wiesel SW, Cuckler JM, Rothman RH. Degenerative spondylolisthesis. To fuse or not to fuse. *Spine* 1985;10:287–9.
6. Herron LD, Trippi AC. L4–5 degenerative spondylolisthesis. The results of treatment by decompressive laminectomy without fusion. *Spine* 1989;14:534–8.
7. Hopp E, Tsou PM. Postdecompression lumbar instability. *Clin Orthop* 1988;227:143–9.
8. Hutter ChG. Spinal stenosis and posterior lumbar interbody fusion. *Clin Orthop Relat Res* 1985;193: 103–14.
9. Lee TCh. Reduction and stabilization without laminectomy for unstable degenerative spondylolisthesis: a preliminary report. *Neurosurgery* 1994;35:1072–6.
10. Lehmann TR, Spratt KF, Tozzi JE. Long-term follow up of lower lumbar fusion patients. *Spine* 1987;12:97–104.
11. Lin PM. Internal decompression for multiple levels of lumbar spinal stenosis: a technical note. *Neurosurgery* 1982;11:546–9.
12. Maroon JC, Kopitnik TA, Schulhof LA, et al. Diagnosis and microsurgical approach to far-lateral disc herniation in the lumbar spine. *J Neurosurg* 1990;72:378–82.
13. Markwelder ThM, Battaglia M. Failed back surgery syndrome. Part II: Surgical techniques, implant choice, and operative results in 171 patients with instability of the lumbar spine. *Acta Neurochir [Wien]* 1993;123:129–34.
14. Ray ChD. New techniques for decompression of lumbar spinal stenosis. *Neurosurgery* 1982;10:587–92.
15. Rompe JD, Eysel P, Hopf Ch, Heine J. Surgical management of central lumbar stenosis—results with decompressive laminectomy only and with comcomitant instrumented fusion with the Cotrel-Dubousset instrumentation. *Neuro-orthopedics* 1995;19:17–31.
16. Shenkin HA, Hash CJ. Spondylolisthesis after multiple bilateral laminectomies and facetectomies for lumbar stenosis. *J Neurosurg* 1979;50:45–7.
17. Turner JA, Ersek M, Herron L, Deyo R. Surgery for lumbar spinal stenosis. Attempted meta-analysis of the literature. *Spine* 1992;17:1–8.
18. Turner JA, Ersek M, Herron L, et al. Patient outcome after lumbar spinal fusions. *JAMA* 1992;268: 907–11.
19. Verbiest H. Stenosis of the lumbar vertebral canal and sciatica. *Neurosurg Rev* 1980;3:75–89.

*Instrumented Fusion of the Degenerative Lumbar Spine: State of the Art, Questions, and Controversies*, edited by M. Šzpalski, R. Gunzburg, D. M. Spengler, and A. Nachemson. Lippincott–Raven Publishers, Philadelphia © 1996.

# 24

# Clinical Trials in Surgery: Methodologic and Statistical Criteria of Validity, with an Example of Meta-Analysis of Randomized Trials in Spine Surgery

## C. Mélot

*Intensive Care Department, Erasme University Hospital, B-1070 Brussels, Belgium*

For many years there has been a heated debate regarding the proper role of randomized and well-controlled trials in surgery. One argument supporting the view that it is both ethical and desirable to perform such surgical trials whenever possible relates to the benefits for society. If a clinical trial involving 100 patients (50 in each of two treatment groups) can evaluate whether a questionable surgical procedure is of value, it is considered unethical to avoid this trial and to subject large numbers of future patients to an operation that might be ineffective, expensive, or even harmful. The history of surgery contains many examples of procedures that gained acceptance and were later shown to be without medical value. Many such operations that have been discarded in recent decades were rejected on the basis of controlled clinical trials. A classic example involved the reputed benefits of the internal mammary artery ligation for improving the clinical status of patients with angina pectoris. The true value of this particular surgery was not adequately assessed until two randomized controlled trials were performed, which included patients with sham operations (1,2). This example, among many others (11), makes one wonder if some surgical procedures used today are essentially no better than placebo or may actually be detrimental to patients.

Over the last few decades there has also been a trend toward emphasizing the role of statistics in the interpretation of investigational data. This focus has been appropriate and has helped to advance the standards of clinical study design, conduct, and interpretation. The proper goal of clinical trials is to obtain evidence that a treatment or a surgical procedure is better than another one in terms of outcomes, costs, and fewer adverse effects.

Clinical studies can be primary data analyses, secondary data analyses, or a combination of both. In studies using primary data, the investigator collects original data and analyzes the results. Case reports, case series, cohort studies, and randomized clinical trials fall into this group (6). Secondary data analyses are usually syntheses or reanalysis of data such as review articles on a subject or meta-analyses. Studies may also be considered as observational studies, in which subjects received no active intervention (e.g., natural history), or experimental studies, in which subjects undergo an intervention.

## STUDY DESIGNS

Study designs can be ordered in such a way that they provide more evidence for the superiority of a new therapeutic procedure. In other words, in the development of a new therapeutic tool, we are moving from a clinical experience published in case reports, case series, or cohort studies to definite clinical evidence of the advantage of the new treatment reported in controlled, randomized trials or meta-analyses of such trials (Fig. 1).

Single case reports are severely limited by the fact that they are confined to one case and to an evaluation by one, usually not disinterested observer, using nonstandard or subjective criteria and having no data for comparison. On the other hand, case reports reporting experiments of nature, properly interpreted, or with compelling findings can be used to develop hypotheses for more detailed studies. In case series, replication of results, which is central to scientific proof, strengthens the impression of efficacy of a medical treatment or a surgical procedure.

A cohort study assembles a group with some common characteristic and follows this group by a standardized protocol over time to determine the frequency of end points. The common characteristic might be the absence of disease or condition of interest, exposure to a common factor (e.g., toxin, medication, or surgical procedure), or the presence of a condition to understand its course. A cohort is similar to traditional case series but requires that zero time is defined, that entry criteria are uniform, and that standardized follow-up is done at regular intervals and that the follow-up rate is as complete as possible. Comparison can be made with a historical control group (i.e., a group of patients assembled before the cohort study group) or with concurrent controls (i.e., a group of patients assembled at the same time as the patients in the study group).

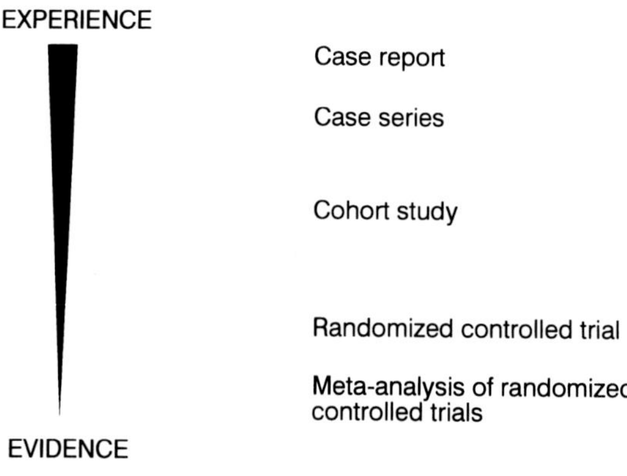



**FIG. 1.** Study designs and meta-analysis: moving from clinical experience to definite evidence of the beneficial effect of a new procedure or treatment.

The gold standard for clinical research is the randomized controlled trial, in which well-defined patients are randomized to treatment or placebo, both patients and physician are blinded to the treatment, and assessment of results is performed blindly and objectively. Randomization is the best technique to balance two groups for known and unknown factors that affect the outcome. Ideally, randomization should occur to the treatment being tested and to a sham or placebo intervention, particularly when the end points are subjective, such as pain.

The advantages and the disadvantages of these designs are summarized in Table 1.

## THE RANDOMIZED CLINICAL TRIAL

The components of a randomized clinical trial are designed to avoid the errors that may arise in the design and conduct of a nonrandomized study, which may bias the results (9). Even so, a randomized clinical trial shares many design features with a prospective, concurrently controlled cohort study. These features include: (a) every component of the randomized clinical trial is determined before the first patient enters the trial, by means of a detailed protocol that is developed to guide the collection of data on all subjects in the study; (b) concurrent comparison group is assembled; and (c) all subjects are followed forward in time (Fig. 2).

The major distinction is that in a prospective cohort study, the treatment to be given is determined by the interaction of physician and patient, whereas in a randomized clinical trial these influences are removed by allocating the treatment randomly. Moreover, in a randomized clinical trial evaluation of a medical therapy, such

**TABLE 1.** *Study designs*

| | Uses | Advantages | Disadvantages |
|---|---|---|---|
| Case report<br>  Single subject | Experiment of nature<br>Suggests association, etiology, course, or effective treatment | Opportunistic<br>Inexpensive<br>Generates questions | No control or comparison |
| Case series<br>  Two or more subjects reported with condition and/or intervention; with or without comparison group | Suggests clinical course, response to intervention | Exploits clinical material<br>Less expensive | Selected patients<br>Biased end point assessment |
| Cohort study<br>  Subjects systematically followed to identify etiologic, prognostic, and risk factors | Identify etiologic, prognosis, risks factors | Prospective<br>Establish causation | Expensive<br>Time-consuming |
| Randomized controlled trial<br>  Eligible patients randomized to two or more interventions and end results are evaluated blindly | Efficacy of treatment | Prospective | Expensive<br>Selected patients and intervention |

From ref. 6.

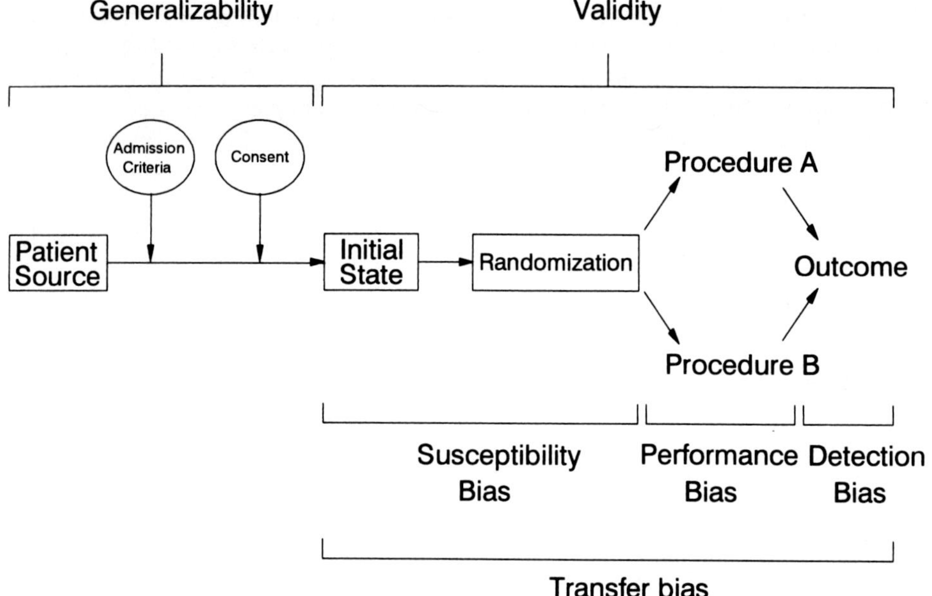


**FIG. 2.** Randomized clinical trial. See text for explanation. (Adapted from ref. 5.)

as a new drug, it is customary that neither the investigator nor the subject knows which agent the subject is receiving (double-blind study design).

In a surgical trial it is not possible to keep the surgeon investigator "blinded" and is rarely possible for the patient to be "blinded." Therefore, it is essential that the information for the initial examination (eligibility or admission criteria) be collected before randomization.

### Bias in Randomized Clinical Trials and Remedial Measures

The essential strength of the randomized clinical trial is its ability to limit the possibility of bias. The term "bias" is used to describe any systematic error arising from the design or conduct of a study. The presence of bias, however, may compromise the validity of the results of the study. There are four major ways in which bias may arise: (a) baseline groups may not be similar (susceptibility or selection bias); (b) procedures may not be performed comparably (performance bias); (c) outcomes for the groups may be measured in a dissimilar manner (detection bias); or (d) study subjects may be lost to follow-up (transfer bias) (9) (Fig. 2).

#### *Susceptibility Bias or Dissimilarity at Initial State*

In evaluations for any feature that is prognostic for a good or bad outcome, superior results in one of the groups may merely reflect the fact that the patients in that group had a better prognosis from the start. The random allocation of patients to a group (randomization) aims to reduce the likelihood of susceptibility bias. Studies using randomization have become the standard for scientific credibility because of the potentially devastating effect of susceptibility bias in studies conducted without this precaution. If an initial feature is a major prognostic factor and the investigator wishes to reduce the likelihood of dissimilarity at the initial state evaluation, stratified randomization may be used.

### *Performance Bias or Unequal Performance of the Procedure*

In comparing two surgical procedures, they must be completed with similar proficiency for both groups. If inexperienced orthopedic residents perform procedure A while experienced senior orthopedic surgeons perform the procedure B, a comparison of outcomes would be unfair. The error resulting from dissimilar levels of skill in performing the procedure is called performance bias.

### *Detection Bias or Dissimilar Detection of Outcome*

Suppose that the surgeon who performed procedure A, examines these patients 1 year later and the surgeon who performed procedure B examines those patients 6 months later. From this time difference in evaluation of the outcome, a detection bias may arise. Moreover, if the two surgeons use their own criteria for measuring the outcome, as well as their own methods of measurement, the outcomes are likely to be evaluated in dissimilar ways for each group of patients. Evaluators who do not know which procedure was performed (i.e., they are blinded) provide a less biased measure of outcome. The classical method to avoid both performance and outcome biases is double blinding, in which neither the study subject nor the individual assessing the outcome knows which therapy has been given. The surgeons clearly know the procedures that they performed. To reduce detection bias in this setting, the outcomes must be measured by someone who does not know which surgical procedure was performed (single blinding). Clearly, double blinding provides the best protection against bias, but single blinding is better than no blinding at all.

### *Transfer Bias or Differential Loss to Follow-Up*

The investigator can measure the outcome only in those subjects who return for evaluation. Patients may leave a study for legitimate reasons or may refuse to return for follow-up. Suppose that 20% of the patients who received procedure A do not return for follow-up because their results are so good and that 20% of the patients who had procedure B do not return because their results are so bad (differential loss to follow-up). The results of the patients who remain in the study may therefore be distorted (transfer bias). The only real protection against transfer bias is to obtain the best possible follow-up.

### Generalizability and Validity of a Randomized Clinical Trial

Even if investigators have completed the most methodologically correct randomized clinical trial and have found a definitive result, they may be chagrined to find that the results are ignored by their colleagues. Among the many potential reasons for this, three merit consideration. These include the population studied, the criteria that limit admission to the study, and the ethical requirement of obtaining informed consent (12).

First, the choice of a particular population as the source of the study subjects determines the spectrum of patients enrolled in a study. If those reading the report of the study believe that this spectrum is not a representative one, they may claim that the results are not generalizable to their own patients.

Second, the admission criteria for the study limit the group to which the study results may be generalized.

A third filter, not under the investigator's control, may further limit generalizability. Subjects must consent to participate in the study, and those who do so may not be representative of the eligible population. If only a small proportion of potential subjects consents to participate and is actually enrolled, the generalizability of results must be questioned.

The distinction between generalizability and validity is an important one. The results of a randomized clinical trial can be generalized only to the type of patient who was enrolled in the study (generalizability is sometimes referred as "external validity"). A valid trial, on the other hand, is one without systematic error or bias, i.e., a trial in which the results are accurate (validity is sometimes referred as "internal validity").

## ALTERNATIVE METHOD OF RANDOMIZATION: THE RANDOMIZED SURGEON DESIGN

The randomized clinical trial offers one approach to answering many orthopedic surgical questions, but it obviously raises several important problems (ethical issues, comparability of surgical procedures, length of follow-up necessary to assess outcome) both for the surgeon and for the patient.

To avoid some of these problems, a new randomized design that is particularly suited to evaluating surgical procedures has been proposed (Fig. 3). Because surgeons are likely to believe in the superiority of one procedure over another, they are more skilled at performing their preferred procedure. In the randomized surgeon design, the surgeons are assigned to one treatment group according to their expertise (13). Patients are still randomized, but they are randomized primarily to a surgeon or group of surgeons and only secondarily to a procedure. In this way the performance bias is minimized. This randomized surgeon design allows the surgeons to remain committed to the favored procedure, to project confidence to the patient, and to perform the surgical procedure at which they are most skilled. Although the surgeon will know the nature of the procedure, this does not prevent a blind assessment of outcome by another observer. The randomized surgeon clinical trial largely removes the source of surgeons' reluctance to participate in randomized clinical trials while maintaining the overall strengths of the classic randomized clinical trial.

## META-ANALYSES OF RANDOMIZED TRIALS

Meta-analysis is the process of formally combining the quantitative results of separate studies to increase the statistical evidence of estimated effects (3,5,10). There is a great need to provide the community with a summary of all available evidence for the effect of a treatment or a surgical procedure. In fact, it is extremely rare in any field of research for a single study alone to provide convincing evidence of an effect, except for large multicenter or randomized controlled trials. When the body of evidence to be summed up includes many trials, and when there is a qualitative and quantitative heterogeneity among studies, the issue of conducting a meta-analysis, as well as its interpretation, becomes complex (3,5). Nevertheless, meta-analysis, if applied and interpreted with care, can provide valuable insight concerning treatment effect. When performing a meta-analysis, potential sources of bias should be controlled (3,5,10).

### Selection Bias

To avoid bias in selecting and rejecting papers, the decision to include a paper should be made by looking only at its methods and not at its results. Treatment effect comparison requires the inclusion of correctly randomized groups for which the only potential difference in outcome must be attributed to the therapeutic effect of the surgical procedure.

### Data Extraction Bias

When papers list a variety of subgroups, end points, or exclusions, it is quite possible that readers may vary in how they interpret the data in a particular study. The ideal way to control for this type of bias is to have the data extracted by more than one observer and then to measure interobserver agreement.

### Publication Bias

The higher likelihood for positive results to be published is well-documented. The tendency not to publish negative studies will introduce a positive bias into results of meta-analyses that are based only on the published literature.

## META-ANALYSIS: AN EXAMPLE IN SPINE SURGERY

Meta-analysis is indicated when a controversy exists concerning the real effect of a given treatment or surgical procedure. We asked the following simple question:

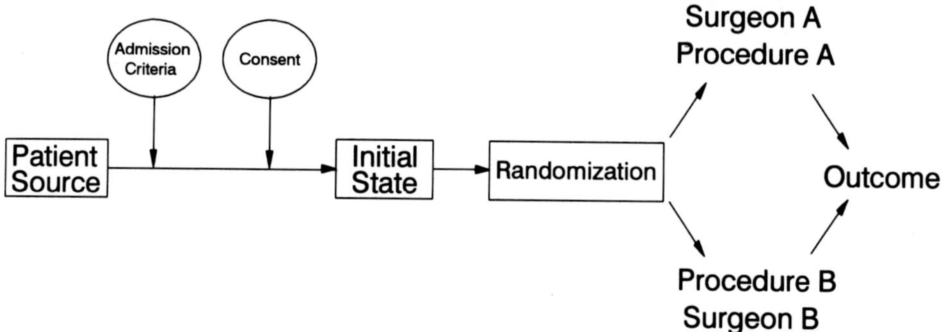


**FIG. 3.** Randomized surgeon design. See text for explanation. (Adapted from ref. 5.)

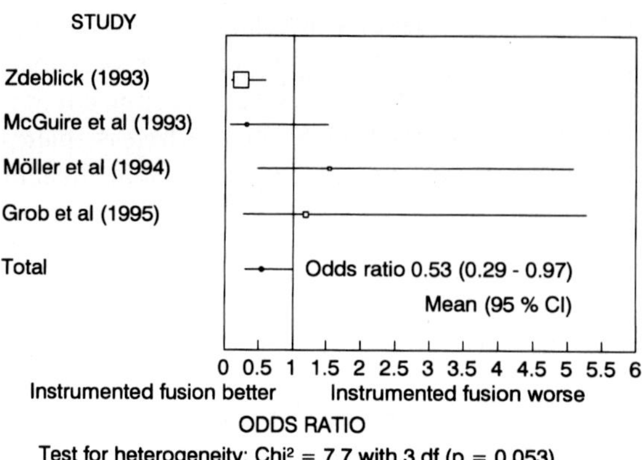


**FIG. 4.** Meta-analysis of four trials that assess pain in randomized groups of instrumented and noninstrumented lumbar fusion.

Does instrumented spine fusion improve pain relief compared with noninstrumented spine fusion? In reviewing the literature, we found four prospective randomized trials concerning patients suffering from low back pain secondary to degenerative lumbar disorders (e.g., degenerative lumbar stenosis, degenerative spondylolisthesis, degenerative disk disease, degenerative scoliosis with spinal stenosis) who underwent either instrumented or noninstrumented spinal fusion (4,7,8,14). Improvement in pain after the surgical procedure was considered as substantial when the results were excellent (no more pain with no activity limitation) or good (occasional pain with no activity limitation). Figure 4 is a graphic display of the meta-analysis: from left to right, the trial identification, the year of publication, the estimated odds ratio (center of the square), and its 95% confidence interval (the horizontal lines). The size of the square is a graphic indication of the amount of statistical information (number of events, i.e., improvement in pain) contributing to the statistical precision of the estimated odds ratio. The solid vertical line placed at odds ratio of 1 indicates equality in pain relief in instrumented and noninstrumented lumbar fusion. An odds ratio between 0 and 1 indicates that instrumented fusion is better for pain relief, and an odds ratio above 1 is in favor of a noninstrumented fusion. The total line refers to the summary estimate, indicating that instrumented fusion seems to be better to improve pain in lumbar degenerative disorders (percent reduction in the odds for pain relief is 47%). Such a graphic display is interesting in many ways: (a) beneficial effect on pain is decreasing in more recent studies where no effects at all were evidenced; (b) the most favorable study for instrumented fusion (14) had a short period of follow-up, which might introduce bias in evaluating the true outcome; and (c) the total odds seems in favor of instrumented fusion, but as the heterogeneity $\chi^2$ is close to the level of significance, these conclusions must be tempered and no definite conclusions can be drawn. Moreover, as the power of the heterogeneity $\chi^2$ is low due to the small sample size of the individual studies, a $p$ value below 0.10 should be considered significant (5). Nonhomogeneity of study outcomes may reflect the fact that the treatment effect varies according to a particular study characteristic, such as the technique used to achieved lumbar fusion.

## REFERENCES


1. Cobb LA, Thomas GI, Dillard DH, Merendino KA, Bruce RA. An evaluation of internal mammary artery ligation by a double-blind technique. *N Engl J Med* 1959;260:1115–8.

 2. Dimond EG, Kittle CF, Crockett JE. Comparison of internal mammary artery ligation and sham operation for angina pectoris. *Am J Cardiol* 1960;5:483–6.
 3. Gelber RD, Goldhirsch A. Meta-analysis: the fashion of summing-up evidence. Part I. Rationale and conduct. *Ann Oncol* 1991;2:461–8.
 4. Grob D, Humke T, Dvorak J. Degenerative lumbar spinal stenosis. Decompression with and without arthrodesis. *J Bone Joint Surg* 1995;77A:1036–41.
 5. L'Abbé KA, Detsky AS, O'Rourke K. Meta-analysis in clinical research. *Ann Intern Med* 1987;107: 224–32.
 6. Liang MH, Andersson G, Bombardier C, et al. Strategies for outcome research in spinal disorders. *Spine* 19(Suppl 18S):2037S–40S.
 7. McGuire RA, Amundson GM. The use of primary internal fixation in spondylolisthesis. *Spine* 1993; 18:1662–72.
 8. Möller H, Hedlund R. Fusion or conservative treatment in adult spondylolisthesis. A prospective randomized study [Abstract]. *Acta Orthop Scand* 1994;65(suppl 260):12.
 9. Rudicel S, Esdaile J. The randomized clinical trial in orthopaedics: obligation or option? *J Bone Joint Surg* 1985;67A:1284–93.
10. Sacks HS, Berrier J, Reitman D, Ancona-Berk VA, Chalmers TC. Meta-analyses of randomized controlled trials. *N Engl J Med* 1987;316:450–5.
11. Spilker B. Surgical trials. In: Spilker B, Ed. *Guide to clinical trials*. New York: Raven Press, 1991:320–8.
12. Van der Linden W. On the generalization of surgical trial results. *Acta Chir Scand* 1980;146:229–34.
13. Van der Linden W. Pitfalls in randomized surgical trials. *Surgery* 1980;87:258–62.
14. Zdeblick TA. A prospective, randomized study of lumbar fusion. Preliminary results. *Spine* 1993;18: 983–91.

*Instrumented Fusion of the Degenerative Lumbar Spine: State of the Art, Questions, and Controversies,* edited by M. Šzpalski, R. Gunzburg, D. M. Spengler, and A. Nachemson. Lippincott–Raven Publishers, Philadelphia © 1996.

# 25

# Fusion of the Lumbosacral Spine: An Excellent Treatment Option for Selected Patients with a Variety of Spinal Disorders

Dan M. Spengler

*Department of Orthopaedics and Rehabilitation, Vanderbilt University Medical Center, Nashville, Tennessee 37232-2550*

The prevalence of low back pain in the United States has been estimated at almost 50% (2,11,12,18). Over 70 percent of individuals experience a significant acute low back episode at some point during their lifetime (2). In addition, all of us develop various structural changes within our spinal motion segments as we age. Given the astonishing prevalence of symptoms and the universal age-related changes that develop within the spine, it is not surprising that a considerable number of Americans undergo lumbar spinal surgery every year. For example, more than 300,000 lumbar discectomy procedures and 70,000 spinal fusion procedures are performed in the United States on an annual basis (11,16). The techniques used to achieve fusion and to enhance solid fusion have evolved over the years. Selected techniques (e.g., pedicle screw-based constructs) have generated a swirl of controversy, with reputable advocates on both sides. Harrington instrumentation was the most popular and reliable of the early spinal instrumentation techniques. Even Harrington had difficulties in promoting his technique because of objections by a number of critics. Ultimately, the Harrington technique became widely accepted for treatment of patients with spinal deformity and selected patients with spinal fractures. Although the results were largely satisfactory, instrument failure rates were reported that involved between 5 and 20% of the patients (11,18). In addition, when the procedure was performed by surgeons who did not have expertise or knowledge of the basic principles, disastrous outcomes were possible and did occur. Harrington instrumentation was never as successful for lumbar spine disorders because of the problem of flatback with a distraction construct across the lumbar lordotic curve.

Newer modular spinal instrumentation systems have now evolved, most of which are based on a pedicle screw as a primary anchor in the lumbar spine. Such systems, although technically exacting, are highly adaptive to a variety of spinal deformities and other disorders. Improved segmental fixation has been shown to result from these newer spinal systems. Complications have also been recognized (3,7,9,19). In general, the complications are not significantly different from those of older forms of spinal instrumentation when proper surgery is performed by an experienced spinal surgeon. In the United States, the FDA has insisted that the pedicle screw be classified as a type III device, which means that the device is investigational and possibly harmful. It can be hoped that the recent advisory panel recommendation to reclassify these devices to class II, based on a cohort study of 3,500 patients and approximately 300 surgeons, will be persuasive to the full committee of the FDA. Until then, surgeons must inform patients of the FDA position so that the patient is aware of the issues and the decision for surgery reflects an informed consent. This chapter discusses the following disorders, which I believe merit consideration for spinal fusion: degenerative spondylolisthesis, spinal stenosis, scoliosis (deformity), segmental hypermobility (instability), and salvage surgery. Clearly, there is no perfect classification scheme for degenerative disorders. Nevertheless, I have selected the above format to more specifically discuss each of these major conditions. Combinations of abnormalities can often be present, e.g., the patient who has degenerative scoliosis with segmental hypermobility, disc herniation, and stenosis. Such patients are addressed in the scoliosis category because the presence of a spinal deformity will dramatically alter the surgical recommendation.

## INDICATIONS FOR SURGICAL MANAGEMENT

### General Indications

In addition to specific surgical indications, a general overview of a conceptual approach to recommend surgical management for lumbar disorders is presented. This approach is applicable to all patients and will be of practical interest to the reader. All patients who present to my office for evaluation complete a questionnaire that reviews pertinent past medical and important social information. Smoking history, litigation, compensation, medications, and general information are included. A pain drawing and pain intensity rating are also completed by the patient (15). The questionnaire is designed to augment the doctor–patient discussion, not to replace such an interaction. During the interview with the patient, I document previous lumbar problems, being as specific as possible to link symptoms to events. Detailed information is also gathered with regard to previous surgical procedures, especially noting the pain-free interval after previous surgeries. Patients who have experienced no pain-free interval after spinal surgery may well have undergone the wrong procedure, or perhaps the correct procedure at the wrong level. Patients are advised in advance to bring past medical records, including operative reports and various imaging studies. Having as much information as possible available on an initial visit allows more rapid decision analysis and more effective care. For example, additional studies can be ordered if necessary, or a surgical procedure can be scheduled, if appropriate, without waiting for prior information. This also reduces the burden on office personnel who assist our patients: fewer phone calls, letters, and faxes.

The medical history is carefully reviewed with all patients to identify the primary care physician and to note any conditions that need to be further investigated before a major spinal procedure is recommended. Medication use must be reviewed to identify potential problems during anesthesia and/or surgery. For example, steroid use may significantly increase the likelihood for infection and may also require that the patient receive a parenteral dose before surgery. Consumption of large doses of salicylates and/or nonsteroidal anti-inflammatory drugs may also adversely affect perioperative bleeding. Patients who have co-morbid conditions require more precise management by the anesthesiologist and the surgical team during the hospital admission. A more accurate length of stay can also be determined, which is most useful in this day of managed care. For example, if a patient has a history of a major cardiac or pulmonary problem, appropriate consultation is arranged before surgery to anticipate the needs of the anesthesiologist and any other special treatment that may be necessary during hospitalization. Such advance planning will reduce the number of delayed or canceled admissions and lead to more optimal surgical management.

Although a comprehensive physical examination is completed on every patient who is evaluated in the office, I will discuss only general findings here. Specific exam features of the degenerative spinal disorders are addressed within each category. Findings that are important to document include hypertension, chronic lung disease, congestive heart failure, peripheral vascular disease, and neuropathies associated with conditions such as diabetes mellitus.

Finally, I believe that each surgeon must establish a good rapport with the patient. If the surgeon does not feel positive about the doctor–patient relationship, I would suggest not performing a major elective spinal procedure. Such an undertaking requires considerable doctor–patient interaction, as well as patient compliance with surgery and the postoperative rehabilitation protocol. A frank and honest discussion must be held that addresses the risk–benefit ratio of the procedure in question, as well as any important cost issues that might arise. The surgeon must clearly understand and listen to the patient's stated goals and expectations of surgical management. Unrealistic patient expectations can lead to many problems, including litigation! Complications should be discussed in general terms, being specific about the more likely complications associated with the specific procedure. For example, if a patient is to undergo a major spinal instrumentation procedure, the worst-case scenario, other than mortality, should be addressed, i.e., during the placement of the instrumentation, nerves could be injured. Mortality should also be discussed to ensure that the patient understands the significance of the intervention. Models illustrating the specific procedure are very helpful during the preoperative discussion. I also encourage patients to obtain second opinions from other surgeons. I want all of my patients to be confident that the surgery is indeed warranted and that my recommendation is reaffirmed by other surgeons who are not associated with my group. Most spinal procedures are recommended to improve pain and "quality of life." Therefore, there is no need to rush. Reflection and additional discussions are often extremely valuable for both patients and surgeons.

In addition to the doctor–patient discussion, our nurse coordinator spends time with the patient and family to provide additional details regarding the procedure, hospitalization, pain management, and rehabilitation. Details of autologous blood transfusions are also provided by the nurse. Our lengths of stay have been lowered considerably because of the advance preparation of our patients. Such information clearly decreases anxiety and facilitates recovery after surgery.

## Degenerative Spondylolisthesis

This condition is one of the more common and least controversial of the conditions to be discussed. Degenerative spondylolisthesis occurs when one vertebra slips forward on the lower vertebra. The key to this diagnosis, which differentiates this condition from isthmic spondylolisthesis, is that the pars interarticularis remains intact in the degenerative condition. Newman discussed the condition in depth in 1955, although Junghanns had first described the condition as pseudospondylolisthesis in 1931. The back and radicular symptoms that result from this condition arise from a combination of stenosis and instability. Operative intervention becomes reasonable if the patient does not respond to nonoperative management and describes a diminished quality of life. Formerly, controversy existed with regard to the type of surgery recommended for patients with degenerative spondylolisthesis. Previous authors have recommended both decompression alone and decompression with fusion (5). Herkowitz and Kurz (10) have contributed significantly to resolution of this controversy by the publication of their prospective study comparing decompression versus decompression and in situ intertransverse process fusion. Relief of back and leg pain was significantly better in the group of patients who underwent concomitant arthrodesis (10). Controversy still remains, however, regarding the use of instrumentation to achieve a solid arthrodesis. Although additional investigations will be necessary to resolve the instrumentation question, I believe that segmental fixation with the use of pedicle screws does enhance the rate of arthrodesis and facilitates patient recovery (Figs. 1 and 2). Zdeblick (21) has demonstrated a higher fusion rate in patients who underwent spinal fusion procedures augmented with rigid pedicle screw fixation systems. Zdeblick recommended instrumentation in patients who underwent spinal fusion for degenerative spondylolisthesis as well as for those who

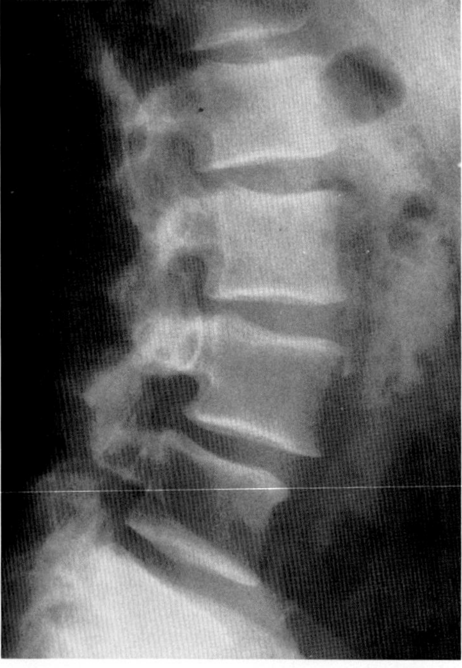

**FIG. 1.** Lateral radiograph of a patient with symptomatic degenerative spondylolisthesis.

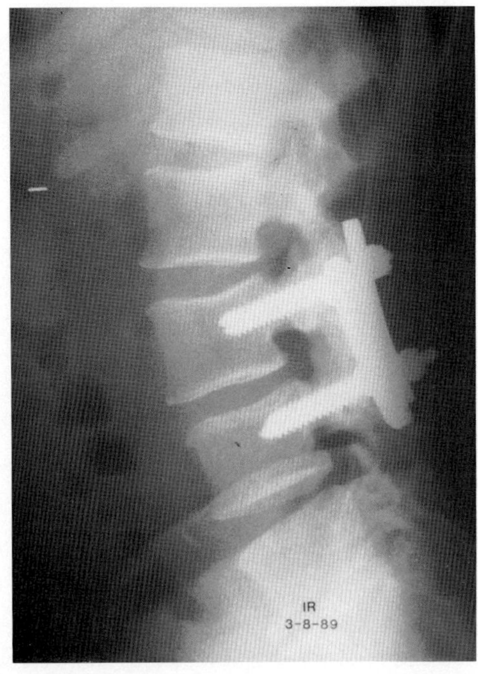


**FIG. 2.** Lateral radiograph of same patient as in Fig. 1 after decompression and posterior lateral fusion with instrumentation.

require revision surgery (21). Although the higher fusion rate is attractive, Herkowitz and Kurz (10) noted that the development of a pseudarthrosis did not preclude a successful result in their patients who underwent intertransverse process arthrodesis. The lack of a single correct recommendation allows the surgeon to individualize the best recommendation for the patient. For example, in a patient with an increased disposition to infection, the surgeon may elect to perform an arthrodesis without instrumentation. In a patient with marked segmental hypermobility on dynamic radiographs, rigid segmental fixation may represent the best approach. The clinical outcome for patients with or without instrumentation ranges from 80 to 96% good to excellent results (1,10,11,13,18,20). These results exclude·patients with degenerative spondylolisthesis who have undergone decompression alone without a concomitant arthrodesis. The specific type of instrumentation to be used in lumbar stabilization procedures should be compatible with the experience of the surgeon. In addition, biomechanical testing studies should be available to document the ability of the construct to withstand physiologic loads and to tolerate reasonable cyclic loading without fatigue failure.

### Lumbar Spinal Stenosis

I will confine this discussion to the most common subset of lumbar spinal stenosis, acquired degenerative lumbar stenosis. This condition is a common cause of low back symptoms, with or without sciatica. Patients with degenerative spinal stenosis are older and have fewer physical findings than patients with lumbar disc herniations. Indeed, most patients with significant stenosis do not exhibit any sciatic tension signs. Decreased sensation and mild weakness of the extensor hallucis longus muscle are common physical findings. Most have increasing pain with walking, which is relieved by resting. Recent studies suggest that the diagnosis of lumbar spinal stenosis can be made when the anteroposterior diameter of the dural sac is 10 mm or less (17). Lateral recess stenosis is present when the recess is 2 mm or less. Although both the MRI scan and the CT myelogram can confirm the diagnosis of stenosis, I prefer to have the CT myelogram available for most patients who elect to have surgery. This technology is changing, however, and MRI alone may well be the only imaging study needed in addition to plain radiographs.

Because patients with degenerative stenosis are usually in an older age range, a thorough evaluation is essential to exclude other causes for low back symptoms, such as tumor and infection (17). In addition, the details of the general patient preoperative assessment discussed earlier must be carefully followed to minimize perioperative risk factors. Because approximately 15% of patients who undergo surgery for spinal stenosis are not improved, the surgeon must have a thorough understanding of the patient's goals and expectations before embarking on a surgical recommendation (17). Unreasonable patient expectations and underlying clinical depression are two common problems that appear to be related to poor outcomes in this patient group.

Once the diagnosis of lumbar spinal stenosis is confirmed, nonoperative treatment can be instituted. Only after failure of an appropriate nonoperative program should surgery be recommended. Nonsteroidal anti-inflammatory drugs or salicylates can be used, although their propensity to cause gastrointestinal bleeding should be borne in mind. I have also been pleased with the results of epidural steroid injections in my patients with underlying spinal stenosis. Clearly, these injections do not alter the space available for the neural elements, but many of my older patients note relief of their symptoms for several months. Once symptom control has been achieved, an aerobic exercise program and trunk-strengthening exercises are initiated. The degree to which such programs are recommended varies according to the goals of the patient and the general medical condition. I must emphasize that the presence of spinal stenosis by itself does not justify surgical intervention. I have followed several patients with high-grade stenosis who continue to enjoy a quality of life that is consistent with their goals and objectives. Surgery should be reserved for the patient who has attempted to improve on a good program but who has an adverse quality of life (8,17).

The specifics of the surgical procedure recommended are determined from the preoperative plain radiographs with lateral flexion–extension films and the MRI and/or CT myelogram. I do not recommend routine spinal fusion unless spinal deformity is present, e.g., scoliosis or spondylolisthesis (5). Fusion should be considered when the preoperative bending films reveal hypermobility of a lumbar motion segment (5). I prefer to see angular motion in excess of 10° or translation in excess of 4 mm. I will also perform a lumbar fusion in any patient in whom the decompression results in the loss of more than one facet joint. In my experience, patients with degenerative lumbar stenosis and a normally aligned spine do not require fusion.

From a technical standpoint, the surgical procedure must include adequate decompression of all involved motion segments and specific foraminotomies of all nerve roots that are involved in either the clinical presentation, weakness on exam, and/or positive electromyography. At the time of surgery, the criteria of MacNab (14) regarding lumbar nerve root mobility are useful. All lumbar roots should be able to be easily displaced 1 cm medially. If not, additional decompression is indicated to achieve this goal. Postoperative management for these patients includes the use of an abdominal binder.

### Degenerative Scoliosis

Patients who have a degenerative spinal deformity in addition to nerve root compression form a subset who are most challenging to manage (4,6,11,20). Almost all of these patients will exhibit evidence of spinal stenosis in addition to the spinal deformity (5). If previous radiographs are available, the progressive nature of the deformity can be appreciated. These patients have symptoms of low back pain, with or without sciatica, which is increased during walking or standing. In the early stages, patients usually note a decrease in their symptoms on sitting or lying supine. The assessment of patients with spinal deformities in addition to nerve root compression is the same as for patients with stenosis. I prefer a CT myelogram in all patients with deformity, since I am better able to interpret these images compared to the MRI. In addition, standing and bending films of the spine are obtained to document the flexibility of the deformity. In my experience, nonoperative treatment approaches are less effective in these patients. Nevertheless, I believe that such strategies should be implemented before a major surgical procedure is recommended. Options for management range from a ''keyhole'' approach for limited decompression without fusion to a major decompression with instrumentation of the entire deformity. Unlike degenerative spondylolisthesis, the ''correct'' surgical approach for patients with spinal deformities remains elusive and awaits further clarification.

In an elderly patient (over the age of 70) with limited goals, focal decompression may be worthwhile to consider. This is especially true when nerve root or cauda equina compression is limited to one motion segment. Patients must understand the objective of this limited approach and should be advised that additional surgery may be necessary if progressive deformity occurs or pain persists. A frank preoperative discussion with the patient to discuss the options and the risk–benefit ratio is particularly useful.

Another option is to perform a limited decompression and a limited fusion, with or without instrumentation. For example, the motion segments at the level of the decompression and the apex of the curve can be stabilized without instrumentation of the entire deformity. This may be an attractive option in a patient with significant co-morbidity factors in whom a more extensive procedure may be life-threatening. This approach can be effective, but sufficient data are not available to totally validate this or any other approach to the patient with lumbar deformity.

The more aggressive option would be to decompress appropriate stenotic segments and also to instrument the entirety of the degenerative curve (Figs. 3 and 4) (4,6). Such approaches must consider both the frontal and the sagittal plane deformity. Although complete correction is not essential, clinical flatback deformities must be avoided. Segmental spinal fixation with rods and pedicle screws offers a reliable construct to stabilize and improve multiplanar deformities (4,6,11,18).

In healthy patients with severe deformities, an anterior approach may be essential to optimize the clinical outcome (4). This procedure is usually combined with a posterior instrumentation at the same time. This combined surgical approach is more commonly required in adult patients with longstanding idiopathic scoliosis, as opposed to patients with degenerative scoliosis acquired as adults.

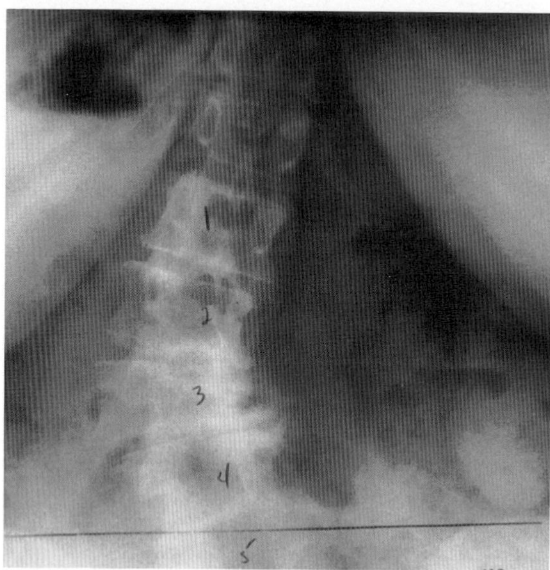

**FIG. 3.** Anteroposterior radiograph of an elderly patient with a symptomatic degenerative scoliosis with stenosis.

## Degenerative Hypermobility (Instability) of the Motion Segment

The instabilities that occur in the functional spinal unit in patients without previous surgery, spondylolisthesis, or deformity are uncommon. Such instabilities are best recognized by a careful assessment of lateral flexion–extension radiographs. Although measurements of translation and angulation of the spinal unit have been criticized, few other strategies exist to objectively document instability. Until predictable and valid techniques that are easy to use in clinical practice are developed, dynamic bending films will probably continue to be used. Angulation over 15° from

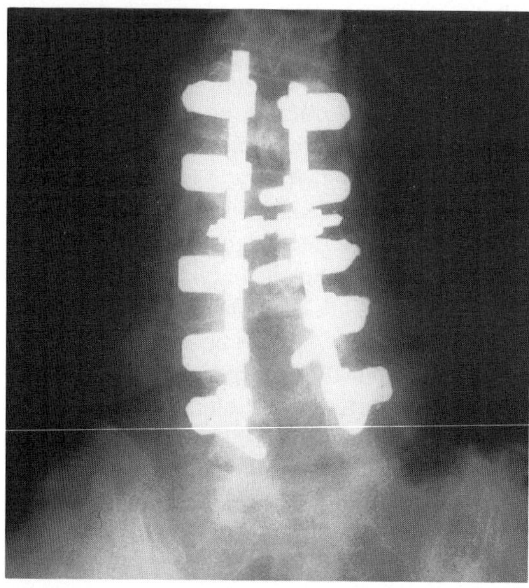

**FIG. 4.** Anteroposterior radiograph of same patient as in Fig. 3 after decompression and an instrumented fusion.

the adjacent disc space or translations in excess of 3 mm have been reported to confirm the diagnosis of segmental instability.

Should clear-cut instability be documented, an evaluation of the spinal canal is required to exclude nerve entrapment or intervertebral disc pathology. Fusion with or without instrumentation can then be recommended, assuming that the spinal canal is clear. Various authors have suggested that posterolateral, posterior lumbar interbody (PLIF), or anterior lumbar interbody fusion (ALIF) be recommended. I prefer the posterolateral intertransverse fusion with instrumentation. I believe that the PLIF has too many potential complications, especially when no reason exists to violate the spinal canal. ALIF is clearly an option, but in men the potential complications that affect sexual function may outweigh any advantages. In situ posterolateral fusion without instrumentation can also be recommended. Nevertheless, Zdeblick (21) has reported a much lower fusion rate in such patients when instrumentation was not used, 45% fusion versus 100% (noninstrumented versus instrumented).

### Revision Surgery of the Lumbar Spine (Salvage)

I will focus this discussion on three common scenarios that are commonly encountered in a clinical spine practice: recurrent disc herniation, postlaminectomy instability, and postfusion instability.

Recurrent disc herniations requiring additional surgery for pain relief occur in approximately 10 to 15% of all patients who undergo primary lumbar disc surgery. In well-selected patients, the reoperation rate should be closer to 2% (17). Multiple recurrences at the same motion segment also occur but are distinctly uncommon. Patients who develop recurrent symptoms after a successful discectomy require careful study to clarify the precise cause of the recurrent symptoms. In my experience, the gadolinium-labeled MRI is the best imaging study to differentiate scar tissue from recurrent disc tissue, because gadolinium creates a tissue enhancement effect that distinguishes scar tissue and disc tissue does not enhance with gadolinium.

When a patient presents with a recurrent disc herniation, nonoperative management is often less effective but worthwhile. Should the patient not improve, a repeat discectomy without spinal fusion is planned unless instability is documented on preoperative radiographs. Should a patient develop more than one recurrence at the same motion segment, I recommend a posterolateral fusion with or without spinal instrumentation, depending on the patient's goals and objectives. I am more inclined to use instrumentation in patients who are older and who have fewer demands. In my experience, the results of patients who have a recurrent disc herniation in the lumbar spine are almost as good as those of patients who undergo a primary lumbar discectomy.

Patients with postlaminectomy instability present with increasing pain complaints involving both the back and the lower extremities (Figs. 5 and 6). Activity aggravates symptoms, and rest decreases the pain. Some patients present shortly after a laminectomy with persistent pain that never responded to treatment, whereas other patients present months to years after an initially successful laminectomy. Careful evaluation is imperative to exclude other causes for referred pain and to exclude recurrent and/or persistent stenosis or disc herniation. Plain radiographs often confirm the diagnosis, especially the flexion–extension views.

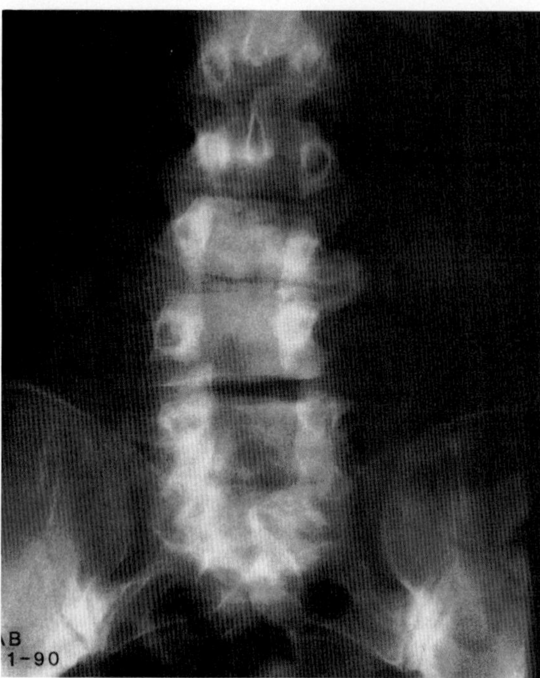

**FIG. 5.** Anteroposterior view of a patient with marked symptoms of instability after an extensive laminectomy.

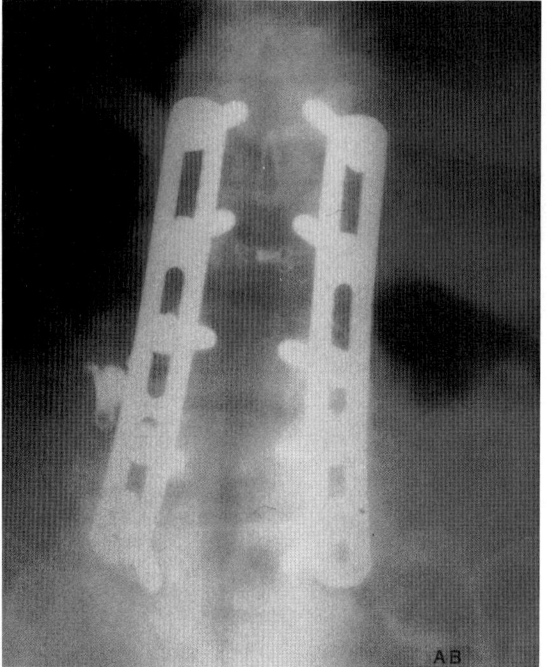

**FIG. 6.** Same patient as in Fig. 5 after VSP plating and posterolateral fusion.

Surgery for this problem should include a posterolateral fusion with instrumentation. In general, a rod construct with pedicle screws works well for patients with multilevel instability after laminectomy. Clinical expectations after major revision surgery are unfortunately less well-documented than surgical results in patients who have been treated primarily. Published complication rates are also higher in this subset of patients, largely due to the altered anatomic landmarks from previous interventions. I believe that intraoperative imaging is useful to reduce malposition of the pedicle screws (Fig. 7). Esses et al. (7) have reported complication rates approaching 50% in patients who underwent revision spinal surgery with the use of pedicle screws.

Patients who exhibit instability after prior surgical fusions present with recurrent back and lower extremity pain symptoms after an interval of pain relief. Although the time elapsed between fusion and subsequent recurrent symptoms is variable, an average time of 2 years is typical. Dynamic bending films and plain radiographs reveal gradual deterioration in the disc above the previous fusion, with or without anterior translation (Figs. 8 and 9). Many of these patients present with rather acute symptoms in spite of the gradual deterioration in the intervertebral disc. These patients do not respond well to nonoperative management, although orthotics and exercise, in addition to mild anti-inflammatory medications, can certainly be tried.

The primary surgical indication revolves around the patient's perceived quality of life (17). Surgical options are best confined to an extension of the instrumentation to include one or two adjacent spinal segments and a posterolateral intertransverse arthrodesis. Decompression may be warranted when the preoperative imaging studies demonstrate significant nerve root compression. Patients with these "transition" syndromes or disc deterioration proximal to a fusion will probably be more commonly encountered because of the increasing number of fusions with spinal instrumentation that are now being performed. Although adjacent segment disc deterioration can occur even in patients with in situ fusions, the rigid instrumentation now being used will most likely accelerate any tendency for this deterioration to occur.

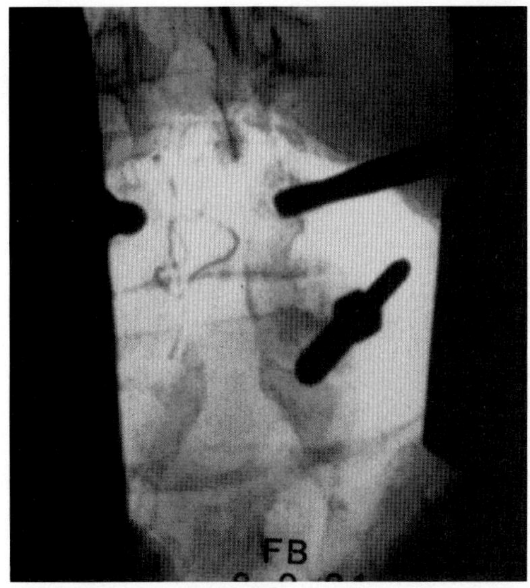

**FIG. 7.** Intraoperative anteroposterior view of pedicle screw insertion during a revision spine procedure. Visualization was excellent.

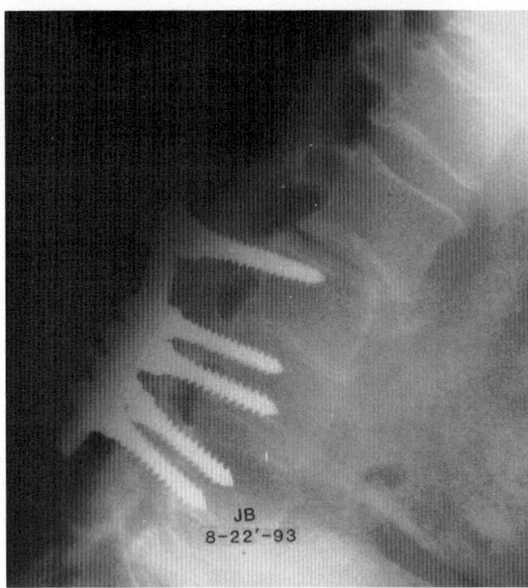

FIG. 8. Lateral radiograph of patient approximately 18 months after successful salvage surgery. Note listhesis above fusion.

During spinal instrumentation procedures, care must be taken to avoid or minimize any injury to the facet joints at the proximal end of the fusion. Although transition syndromes can occur distal to rigid instrumentation in certain patients who have undergone fusions for idiopathic scoliosis, I have not seen a convincing case of this problem occurring at the lumbosacral junction below a floating fusion. If a major decompression is required at the lumbosacral junction, fusion with instrumentation should include this segment.

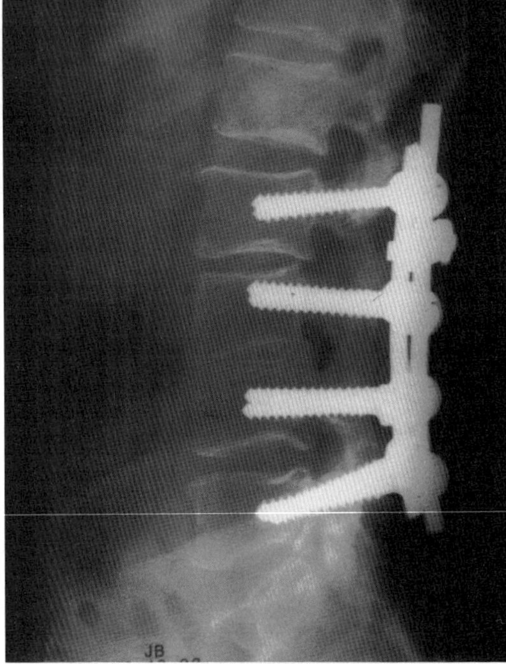

FIG. 9. Lateral radiograph of same patient as in Fig. 8 following reinstrumentation and addition of one cephalad motion segment.

## Complications of Lumbar Spine Surgery

Major spine surgery can be performed in excellent fashion yet complications still occur. The surgeon must anticipate complications and act swiftly to minimize their impact. Naturally, the primary goal is to avoid complications, but realistically, being prepared is good advice. The most dreaded complication, other than mortality, is neurologic worsening after a surgical procedure. If a cauda equina type syndrome occurs gradually or acutely after a spinal procedure, the patient must be promptly evaluated and treated. If an epidural hematoma is suspected, prompt evacuation may result in near-complete resolution of symptoms, although some patients do not recover despite prompt treatment. The decision to proceed directly to the operating room or to first order an imaging study depends on the clinical evaluation at the time of decision analysis. If all of the clinical parameters point to a hematoma, such as a large, swollen wound, prompt evacuation without a study may represent an excellent choice. If any doubt exists, however, a lumbar myelogram with a postmyelogram CT scan should be obtained to confirm the diagnosis. Because MRIs are very difficult for me to interpret during the immediate postoperative period, I prefer the myelogram in this setting. If pedicle screws were used during the procedure and the patient awakens with severe sciatica, a CT scan followed by removal of the offending screw should be planned. Pain will probably be improved by removal of the screw (9).

Wound infections occur more commonly in patients who undergo major spinal instrumentation procedures. Our recent incidence of infection in 100 consecutive patients was 3%, which is higher than we encounter in noninstrumented patients. Preoperative antibiotics and thorough wound debridement with pulse lavage has helped to reduce our rate of infections from an initial high of approximately 10%. When infections are recognized, early aggressive wound debridement and identification of the offending organism represents the best management approach. In general, I prefer not to remove instrumentation until an arthrodesis has been achieved.

Dural tears are often encountered during spinal revision surgery. Most commonly, such tears occur during exposure of the nerve roots or during midline decompression of the cauda equina. Small spicules of bone and/or adhesions between the laminectomy membrane or ligamentum flavum and the dura are usually responsible. Repair with fine nonresorbable suture, with or without a graft, is usually successful. On occasion, no repair is necessary (e.g., if only a small puncture wound is encountered). Patients must be observed for evidence of ongoing drainage. Repeat surgery for a cerebrospinal fluid leak has seldom been required in my experience.

Other complications that should be anticipated include various nerve entrapment syndromes from positioning the patient in the prone position for long procedures. Attention must be paid to the ulnar nerves at the elbow, the brachial plexus, and the lateral femoral cutaneous nerve, to cite the more commonly encountered clinical situations. Fortunately, most but not all of these conditions are transient and improve over time.

Although other complications can be encountered in dealing with these patients (e.g., urinary tract infections, pulmonary problems, cardiovascular conditions), my purpose was to highlight selected complications.

## POSTOPERATIVE MANAGEMENT

Patients who are scheduled for spine surgery are managed by critical care pathways that have been created by physicians working with nurses. The goals for these pathways are to ensure an excellent standard of care and to reduce the length of hospital stay to the minimal number of days consistent with quality outcome. Patients are informed before admission about what will happen on each day of the hospitalization. The tentative date for discharge is also identified. If variances occur, the patient is maintained in the hospital until all potential problem situations are resolved. At present, patients for elective lumbar discectomy are being discharged on the first day after surgery. Patients who have undergone spinal instrumentation and fusion are staying 3 to 4 days. We anticipate that this number will also continue to decrease over time.

Patients who have undergone discectomy or intertransverse process fusions without instrumentation are provided with a lumbar corset for the first month. Patients who have undergone spinal instrumentation procedures are placed in a molded polypropylene orthosis for approximately 2 to 3 months. If the lumbosacral articulation is instrumented, a pantaloon thigh extension is provided for the first 6 weeks. Objectives are to limit patient activity initially and to reduce the chance for implant failure.

Aerobic activity (e.g., walking, bicycling, swimming) is initiated in earnest approximately 4 weeks after discectomy and 8–12 weeks after spinal instrumentation. Trunk flexion–extension exercises using resistive equipment round out the specific back rehabilitation protocol. Patient compliance with the protocol can be monitored by use of a dynamometer. Patients are followed for 12 months after discectomy and for 2 years after an instrumented spine fusion.

An active lifestyle is encouraged, and few restrictions are placed on patients who do not engage in medium or heavy labor. Patients who are gainfully employed in occupations that require heavy lifting are advised to reevaluate their interests and to seek employment that requires less physical effort.

## SUMMARY

I have reviewed the indications and expectations for surgical procedures for the following degenerative conditions that affect the lumbar spine: degenerative spondylolisthesis, stenosis, scoliosis, segmental instability, and revision surgery (salvage). By using appropriate patient selection parameters and exercising good surgical judgement, the surgeon is provided with a basis for use of his or her skill in a positive way to assist the patient with a lumbar spine disorder. Although complications will occur, prompt recognition will facilitate resolution of these problems. Even though many patients will not return to their original jobs, an improved quality of life should result for most patients.

## REFERENCES

1. Bernhardt M, Swartz DE, Clothiaux PL, Crowell RR, White HA. Posterolateral lumbar and lumbosacral fusion with and without pedicle screw internal fixation. *Clin Orthop Relat Res* 1992;284: 109–15.
2. Biering-Sorenson F. Low back trouble in a general population of 30-, 40-, 50-, and 60-year-old men and women. *Dan Med Bull* 1982;29:289–99.
3. Blumenthal S, Gill K. Complications of the Wiltse pedicle screw system. *Spine* 1993;18:1867–71.
4. Boachie-Adjer O, Dendrinos G, Ogilvie JW, Bradford DS. Management of adult spinal deformity with combine anterior-posterior arthrodesis and Luque-Galveston instrumentation. *J Spinal Dis* 1991;4: 131–41.

 5. Bridwell KH, Sedgewick TA, O'Brien MF, et al. Role of fusion and instrumentation in the treatment of degenerative spondylolisthesis with spinal stenosis. *J Spinal Dis* 1993;6:461–72.
 6. Devlin VJ, Boachie-Adjer O, Bradford D, et al. Treatment of adult spinal deformity with fusion to the sacrum using CD instrumentation. *J Spinal Dis* 1991;4:1–14.
 7. Esses SI, Sachs BL, Dreyryin V. Complications associated with the technique of pedicle screw fixation. *Spine* 1993;18:2231–8.
 8. Frymoyer JW. The role of spine fusion. *Spine* 1987;6:284–90.
 9. Gertzbein SD, Robbins SE. Accuracy of pedicular screw placement in vivo. *Spine* 1990;15:11–4.
10. Herkowitz HN, Kurz LT. Degenerative lumbar spondylolisthesis with spinal stenosis. *J Bone Joint Surg* 1991;73A:802–8.
11. Herkowitz HN, Sidhu KS. Lumbar spine fusion in the treatment of degenerative conditions: current indications and recommendations. *J Am Acad Orthop Surg* 1995;3:123–35.
12. Holbrook TL, Grazier K, Kelsey JL, Stauffer RN. *The socioeconomic impact of selected musculoskeletal disorders*. Chicago: American Academy of Orthopedic Surgery, 1984.
13. Lenke LG, Bridwell KH, Bullis D, et al. Results of in situ fusion for isthmic spondylolisthesis. *J Spinal Dis* 1992;5:433–42.
14. MacNab I. Negative disc exploration. *J Bone Joint Surg* 1971;53A:891–903.
15. Ransford AO, Cairns D, Mooney V. The pain drawing as an aid to the psychological evaluation of patients with low back pain. *Spine* 1976;1:127–33.
16. Rutkow IM. Orthopaedic operations in the United States 1979–1983. *J Bone Joint Surg* 1986;68A:716–9.
17. Spengler DM. Degenerative stenosis of the lumbar spine. *J Bone Joint Surg* 1987;69A:305–8.
18. Vaccaro AR, Garfin SR. Pedicle-screw fixation in the lumbar spine. *J Am Acad Orthop Surg* 1995;3:263–74.
19. Weinstein JN, Sprait KF, Spengler D, Brick G. Spinal pedicle fixation. *Spine* 1988;13:1012–8.
20. West JL, Bradford DS, Ogilvie JW. Results of spinal arthrodesis with pedicle screw-plate fixation. *J Bone Joint Surg* 1991;73A:1179–84.
21. Zdeblick TA. A prospective, randomized study of lumbar fusion. Preliminary results. *Spine* 1993;18:983–91.

*Instrumented Fusion of the Degenerative Lumbar Spine: State of the Art, Questions, and Controversies*, edited by M. Szpalski, R. Gunzburg, D. M. Spengler, and A. Nachemson. Lippincott–Raven Publishers, Philadelphia © 1996.

# 26

# Instrumented Fusion of The Lumbar Spine For Degenerative Disorders: A Critical Look

Alf L. Nachemson

*Department of Orthopaedics, Göteborg University, Sahlgren Hospital, S-413 45 Göteborg, Sweden*

This critique concentrates on instrumented lumbar fusion operations in the so-called degenerative disorders. In my view, there is little, if any, support for such procedures in patients with chronic low back pain alone. Even for those with low back pain and leg pain, the support for instrumented fusion is indeed meager, despite the efforts made by the authors of the preceding chapters and several publications during the past 3 years (1,18,38,48,77,90,93,116,136,149). My doubts have been reinforced by the contributions from the biostatistician (96) and the radiologists (112) in the preceding chapters.

## CAN THE PAINFUL DISC BE DIAGNOSED AND FUSION RESULTS PREDICTED?

With the exception of the diagnoses of disc hernia and spinal stenosis, very few studies have validated preoperative diagnostic testing to determine the source of chronic low back pain or to predict the outcome of fusion in patients with degenerative disc disorders (Table 1). Discography was found to be of no value in the study by Esses et al. (39), who found some information to be gained from external fixators, alternatively fixed or loosened with the patient blinded. Their findings were corroborated by Ordeberg et al. (111) but not by Soini et al. (127). All of these authors found the method to pose considerable risk.

Although most of us believe that the lumbar disc may be the source of low back pain in many patients, ultimate proof of this does not exist (11,22,55). Studies by Kuslich et al. (80) certainly confirmed previous observation by British researchers (126) that one-third of patients with sciatica who had nerve roots painful on touch also had pain in the posterior annulus. Perhaps in the future these patients with painful annula can be identified by some valid preoperative test. To ascertain the validity of any such tests, including discography, prospective randomized trials must

**TABLE 1.** *Predictive value of some preoperative diagnostic tests for clinical outcomes of spinal fusion in patients with chronic nonspecific low back (±leg) pain*

|  | Prospective studies | Retrospective studies |
| --- | --- | --- |
| X-ray, with flexion–extension views, MRI, CT | Neg (70,76,130) | Neg (6,52,69,102) |
| Brace, corset | Neg (3) | |
| Cast (one leg included) | Pos (29) | |
| Facet blocks | | Neg (41,67) |
| Discography | Neg (39) | Neg (9,46,65,68,107,119) |
| External transpedicle fixator | Pos (39,111) | Neg (127) |
| Psychosocial testing | Pos (15,59,128,141) | Pos (16,54,139) |
| Nerve root blocks (only when root canal stenosis is suspected) | Pos (137) | |

be performed in which the decision to fuse a supposedly painful lumbar segment is made regardless of the outcome of the diagnostic study (19,98,101,145,148). Thus far, only negative results exist regarding ordinary x-rays (6,52,53,76,102,130,143), including flexion–extension views, preoperative brace test (2,3), facet blocks (41,67), MRI studies (15,69,70), and discography (9,46,65,107,119). The study of Colhoun et al. (28) cannot be regarded as proof because the authors switched categories after randomization and had an incomplete follow-up. Hess et al. (65), in a large retrospective study, found no supporting evidence for discography, and Esses et al. (39) refuted this diagnostic procedure in a prospective trial.

We simply do not know the origin of low back pain and we have difficulty in pinpointing its exact cause in each individual patient (12,13,63,66,122). Modern pain research has clearly demonstrated that, in chronic pain patients, sensitized cells of the cord can themselves generate pain from minor nociception arising anywhere in the lumbar motion segment. Nociceptive impulses can arise from the outer part of the disc, from the ligaments, from the facet joints, from the muscles, and perhaps also from the vertebrae (7), since they have recently been shown to possess substance P-reactive nerve endings. Previously sensitized NMDA receptors in the cord often exist in patients with chronic pain syndromes, further complicating our ability to pinpoint the origin of nociception (144).

On the other hand, we are much better at understanding and diagnosing the psychosocial factors that influence both individual success and return to work after fusion operations, as well as other treatment modalities for chronic back pain (15,16,20,54,59,61,78,79,109,113,114,125,138–142). The predictive value of these factors is of such clear importance and emanates from such a large body of information that psychosocial evaluations should be the first evaluations performed by spine surgeons contemplating operations in patients with back and leg pain of uncertain origin. In addition, such evaluations probably should also be performed in patients with low back and leg pain caused by disc herniation (15,128), spinal and/or root canal stenosis, and spondylolisthesis, if no "red flags" (6) are present.

## YELLOW FLAG EXAMINATIONS

A patient's health beliefs, coping abilities, work and social environment, and insurance coverage all influence the success or failure of any treatment for low back pain. In taking the history, spine surgeons must elucidate not only the extent of the pain but also the "yellow flags" that indicate distress and illness behavior (Table 2).

**TABLE 2.** *Psychosocial "yellow flag" history points of predictive value for results of both conservative and operative treatment in patients with subacute or chronic low back pain*

| Major points | Minor points |
| --- | --- |
| Poor health beliefs | Sleep disturbance |
| Never pain free | Hopelessness |
| Fear of activity/moving | Living alone |
| Previous long disability from low back pain | Very supportive spouse |
| Frequent emergency treatments | Heavy smoking |
| Whole body part numbness | Drug abuse |
| Whole extremity giving way | Job dissatisfaction |
| | Job changes |
| | Fear of lay-off |
| | Employer blame |
| | Legal involvement |
| | Poor sex life |

From refs. 15,16,20,54,57–59,61,78,79,109,113,114,125,138–142.

Their validity in predicting the outcome of surgery has repeatedly been proven (15,57–59,128,139,142), unlike most other preoperative tests in common use.

The examination must include a pain drawing that can be evaluated for symptom magnification (109), the Waddell tests (138–142), and the UAB pain behavior rating scale (78,110) for illness behavior. In most cases, high scores on these tests predict unsuccessful surgical outcomes, even for sciatica caused by disc herniation (128). These results demonstrate the importance of central influences on the expression of subjective pain and their effects on the pain gates in the cord (147).

Further diagnostic studies should be performed only if psychosocial deterrents to a good outcome are minor. In such instances, studies such as double-blind facet blocks (122), nerve root blocks (137), external fixators (39), plaster casts (29), or stereophotogrammetric evaluation (3,123,131) can be used according to the surgeon's belief of the origin of the pain.

## BONY HEALING AFTER FUSION

Many studies have underscored the difficulties of evaluating the occurrence of bony fusion (76,112). At present, only two reliable methods are available: exploration and visual examination of the fusion mass, which is expensive and not usually performed except in patients with persisting pain, and stereophotogrammetry (3,4, 75,123,131). This last method, which has been used in several studies, including one that examined Steffee plate fusions (131), involves the insertion of three small 0.8-mm diameter tantalum ball bearings in each of the vertebrae included in the fusion for later exact x-ray evaluation of mobility. It is my conviction that this should be a routine procedure in all fusion operations. It is the only way, short of reexploration, by which we later can evaluate whether we obtained a good fusion or, if pain recurs, whether a pseudarthrosis could possibly be the cause of pain.

## RESULTS OF INSTRUMENTED FUSION OPERATION

No good clinical studies exist (8,134,135) that demonstrate satisfactory outcomes of fusion operations performed for disc degeneration presumed to cause low back pain, at least not in the industrialized world in which liberal insurance systems exist (16,49,104,151). The few existing small, randomized, controlled trials (60,99) (RCTs) do not indicate that adding pedicular screws to these operations enhances results. The Zedeblick study (150) was invalidated by several factors: various diagnoses of patients, changes of group allotment after randomization, personal follow-up by treating physician [biased follow-up (120)], and too short a follow-up period. This is true also for many nonrandomized follow-up studies in this book and elsewhere (88,132,146). Even in spinal stenosis, in which fusion may be indicated (44) after total laminectomy and facetectomy to retain disc height, if still preserved at the stenosed level, the two existing randomized trials (60,64) do not favor pedicle screws, nor do many retrospective studies (5,25,72–74,151). Nevertheless, it is likely that their introduction into this area of "degenerative disc diseases" forms the basis for the increase of the overall fusion rates in many industrialized countries (24,32) (Fig. 1).

The use of pedicle screws has created a lively debate in spine surgery circles, as mentioned above. Some mechanical advantages of their use have been demonstrated in certain unstable vertebral fracture (37,95,97) that are beyond the scope of this review. However, pedicle screws have also been associated with nerve damage, vascular injuries, dural tears, and an increased rate of surgical removal. Overall, the rates of these and other complications are between 20 and 25% (10,14,33,36,40,43, 84,91,108). In response to the risks involved in the placement of pedicle screws, very expensive computer-assisted intraoperative systems are now marketed (105), possibly adding further to the astronomical costs of this uncertain area of spine surgery. Other methods for avoidance of severe nerve root complications have also been described (21,27,42,83,89,133). Fusion operations by any method are also followed by increased stresses on adjacent segments that later enhance degenerative changes of aging (82,147).

It appears strange that more than 100 pedicle screw systems are now marketed without any true scientific proof of their benefit in degenerative spinal disorders. The FDA in the United States (48) is also considering releasing these systems for some of these disorders, based on a retrospective, not unbiased, case series by members of the North American Spine Society, who contributed their own cases, followed nonsystematically by the surgeons themselves (149).

New technology, such as pedicle screws and plates, always excites surgeons. Early enthusiastic reports by the inventors of any new method in medicine usually demonstrate better than 90% success rates. These are usually followed by controlled

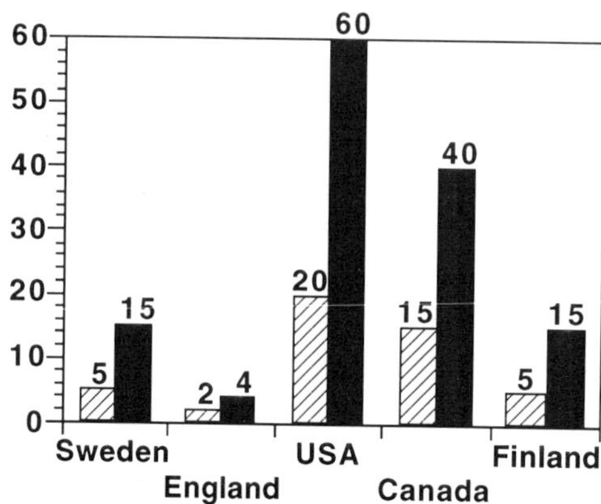

FIG. 1. Rate of lumbar fusion (number per 100,000 population) in some countries, 1989 □ and 1994 ■.

case series, performed by others, that show 60 to 70% good results. Thereafter, prospective clinical cohort studies often end up showing that only 50% of patients treated with the new methods have excellent or good results. Finally, the larger RCTs may show that only 30 to 40% of patients achieve good outcomes. A case in point is automated percutaneous lumbar discectomy, which still is marketed and is used on thousands of patients around the world, despite the poor results reported (23,34,118,129).

Unfortunately, many extensive conservative treatment programs for chronic low back pain patients have also failed to demonstrate clinical efficacy or societal effectiveness (30,35,45). Such programs usually demonstrate a 60% success rate (92), but these treatments have the advantage of avoiding severe complications and risks for repeated surgery. If such more elaborate nonoperative exercise programs are applied to patients with subacute back pain, both efficacy and effectiveness can be demonstrated (85,86).

## INSTABILITY

Instability is difficult to diagnosis by noninvasive methods (31,52,53,102,130). It can be suspected in spondylolisthesis in the younger (below the age of 40) population. There is some evidence that patients with spondylolisthesis who have back and leg pain benefit from fusion operations (17,47,51,52,71,115). But, again, there is not support from scientifically admissible studies (RCTs) that addition of pedicle screws enhances the results (94,99).

## FAILED BACK SURGERY

Repeat surgeries, except for patients with a new disc herniation after a 1-year period of freedom from pain after the first surgery (103,124), should be abandoned. Poor results are repeatedly reported in the literature, with the majority of patients having either the same or worse results than they had before the repeat surgery (81,87,106,138,146). "You can't unscrew what was screwed up by screwing it again," as I heard one failed back surgery patient say. In fairness, the patient should be aware that the chance of success with a new surgical attempt is less than 50% and that there is a 20 to 30% risk of worsening and a 20 to 25% complication rate.

Surgeons must pay more attention to pain behavior, as elucidated by the "yellow flag" history (see Table 2) and perform examinations to detect illness behavior which, when present to a significant degree, precludes good result from fusion surgery in so-called degenerative disc disorders for primary and particularly for repeated fusion operations.

## ACTIONS FOR THE FUTURE

With spiraling health care costs in many industrialized nations and increasing budget deficiencies, politicians and insurers are trying to find ways to diminish overall health care expenses while at the same time maintaining or even improving the quality of care. This necessitates careful evaluation of different methods of treatment in all fields, including orthopedics (8,56,103,104,117,121).

Attempts by government organizations to evaluate the effectiveness of treatments for back pain have resulted in the so-called clinical guidelines that have been developed in several countries since 1987 (6,26,62,100,103). A more ambitious project has been initiated by the Cochrane Collaboration (50), which is attempting to compile all available randomized controlled trials in all areas of medicine and surgery and then to evaluate treatment effectiveness by meta-analytical methods. This process will take some years, but when it is completed it will offer physicians and politicians on-line access to valuable data.

In the future, spine surgeons will compete for resources with knee and hip replacement surgeons, who have already demonstrated effectiveness through good outcome studies. As stated previously, there is at present no scientific evidence for benefit of spine fusion in so-called degenerative disc disease, and even less a case for expensive instrumentation. A few exceptions have been mentioned in this text, e.g., some operations for spondylolisthesis and spinal stenosis.

It must be emphasized that the cost of good clinical research in this area is indeed small compared to the price of patients' suffering and the societal costs of inefficient care and disability. While we await the results of the randomized controlled studies that are now under way in some countries, we should, as spine surgeons, refrain from the use of instrumented spine fusions in patients with chronic low back pain presumably due to some poorly defined degenerative disorder.

## REFERENCES


1. Anderson GBJ, Weinstein JN. Introduction to focus issue on fusion. *Spine* 1995;205:75–6.
2. Axelsson P, Johnsson R, Strömqvist B. Effect of lumbar orthosis on intervertebral mobility. A roentgen stereophotogrammetric analysis. *Spine* 1992;17:678–81.
3. Axelsson P, Johnsson R, Strömqvist B, Nilsson LT, Akesson M. Orthosis as prognostic instrument in lumbar fusion: no predictive value in 50 cases followed prospectively. *J Spinal Dis* 1995;8:284–8.
4. Axelsson P, Johnsson R, Strömqvist B. Mechanics of the external fixation test in the lumbar spine. A roentgen stereophotogrammetric analysis. *Spine* [*in press*].
5. Bernhardt M, Swartz DE, Clothiaux PL, Crowell RR, White AA. Posterolateral lumbar and lumbosacral fusion with and without pedicle screw internal fixation. *Clin Orthop* 1992;284:109–15.
6. Bigos S, Bowyer O, Braen G, et al. *Acute low back problems in adults. Clinical practice guideline No 14.* AHCPR Publication No 95-0642. Rockville, MD. Agency for Health Care Policy and Research, Public Health Service, US Department of Health and Human Services, December 1994.
7. Bjurholm A, Kreicbergs A, Brodin E, Schultzberg M. Substance P- and CGRP-immunoreactive nerves in bone. *Peptides* 1988;9:165–71.
8. Bloch R. Methodology of clinical back pain trials. *Spine* 1987;12:430–2.
9. Block AR, Guyer RD, Hochschuler SH, Ohnmeiss DD, Vanharanta H. Discographic pain report: influence of psychological factors. *Spine* 1996;21:334–8.
10. Blumenthal S, Gill K. Complications of the Wiltse pedicle screw fixation system. *Spine* 1993;18:1867–71.
11. Bogduk N. The sources of low back pain. In: Jayson MIV, ed. *The lumbar spine and back pain.* 4th ed. Edinburgh: Churchill Livingstone, 1992:61–88.
12. Bogduk N. Focus article: diskography. *APS J* 1994;3:149–54.
13. Bogduk N. Rebuttal [Reply]. *APS J* 1994;3:166–7.
14. Boos N, Marchesi D, Aebi M. Survivorship analysis of pedicular fixation systems in the treatment of degenerative disorders of the lumbar spine: a comparison of Cotrel-Dubousset instrumentation and the AO internal fixator. *J Spinal Dis* 1992;5:403–9.
15. Boos N, Rieder R, Schade V, Spratt KF, Semmer N, Aebi M. The diagnostic accuracy of MRI, work perception and psychosocial factors in identifying symptomatic disc herniations. *Spine* 1995;24:2613–25.
16. Bosacco SJ, Berman AT, Bosacco DN, Levenberg RJ. Results of lumbar disk surgery in a city compensation population. *Orthopedics* 1995;18:351–5.
17. Bradford DS, Boachie-Adjei O. Treatment of severe spondylolisthesis by anterior and posterior reduction and stabilization. A long-term follow-up study. *J Bone Joint Surg* 1990;72-A:1060–6.
18. Brantigan JW. A surgeon's perspective of medical device regulation. *J Spinal Dis* 1995;8:396–412.

19. Burchiel KJ, Frank EH, Keenen TL. A plea for prospective studies on diskography [Commentary]. *APS J* 1994;3:160–2.
20. Burton AK, Tillotson KM, Main CJ, Hollis S. Psychosocial predictors of outcome in acute and subchronic low back trouble. *Spine* 1995;20:722–8.
21. Calancie B, Madsen P, Lebwohl N. Stimulus-evoked EMG monitoring during transpedicular lumbosacral spine instrumentation: initial clinical results. *Spine* 1994;19:2780–6.
22. Campbell JN, Belzberg AJ. Use of disk distension to diagnose pain of spinal origin [Commentary]. *APS J* 1994;3:157–9.
23. Chatterjee S, Foy PM, Findlay GF. Report of a controlled clinical trial comparing automated percutaneous lumbar discectomy and microdiscectomy in the treatment of contained lumbar disc herniation. *Spine* 1995;20:734–8.
24. Cherkin DC, Deyo RA, Loeser JD, Bush T, Waddell G. An international comparison of back surgery rates. *Spine* 1994;19:1201–6.
25. Cinotti G, Spratt KF, Weinstein JN. Instrumented and non-instrumented fusion. A minimum 5-year follow up. Presented at the 6th annual meeting of the European Spine Society, Noordwijk aan Zee, The Netherlands, Sept. 14–16, 1995.
26. Clinical Standards Advisory Group. Back pain. Report of a CSAG Committee on Back Pain. Chaired by Michael Rosen. London: HMSO, May 1994.
27. Coe JD, Warden KE, Herzig MA, McAfee PC. Influence of bone mineral density on the fixation of thoracolumbar implants: a comparative study of transpedicular screws, laminar hooks, and spinous process wires. *Spine* 1990;15:902–7.
28. Colhoun E, McCall IW, Williams L, Cassar Pullicino VN. Provocation discography as a guide to planning operations on the spine. *J Bone Joint Surg* 1988;70-B:267–71.
29. Curcin A, Rosenthal MS. Cast immobilization of the lumbar spine predicts symtomatic outcome of fusion surgery [Abstract]. *Proc Am Acad Orthop Surg* 1996:216.
30. Cutler RB, Fishbain DA, Rosomoff HL, Abdel-Moty E, Khalil TM, Steele-Rosomoff R. Does nonsurgical pain center treatment of chronic pain return patients to work? A review and meta-analysis of the literature. *Spine* 1994;19:643–52.
31. Danielson B, Frennered K, Selvik G, Irstam L. Roentgenologic assessment of spondylolisthesis. II. An evaluation of progression. *Acta Radiol* 1989;30:65–8.
32. Davies H. Increasing rates of cervical and lumbar spine surgery in the United States, 1979–1990. *Spine* 1994;19:1117–24.
33. Davne SH, Myers DL. Complications of lumbar spinal fusion with transpedicular instrumentation. *Spine* 1992;17(suppl 6S):S184–9.
34. Delamarter RB, Howard MW, Goldstein T, Deutsch AL, Mink JH, Dawson EG. Percutaneous lumbar discectomy. Preoperative and postoperative magnetic resonance imaging. *J Bone Joint Surg* 1995;77-A:578–84.
35. Deyo RA, Cherkin D, Conrad D, Volinn E. Cost, controversy, crisis: low back pain and the health of the public. *Annu Rev Public Health* 1991;12:141–56.
36. Deyo RA, Cherkin DC, Loeser JD, Bigos SJ, Ciol MA. Morbidity and mortality in association with operations on the lumbar spine. The influence of age, diagnosis and procedure. *J Bone Joint Surg* 1992;74-A:536–43.
37. Dickman CA, Yahiro MA, Lu HTC, Melkerson MN. Surgical treatment alternatives for fixation of unstable fractures of the thoracic and lumbar spine: a meta-analysis. *Spine* 1994;19(Suppl 20S):2266S–73S.
38. Ducker TB. Spinal implants [Editorial]. *J Spinal Dis* 1995;8:395.
39. Esses SI, Botsford DJ, Kostuik JP. The role of external spinal skeletal fixation in the assessment of low back disorders. *Spine* 1989;14:594–601.
40. Esses SI, Sachs BL, Dreyzin V. Complications associated with the technique of pedicle screw fixation: a selected survey of ABS members. *Spine* 1993;18:2231–9.
41. Esses SI, Moro JK. The value of facet blocks in patient selection for lumbar fusion. *Spine* 1993;18:185–90.
42. Farber GL, Place HM, Mazur RA, Jones DEC, Damiano TR. Accuracy of pedicle screw placement in lumbar fusions by plain radiographs and computed tomography. *Spine* 1995;20:1494–9.
43. Farcy JPC, Rawlins BA, Glassman SD. Technique and results of fixation to the sacrum with iliosacral screws. *Spine* 1992;17(suppl 6S):S190–5.
44. Feffer HL, Wiesel SW, Cuckler JM, Rothman RH. Degenerative spondylolisthesis: to fuse or not to fuse. *Spine* 1985;10:287–9.
45. Flor H, Fydrich T, Turk DC. Efficacy of multidisciplinary pain treatment centers: a meta-analytic review. *Pain* 1992;49:221–30.
46. Fluke MM. Letter to the editor. *Spine* 1995;20:501–4.
47. Flynn JC, Hoque MA. Anterior fusion of the lumbar spine. End-result study with long-term follow-up. *J Bone Joint Surg* 1979;61-A:1143–50.
48. Food and Drug Administration, Department of Health and Human Services. Orthopedic devices:

classification, reclassification, and codification of pedicle screw spinal systems. *Fed Reg* 1995;60: 51946–62.

49. Franklin GM, Haug J, Heyer NJ, McKeefrey SP, Picciano JF. Outcome of lumbar fusion in Washington State workers' compensations. *Spine* 1994;19:1897–904.

50. Freemantle N, Grilli R, Grimshaw, Oxman A. Implementing findings of medical research: the Cochrane Colloboration on Effective Professional Practice. *Qual Health Care* 1995;4:45–7.

51. Frennered AK, Danielson BI, Nachemson AL, Nordwall AB. Midterm follow-up of young patients fused in situ for spondylolisthesis. *Spine* 1991;16:409–16.

52. Frennered K. Symptomatic lumbar spondylolisthesis in young patients. A clinical and radiological follow-up after non-operative and operative treatment [Thesis]. Göteborg University, Sweden, 1991.

53. Friberg O. Lumbar instability: a dynamic approach by traction-compression radiography. *Spine* 1987;12:119–29.

54. Frymoyer JW. Predicting disability from low back pain. *Clin Orthop* 1992;279:101–9.

55. Frymoyer JW. Quality: an international challenge to the diagnosis and treatment of disorders of the lumbar spine. *Spine* 1993;18:2147–52.

56. Gartland JJ. Orthopaedic clinical research. Deficiencies in experimental design and determination of outcome. *J Bone Joint Surg* 1988;70-A:1357–63.

57. Greenough CG, Fraser RD. The effects of compensation on recovery from low-back injury. *Spine* 1989;14:947–55.

58. Greenough CG, Taylor LJ, Fraser RD. Anterior lumbar fusion. A comparison of noncompensation patients with compensation patients. *Clin Orthop* 1994;300:30–7.

59. Greenough CG. Outcome assessment of lumbar spinal fusion. In: Szpalski M, Gunzberg R, Spengler DM, Nachemson A, eds. *Instrumented fusion of the degenerative lumbar spine: state of the art, questions, and controversies.* New York: Lippincott-Raven Publishers, 1996:45–54 (this volume).

60. Grob D, Humke T, Dvorak J. Degenerative lumbar spinal stenosis. Decompression with and without arthrodesis. *J Bone Joint Surg* 1995;77-A:1036–41.

61. Guest GH, Drummond PD. Clinical section. Effect of compensation on emotional state and disability in chronic back pain. *Pain* 1992;48:125–32.

62. *Guidelines for the management of back-injured employees.* Workover Corporation, South Australia, October 1993.

63. Heggeness MH, Doherty BJ. Discography causes end plate deflection. *Spine* 1993;18:1050–3.

64. Herkowitz HN, Kurz LT. Degenerative lumbar spondylolisthesis with spinal stenosis. A prospective study comparing decompression with decompression and intertransverse process arthrodesis. *J Bone Joint Surg* 1991;73-A:802–8.

65. Hess WF, Jackson RP, Ebelke DK, Crawley SA, Arnett KW. Pain response by discography as a predictor of clinical outcome in patients with solid posterolateral lumbosacral fusion. Presented at the 27th annual meeting of the Scoliosis Research Society, Kansas City, MO, 1992.

66. Hirsch C, Ingelmark B-E, Miller M. The anatomical basis for low back pain: studies on the presence of sensory nerve endings in ligamentous, capsular and intervertebral disc structures in the human lumbar spine. *Acta Orthop Scand* 1963;33:1–17.

67. Jackson RP, Cain JE Jr, Jacobs RR, Cooper BR, McManus GE. The neuroradiographic diagnosis of lumbar herniated nucleus pulposus: I. A comparison of computed tomography (CT), myelography, CT-myelography, discography, and CT-discography. *Spine* 1989;14:1356–61.

68. Jackson RP, Cain JE Jr, Jacobs RR, Cooper BR, McManus GE. The neuroradiographic diagnosis of lumbar herniated nucleus pulposus: II. A comparison of computed tomography (CT), myelography, CT-myelography, and magnetic resonance imaging. *Spine* 1989;14:1362–7.

69. Jackson RP, Jacobs RR, Montesano PX. Facet joint injection in low-back pain. A prospective statistical study. *Spine* 1988;13:966–71.

70. Jensen MC, Brant-Zawadzki MN, Obuchowski N, Modic MT, Malkasian D, Ross JS. Magnetic resonance imaging of the lumbar spine in people without back pain. *N Engl J Med* 1994;331:69–73.

71. Johnson JR, Kirwan EO. The long-term results of fusion in situ for severe spondylolisthesis. *J Bone Joint Surg* 1983;65-B:43–6.

72. Johnsson KE. Lumbar spinal stenosis. A retrospective study of 163 cases in southern Sweden. *Acta Orthop Scand* 1995;66:403–5.

73. Johnsson KE, Willner S, Johnsson K. Postoperative instability after decompression for lumbar spinal stenosis. *Spine* 1986;11:107–10.

74. Johnsson KE, Rosén J, Udé A. The natural course of lumbar spinal stenosis. *Clin Orthop* 1992;279: 82–6.

75. Johnsson R, Selvik G, Strömqvist B, Sundén G. Mobility of the lower lumbar spine after posterolateral fusion determined by roentgen stereophotogrammetric analysis. *Spine* 1990;15:347–50.

76. Kant AP, Daum WJ, Dean SM, Uchida T. Evaluation of lumbar spine fusion. Plain radiographs versus direct surgical exploration and observation. *Spine* 1995;20:2313–7.

77. Katz JN, Spratt KF, Andersson GBJ, et al. Epidemiology introduction: 1995 focus issue meeting on fusion [Editorial]. *Spine* 1995;20(suppl 24S):76S–7S.

78. Keefe FJ, Block AR. Development of an observation method for assessing pain behavior in chronic low back pain patients. *Behav Ther* 1982;13:363–75.
79. Klenerman L, Slade PD, Stanley IM, et al. The prediction of chronicity in patients with an acute attack of low back pain in a general practice setting. *Spine* 1995;20:478–84.
80. Kuslich SD, Ulstrom CL, Michael CJ. The tissue origin of low back pain and sciatica: a report of pain response to tissue stimulation during operations on the lumbar spine using local anesthesia. *Orthop Clin North Am* 1993;22:181–7.
81. Lauerman WC, Bradford DS, Ogilvie JW, Transfeldt EE. Results of lumbar pseudarthrosis repair. *J Spinal Dis* 1992;5:149–57.
82. Lehmann TR, Spratt KF, Tozzi JE, et al. Long-term follow-up of lower lumbar fusion patients. *Spine* 1987;12:97–104.
83. Lenke LG, Padberg AM, Russo MH, Bridwell KH, Gelb DE. Triggered electromyographic threshold for accuracy of pedicle screw placement: an animal model and clinical correlation. *Spine* 1995; 20:1585–91.
84. Licht NJ, Rowe DE, Ross LM. Pitfalls of pedicle screw fixation in the sacrum: a cadaver model. *Spine* 1992;17:892–6.
85. Lindstrom I. Back health clinic in the community. A prospective cohort study with controls. Personal communication, 1995.
86. Lindström I, Öhlund C, Eek C, et al. Mobility, strength and fitness after a graded activity program for patients with subacute low back pain. *Spine* 1992;17:641–52.
87 Long DM, Filtzer DL, BenDebba M, Hendler NH. Clinical features of the failed back syndrome. *J Neurosurg* 1988;69:61–71.
88. Lorenz M, Zindrick M, Schwaegler P, et al. A comparison of single-level fusions with and without hardware. *Spine* 1991;16(suppl 8S):S455–8.
89. Maguire J, Wallace S, Madiga R, Leppanen R, Draper V. Evaluation of intrapedicular screw position using intraoperative evoked electromyography. *Spine* 1995;20:1068–74.
90. Mardjetko SM, Connolly PJ, Shott S. Degenerative lumbar spondylolisthesis: a meta-analysis of literature 1970–1993. *Spine* 1994;19(suppl 20S):2256S–65S.
91. Matsuzaki H, Tokuhashi Y, Matsumoto F, Hoshino M, Kiuchi T, Toriyama S. Problems and solutions of pedicle screw plate fixation of lumbar spine. *Spine* 1990;15:1159–65.
92. Mayer TG, Gatchel RJ, Mayer H, Kishino ND, Keeley J, Mooney V. A prospective two year study of functional resoration in industrial low back injury. An objective assessment procedure. *JAMA* 1987;258:1763–7.
93. McAfee PC, Weiland DJ, Carlow JJ. Survivorship analysis of pedicle spinal instrumentation. *Spine* 1991;16(suppl 8S):S422–7.
94. McGuire RA, Amundson GM. The use of primary internal fixation in spondyolisthesis. *Spine* 1993; 18:1662–72.
95. McLain RF, Sparling E, Benson DR. Early failure of short-segment pedicle instrumentation for thoracolumbar fractures. *J Bone Joint Surg* 1993;75-A:162–7.
96. Mélot C. Clinical studies of surgical results: methodological and statistical criteria of validity. In: Szpalski M, Gunzburg R, Spengler DM, Nachemson A, eds. *Instrumented fusion of the degenerative lumbar spine: state of the art, questions, and controversies.* New York: Lippincott-Raven Publishers, 1996:281–9 (this volume).
97. Mick CA, Carl A, Sachs B, Hresko MT, Pfeifer BA. Burst fractures of the fifth lumbar vertebra. *Spine* 1993;18:1878–84.
98. Modic MT. Controversy lumbar discography. *Spine* 1996;21:403–4.
99. Möller H, Hedlund R. Fusion or conservative treatment in adult spondylolisthesis—a prospective randomised study. *Acta Orthop Scand* 1994;65(suppl 260):12.
100. Nachemson A with Spitzer WO, et al. Scientific approach to the assessment and management of activity-related spinal disorders. A monograph of clinicians. Report of the Quebec Task Force on Spinal Disorders. *Spine* 1987;12(suppl 1):S1–S59.
101. Nachemson A. Editorical comment. Lumbar discography—where are we today? *Spine* 1987;14: 555–7.
102. Nachemson AL. Instability of the lumbar spine. Pathology, treatment, and clinical evaluation. *Neurosurg Clin North Am* 1991;2:785–90.
103. Nachemson AL. Newest knowledge of low back pain. A critical look. *Clin Orthop* 1992;279:8–20.
104. Nachemson A. Chronic pain—the end of the welfare state. *Qual Life Res* 1994;3(suppl 1):S11–7.
105. Nolte L-P, Zamorano LJ, Jiang Z, Wang Q, Langlotz F, Berlemann U. Image-guided insertion of transpedicular screws: a laboratory set-up. *Spine* 1995;20:497–500.
106. North RB, Campbell JN, James CS, et al. Failed back surgery syndrome: 5-year follow-up in 102 patients undergoing repeated operation. *Neurosurgery* 1991;28:685–91.
107. O'Donnell JL, Kuchle JW. Can discography predict lumbar pseudarthrosis [Abstract]? *Proc Am Acad Orthop Surg* 1996:215. Program page 215.
108. Ohlin A, Karlsson M, Düppe H, Hasserius R, Redlund-Johnell I. Complications after transpedicular stabilization of the spine. A survivorship analysis of 163 cases. *Spine* 1994;19:2774–9.

109. Ohlund C, Eek C, Palmblad S, Areskoug B, Nachemson A. Quantified pain drawing in subacute low back pain. Validation in a nonselected outpatient industrial sample. *Spine* [*in press*].
110. Ohlund C, Lindström I, Areskoug B, Eek C, Peterson L-E, Nachemson A. Pain behavior in industrial subacute low back pain. Part I. Reliability: concurrent and predictive validity of pain behavior assessments. *Pain* 1994;58:201–9.
111. Ordeberg G, Enskog J, Sjostrom L. Diagnostic external fixation of the lumbar spine. *Acta Orthop Scand* 1993;64(suppl 251):94–6.
112. Parizel PM, Van Goethem JW, van den Hauwe L, et al. Imaging of spinal implants and radiological assessment of fusion. In: Szpalski M, Gunzburg R, Spengler DM, Nachemson A, eds. *Instrumented fusion of the degenerative lumbar spine: state of the art, questions, and controversies*. New York: Lippincott-Raven Publishers, 1996:25–33 (this volume).
113. Philips HC. Avoidance behaviour and its role in sustaining chronic pain. *Behav Res Ther* 1987;25: 273–9.
114. Polatin P, Kinney RK, Gatchel RJ, Lillo E, Mayer TG. Psychiatric illness and chronic low back pain: the mind and the spine—which goes first? *Spine* 1993;18:66–71.
115. Poussa M, Schlenzka D, Seitsalo S, Ylikoski M, Hurri H, Österman K. Surgical treatment of severe isthmic spondylolisthesis in adolescents. Reduction or fuion in situ. *Spine* 1993;18:894–901.
116. Rechtine G. Whistler report: a survey of current indications for spinal instrumentation. *J Spinal Dis* 1995;8:422–4.
117. Relman AS. Assessment and accountability: the third revolution in medical care. *N Engl J Med* 1988;319:1220–2.
118. Revel M, Payan C, Vallee C, et al. Automated percutaneous lumbar discectomy versus chemonucleolysis in the treatment of sciatica: a randomized multicenter trial. *Spine* 1993;18:1–7.
119. Rhyne AL, Smith SE, Wood KE, Darden BV. Outcome of unoperated discogram positive low back pain. *Spine* 1995;20:1997–2000.
120. Roberts N, Smith R, Bennett S, Cape J, Norton R, Kilburn P. Health beliefs and rehabilitation after lumbar disc surgery. *J Psychosom Res* 1984;28:139–44.
121. Rudicel S, Esdaile J. The randomized clinical trial in orthopaedics: obligation or option? *J Bone Joint Surg* 1985;67-A:1284–93.
122. Schwarzer AC, Aprill CN, Derby R, Fortin J, Kine G, Bogduk N. The relative contributions of the disc and zygapophyseal joint in chronic low back pain. *Spine* 1994;19:801–6.
123. Selvik G. Roentgen stereophotogrammetry. A method for the study of the kinematics of the skeletal system. *Acta Orthop Scand* 1989;60(suppl 232):1–51.
124. Silvers HR, Lewis PJ, Asch HL, Clabeaux DE. Lumbar diskectomy for recurrent disk herniation. *J Spinal Dis* 1994;7:408–19.
125. Slade PD, Troup JDG, Letham J, Bentley G. The fear-avoidance model of exaggerated pain perception. Part 2: Preliminary studies of coping strategies for pain. *Behav Res Ther* 1983;21:409–16.
126. Smyth MJ, Wright V. Sciatica and the intervertebral disc. An experimental study. *J Bone Joint Surg* 1958;40-A:1401–18.
127. Soini JR, Seitsalo SK. The external fixation test of the lumbar spine. 30 complications in 25 to 100 consecutive patients. *Acta Orthop Scand* 1993;64:147–9.
128. Spengler DM, EA Ouellette, Battiè M, Zeh J. Elective discectomy for herniation of a lumbar disc. Additional experience with an objective method. *J Bone Joint Surg* 1990;72-A:230–7.
129. Stevenson RC, McCabe CJ, Findlay AM. An economic evaluation of a clinical trial to compare automated percutaneous lumbar discectomy with microdiscectomy in the treatment of contained lumbar disc herniation. *Spine* 1995;20:739–42.
130. Stokes IAF, Frymoyer JW. Segmental motion and instability. *Spine* 1987;12:688–91.
131. Stromqvist B, Johnsson R, Axelsson P. Stability of lumbar fusin with Steffee plates. Roentgen stereophotogrammetric analysis. Presented at the 10th annual conference of the North American Spine Society, Washington, DC, Oct. 18–21, 1995.
132. Temple HT, Kruss RW, van Dam BE. Lumbar and lumbosacral fusion using Steffee instrumentation. *Spine* 1994;19:537–41.
133. Toleikis JR, Carlvin AO, Shapiro DE, Schafer MF. The use of dermatomal evoked responses during surgical procedures that use intrapedicular fixation of the lumbosacral spine. *Spine* 1993;18:2401–7.
134. Turner JA, Ersek M, Herron L, Deyo R. Surgery for lumbar spinal stenosis: attempted meta-analysis of the literature. *Spine* 1992;17:1–8.
135. Turner JA, Ersek M, Herron L, et al. Patient outcomes after lumbar spinal fusions. *JAMA* 1992; 268:907–11.
136. Vaccaro AR, Gardin SR. Pedicle-screw fixation in the lumbar spine. *J Am Acad Orthop Surg* 1995;3:263–74.
137. Van Akkerveeken PF. Lateral stenosis of the lumbar spine. A new diagnostic test and its influence on management of patients with pain only [Thesis]. Rijksuniversiteit of Utrecht, The Netherlands, 1989.
138. Waddell G. Biopsychosocial analysis of low back pain. *Baillieres Clin Rheumatol* 1992;6:523–57.

139. Waddell G, Kummell EG, Lotto WN, Graham JD, Hall H, McCulloch JA. Failed lumbar disc surgery and repeat surgery following industrial injuries. *J Bone Joint Surg* 1979;61-A:201–7.
140. Waddell G, Main CJ, Morris EW, DiPaola M, Gray ICM. Chronic low back pain, psychological distress and illness behavior. *Spine* 1984;9:209–13.
141. Waddell G, McCulloch JA, Kummel E, Venner RM. Nonorganic physical signs in low back pain. 1979 Volvo Award in clinical science. *Spine* 1980;5:117–23.
142. Waddell G, Newton M, Henderson I, Somerville D, Main CJ. A fear-avoidance beliefs questionnaire (FABQ) and the role of fear-avoidance beliefs in chronic low back pain and disability. *Pain* 1993;52:157–68.
143. Wall MS, Oppenheim WL. Measurement error of spondylolisthesis as a function of radiographic beam angle. *J Pediatr Orthop* 1995;15:193–8.
144. Wall PD, Melzack R. *Textbook of pain.* Edinburgh: Churchill Livingstone, 1989.
145. Walsh TR, Weinstein JN, Spratt KF, Lehmann TR, Aprill C, Sayre H. Lumbar discography in normal subjects. A controlled, prospective study. *J Bone Joint Surg* 1990;72-A:1081–8.
146. Wetzel FT, LaRocca SH, Lowery GL, Aprill CN. The treatment of lumbar spinal pain syndromes diagnosed by discography: lumbar arthrodesis. *Spine* 1994;19:792–800.
147. Whitecloud TS, Davis JM, Olive PM. Operative treatment of the degenerated segment adjacent to a lumbar fusion. *Spine* 1994;19:531–6.
148. Wilson PR. Diskography is still investigational [Commentary]. *APS J* 1994;3:163–5.
149. Yuan HA, Garfin SR, Dickman CA, Mardjetko SM. A historical cohort study of pedicle screw fixation in thoracic, lumbar, and sacral spinal fusions. *Spine* 1994;19(suppl 20S):2279S–96S.
150. Zdeblick TA. A prospective, randomized study of lumbar fusion. Preliminary results. *Spine* 1993;18:983–91.
151. Zucherman J, Hsu K, Picetti G, White A, Wynne G, Taylor L. Clinical efficacy of spinal instrumentation in lumbar degenerative disc disease. *Spine* 1992;17:834–7.

# Subject Index